THE
DICTATED WORD

DELMAR
CENGAGE Learning

Australia Canada Mexico Singapore Spain United Kingdom United States

THE
DICTATED WORD

PATRICIA A. IRELAND, CMT, FAAMT

CARRIE K. STEIN, CMT

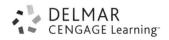
DELMAR
CENGAGE Learning™

Australia Canada Mexico Singapore Spain United Kingdom United States

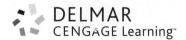

The Dictated Word
Patricia A. Ireland, CMT, FAAMT,
Carrie K. Stein, CMT

Vice President, Career and Professional Editorial: Dave Garza

Director of Learning Solutions: Matthew Kane

Senior Acquisitions Editor: Sherry Dickinson

Managing Editor: Marah Bellegarde

Product Manager: Natalie Pashoukos

Editorial Assistant: Anthony Souza

Vice President, Career and Professional Marketing: Jennifer McAvey

Marketing Director: Wendy Mapstone

Senior Marketing Manager: Nancy Bradshaw

Marketing Coordinator: Erica Ropitzky

Production Director: Carolyn Miller

Production Manager: Andrew Crouth

Senior Content Project Manager: James Zayicek

Senior Art Director: David Arsenault

Senior Technology Product Manager: Mary Colleen Liburdi

For product information and technology assistance, contact us at
Professional & Career Group Customer Support, 1-800-648-7450

For permission to use material from this text or product,
submit all requests online at **cengage.com/permissions.**
Further permissions questions can be e-mailed to
permissionrequest@cengage.com.

Example: Microsoft® is a registered trademark of the Microsoft Corporation.

Library of Congress Control Number: 2007941007

ISBN-13: 978-1-4354-2020-5
ISBN-10: 1-4354-2020-9

Delmar
5 Maxwell Drive
Clifton Park, NY 12065-2919
USA

Cengage Learning products are represented in Canada by Nelson Education, Ltd.

For your lifelong learning solutions, visit **delmar.cengage.com**

Visit our corporate website at **cengage.com**.

Notice to the Reader
Publisher does not warrant or guarantee any of the products described herein or perform any independent analysis in connection with any of the product information contained herein. Publisher does not assume, and expressly disclaims, any obligation to obtain and include information other than that provided to it by the manufacturer. The reader is expressly warned to consider and adopt all safety precautions that might be indicated by the activities described herein and to avoid all potential hazards. By following the instructions contained herein, the reader willingly assumes all risks in connection with such instructions. The publisher makes no representations or warranties of any kind, including but not limited to, the warranties of fitness for particular purpose or merchantability, nor are any such representations implied with respect to the material set forth herein, and the publisher takes no responsibility with respect to such material. The publisher shall not be liable for any special, consequential, or exemplary damages resulting, in whole or part, from the readers' use of, or reliance upon, this material.

Printed in the United States of America
1 2 3 4 5 6 7 12 11 10 09

CONTENTS

SECTION 1

MEDICAL REPORTS

SECTION 2

RADIOLOGY REPORTS

SECTION 3

SURGICAL REPORTS

Note: The numbers listed in the Table of Contents are not consecutive because some reports (M-8; M-22; M-33; M-35; M-49; M-53; M-58; M-98; S-22; S-35; S-41; S-48; S-51; S-53; S-55; S-57; and S-69) had to be deleted from the final count due to technical difficulties.

Key: M = medical
        R = radiology
        S = surgical

PREFACE

We are excited about *The Dictated Word* in that we feel it fills a void in the teaching of medical transcription. We heard the call from medical instructors and students everywhere: They want reports to transcribe, and they want reality. *The Dictated Word* answers this call, providing over 15 hours of physician-dictated medical, surgical, and radiology reports. A valuable addendum, it will fit in with any medical transcription curriculum, offering a variety of medical reports—beginning and advanced—as dictated by physicians.

HOW TO USE THIS TEXT

The reports are listed by ID number in the table of contents and by specialty in the index. This cross-indexing allows both student and instructor to find a specific medical specialty to fit in with the curriculum, a potential employment opportunity, or a particular field of research.

The physician dictations are available as MP3 files on the CDs in the back of the book. Instructors can use the individual reports for their own purposes, be it for extra credit, testing, as an addition to the curriculum, or as extra practice for the MT student.

APPENDICES

- "Common Dictation Errors" illustrates how transcriptionists use medical language and editing skills to correct common dictation errors
- "The Joint Commission's Official Do Not Use List"
- A comprehensive table that lists the total run times for each dictated report

FEATURES

- Authentic physician dictation comprised of doctors, nurse practitioners, and physician assistants.
- A flexible design that fits in with any medical transcription curriculum.
- Differing levels of medical reports, from entry level to advanced.
- The basic four, which consists of History & Physical Exams, Operative Notes, Discharge Summaries, and Consults, as well as Radiology reports that includes a variety of medical specialties and body systems.

ACKNOWLEDGMENTS

We are deeply grateful to our reviewers for their valuable assistance in critiquing the contents of *The Dictated Word*.

• Carol Crumrine, a multispecialty medical transcriptionist since 1969.
• Linda Innis, MSN, CFNP, an emergency room nurse and certified family nurse practitioner.

We also thank our team at Delmar Cengage Learning, without whom none of this would be possible.

Patricia A. Ireland, CMT, FAAMT   Carolyn K. (Carrie) Stein, CMT

"I touch the future. I teach."
Christa McAulifffe
American schoolteacher
(1948-1986)

SECTION 1

MEDICAL REPORTS

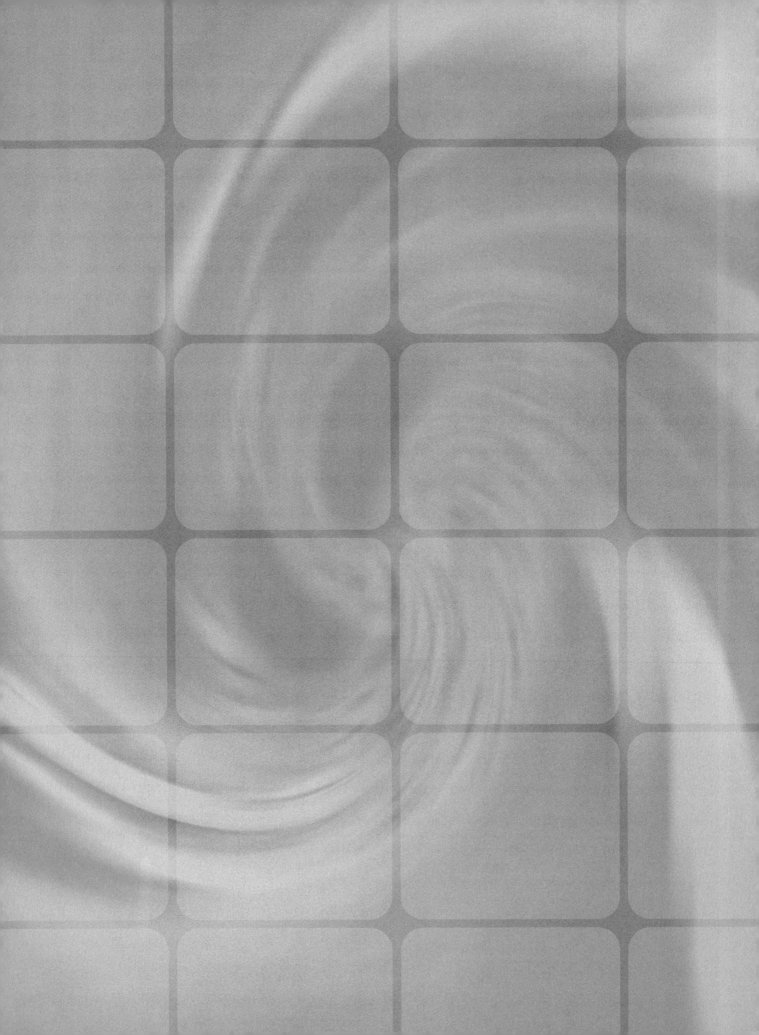

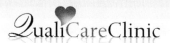

Bone Marrow Transplant Clinic

Patient Name: E. Sinks McClarty   **PCP:** Solomon T. Fisher, MD

Date of Exam: 06/19/----   **Age/Sex:** 45/M   **ID#:** M-1

INTRODUCTION: The patient is a 45-year-old male who is 11 days status post high-dose melphalan and autologous stem cell rescue for myeloma. The patient is being seen today for his first day after discharge from the hospital.

HISTORY: The patient states that he feels well today. He denies nausea, vomiting, or diarrhea. Patient denies shortness of breath or chest pain. The patient does state that he still feels fatigued but has no other complaints at this time.

REVIEW OF SYSTEMS: Patient denies headaches, shortness of breath, chest pain, abdominal cramping, nausea, vomiting, diarrhea. Patient has no skin rashes. He is having no problems with his line at this time.

CURRENT MEDICATIONS
1. Acyclovir 800 mg p.o. b.i.d.
2. Septra DS 1 p.o. q. Monday, Wednesday, Friday.
3. Magnesium oxide 400 mg p.o. q.12 h.
4. Norvasc 5 mg p.o. daily.
5. Lopressor 50 mg p.o. b.i.d.
6. Lantus insulin 12 units subcu q.h.s.
7. Duragesic patch 15 mcg q.3 days.
8. Neupogen 590 mcg subcu in clinic today.
9. Flagyl 500 mg p.o. t.i.d. through tomorrow.
10. Percocet p.r.n.
11. Imodium p.r.n.
12. The patient is also on insulin sliding scale at home.

ALLERGIES: NKDA.

PHYSICAL EXAMINATION

VITAL SIGNS: Blood pressure 101/69, temperature 100.1, heart rate 81, pulse oximetry 99% on room air. **GENERAL EXAMINATION:** No acute distress. **HEENT:** Normocephalic, atraumatic. Oropharynx pink without mucosal changes. **NECK:** Supple without adenopathy. **LUNGS:** Clear to auscultation bilaterally. **CARDIOVASCULAR:** Regular rate and rhythm with normal S1 and S2. **EXTREMITIES:** The patient does have +1 bilateral pedal edema. **SKIN:** No rashes or skin changes at this time. **ABDOMEN:** Soft, nontender, nondistended. Bowel sounds x4.

LABORATORY DATA: White blood cells 5.9, hemoglobin 9, hematocrit 25.6, platelet count pending. Glucose 101, BUN 6, creatinine 0.6, sodium 139, potassium 3.4, chloride 110, bicarbonate 19, calcium 6.8, total protein 5.7, albumin 2.8, alk phos 58, AST 8, total bilirubin 0.2, ALT 10, magnesium 1.4.

(Continued)

ID#: M-1   PAGE 2

IMPRESSION
The patient is a 45-year-old male who is day +11 status post autologous peripheral blood stem cell transplant for his multiple myeloma. The patient is doing pretty well at this time. He is on a study for which he will be getting his Neupogen today.

PLAN
1. Neupogen 590 mcg subcutaneously today.
2. Patient is to return to clinic on 07/13/----.
3. Continue all of his home medications.
4. Awaiting platelet count to determine whether or not he needs platelets today.

_____
Solomon T. Fisher, MD
Hematology/Oncology

STF:cks
D:06/19/----
T:06/20/----

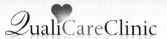

QualiCareClinic

<u>**Physical Medicine and Rehabilitation Consultation**</u>

Patient Name: Valerie Smith   **PCP:** Susan McGinnis, MD

Date of Consultation: 03/10/----   **Age/Sex:** 49/F   **ID#:** M-2

REASON FOR CONSULTATION: Recurrent back pain with intermittent right sciatica.

HISTORY OF PRESENT ILLNESS: Ms. Smith is a 49-year-old female who presents to me with an acute exacerbation of her chronic intermittent back pain with some associated right radicular/neurogenic leg pain. The patient states that initially she had a severe back pain episode in 1983. Then her first combined back pain with sciatica occurred in 1986. She subsequently underwent a myelogram, which demonstrated combined congenital and acquired spinal stenosis at L4-5 and less so at L5-S1. Eventually her sciatica pain improved, but she has had recurrent bouts of back pain, slightly worse on the right, over subsequent years. She had a recent exacerbation at the beginning of this week in which she awakened with no precipitating injury, activity, or other known variable. She presents today indicating that while sitting, her back pain represents 100% of her pain; but while standing and walking, the back pain represents only about 70% of her total pain, with the right lateral thigh pain and occasionally slightly further than her knee representing the other 30% of her pain. Her pain is generally aggravated with any type of activity, particularly stooping, bending, and lifting, as well as with prolonged standing and walking. The pain is a combination of a dull ache across her back and a slightly sharper shooting pain down the right leg. Her pain severity ranges now from a 4/10 to a 9/10.

NEUROLOGIC REVIEW OF SYSTEMS: Remarkable for the intermittent right sciatica in a predominantly L5 distribution. She will have some associated numbness and paresthesias on the right lateral ankle and foot, dorsal region, in a partial L5 dermatomal distribution. She occasionally feels some weakness in the right leg, particularly when the sciatica pain has worsened. Denies bowel or bladder changes or incontinence.

CONSTITUTIONAL REVIEW OF SYSTEMS: Unremarkable for fevers, chills, night sweats, malaise, weight loss, history of malignancy, or recent infection.

Treatment for this back pain has consisted only of some analgesic medications. Patient has had no recent physical therapy and has had no injections for this back problem. Furthermore, she is unable to do any specific exercises at this time, although she does attempt to do some low-impact cardiovascular conditioning when the pain is not exacerbated.

PAST HISTORY: Probable viral myocarditis with secondary residual cardiomyopathy (ejection fraction ranging from 35% to 45%), associated intermittent ventricular tachycardia, and hyperlipidemia.

PAST SURGICAL HISTORY: Noncontributory.

SOCIAL HISTORY: Denies tobacco use and alcohol use. Her current job is that of a linguist with the Defense Language Institute.

MEDICATIONS: Current analgesics consist of Skelaxin 800 mg 1 tablet p.o. t.i.d. p.r.n., tramadol 1 to 2 tablets q.i.d. p.r.n. (generally uses only one of these tablets daily). Other meds include Coreg, ramipril, Zocor, and aspirin.

PHYSICAL EXAMINATION

GENERAL APPEARANCE: Well-nourished, well-developed female in mild distress, alert and oriented x4, pleasant, cooperative, and appropriate.

(Continued)

Spine
- Posture/Inspection: Obvious list/shift to the right while sitting, particularly more evident while standing.
- Lumbopelvic AROM: Patient has aggravation of the lumbosacral-area back pain with flexion greater than 60 degrees, even more so with extension, particularly on the right side, in which she has exacerbation of the right lumbosacral area with greater than 10 degrees.
- Palpation: Tenderness is noted over the lumbosacral region.

Neurologic

Gait: Able to do heel-toe and tandem walking for a few steps.

Motor: Five out of five in all muscle groups in the lower extremities.
- Sensory: There is diminished light touch and pinprick evident on the right lateral ankle and foot, dorsum, in a partial L5 dermatome; the remaining portions of the lower extremities are intact to light touch and pinprick.
- Reflexes: Patella is 2+ and symmetric. Achilles 2- and symmetric with a normal flexion response to Babinski testing.
- Nerve tension signs: There is a positive reproduction of some of the right buttock and lateral leg thigh pain with a right straight-leg raise; however, this does not go beyond that of the popliteal fossa. The left side is unremarkable.

Extremities/Vascular

There is normal temperature and coloration of the distal legs and feet, with palpable dorsalis pedis pulses and without cyanosis or edema.

X-RAY DATA: CT myelogram done in the late 1980s demonstrated some combined degenerative and congenital L4-5 greater than L5-S1 canal stenosis with some disk protrusions at L4-5 greater than L5-S1 and facet arthropathy.

ASSESSMENT

Recurrent right L4-5 greater than L5-S1 herniated nucleus pulposus (HNP), protrusion type, with associated canal stenosis and secondary mechanical low back pain as well as intermittent right L5 neurogenic leg claudication.

PLAN
1. Naprosyn 500 mg 1 tablet b.i.d.
2. Vicodin 1 to 2 tablets q.i.d. p.r.n. increased pain along with the Skelaxin p.r.n. difficulty with sleep.
3. Will obtain x-rays of her lumbosacral spine today.
4. Lumbosacral magnetic resonance imaging scan (MRI) to better assess the soft tissue, disk, and neural structures as well as the severity of the canal stenosis.
5. Physical therapy for core stabilization.
6. Patient will return to clinic after obtaining the MRI, as well as start a physical therapy program.

Jean W. Mooney, PA
Physical Medicine and Rehabilitation

JWM:cks
D:03/10/----
T:03/10/----

c: Susan McGinnis, MD, Family Practice

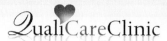

Orthopedic Clinic

Patient Name: Natalie Birch   **PCP:** Reed Phillips, MD

Date of Exam: 12/5/----   **Age/Sex:** 13 months/F   **ID#:** M-3

CHIEF COMPLAINT: She is here for followup status post left buckle fracture.

HISTORY: This is a 13-month-old who fell from a crib at a height of 3 to 4 feet on 11/21/----. She was evaluated in the ED at Hillcrest Medical Center and treated with a long arm cast, status post buckle fracture of the left distal wrist. The patient was seen in followup 1 week ago and was progressing well at the time. She presents today for routine evaluation. The father of the child is with the patient today and states that she has been doing very well since last the appointment, without any changes.

Past medical history is significant for a patent ductus arteriosus.

PAST SURGICAL HISTORY: She has no past surgical history.

MEDICATIONS: She is not on any medications.

ALLERGIES: She has no known drug allergies.

PHYSICAL EXAMINATION

The patient is alert and oriented x3, is sitting comfortably in her father's arms. The skin and surrounding tissues adjacent to the cast are without abnormalities. There is no erythema, edema, cracks, fissures, or discharge. Her capillary refill is less than 2 seconds, and she has full, active range of motion in the fingers of both hands.

ASSESSMENT/PLAN

The patient is a 13-month-old female with a buckle fracture of the left wrist who seems to be doing quite well. We will continue with a long arm cast and will see patient back in followup in 2 weeks. We will conduct x-rays out of the cast at that time, and if she has no pain, we will discontinue the cast and follow the patient on an as-needed basis. The patient is to return to clinic sooner should symptoms worsen.

_____

Raquel Rodriguez, MD
Orthopedic Surgery

RR:cks
D:12/6/----
T:12/6/----

c: Reed Phillips, MD, Pediatrics

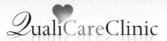

Emergency Department Treatment Record

Patient Name: Braden L. Webb   **PCP:** N/A

Date of Exam: 05/28/----   **Age/Sex:** 26/M   **ID#:** M-4

CONSULTING SERVICE: Endocrinology Service.

HISTORY OF PRESENT ILLNESS: This is a 26-year-old active-duty male airman basic, week 0, day 2, who presents to the emergency department stating that he has had a little bit of polyuria and polydipsia over the past 24 hours. Patient states in addition he feels he has had some minor dysuria. Patient states that he feels as if he has to void; however, when he attempts to, he is able to produce only a little bit of urine at a time. Denies abdominal pain, fevers, chills, stating that he has had no previous urinary problems.

REVIEW OF SYSTEMS in the ED, all other systems negative.

PAST MEDICAL HISTORY: Negative.

PAST SURGICAL HISTORY: Negative.

MEDICATIONS: None.

ALLERGIES: No known drug allergies.

SOCIAL HISTORY: Denies alcohol, tobacco, and illicit drug use.

PHYSICAL EXAMINATION

VITAL SIGNS on presentation: Pulse 96, blood pressure 144/74, respiratory rate 16, temperature 98.0, O2 saturation 98% on room air. GENERAL APPEARANCE: Awake, alert, oriented x3. He is in no acute distress, is resting comfortably in bed, talking with his battle buddy. HEENT: Normocephalic, atraumatic. Extraocular movements intact. Pupils are equal, round, and reactive to light and accommodation. Mucous membranes moist and pink. Negative oropharyngeal erythema or exudate. PULMONARY: Clear to auscultation bilaterally. CARDIAC: Regular. Negative murmur. ABDOMEN: Soft, nontender. No distended bladder palpated. Normoactive bowel sounds. Negative rebound, negative guarding. Negative masses appreciated. EXTREMITIES: Negative clubbing, cyanosis, or edema.

TEST RESULTS: CBC within normal limits. Chem-7: Sodium 136, potassium 3, chloride 101, bicarb 8, BUN 12, creatinine 0.9, glucose 290. TSH within normal limits. LFTs within normal limits with the exception of a total bilirubin of 1.4. Serum ketones positive. Urinalysis shows 3+ glucose, 4+ ketones, trace blood, 1+ protein. Chest x-ray: No acute disease. CT abdomen/pelvis, noncontrast, shows a mildly distended urinary bladder. Official read is pending at this time.

(Continued)

ID#: M-4   PAGE 2

EMERGENCY DEPARTMENT COURSE/MEDICAL DECISION MAKING: The patient was seen and examined. His Dextrostix by Triage showed a glucose of approximately 290 in a patient who denies previous history of diabetes. H&P revealed polyuria, polydipsia, and while the patient's mucous membranes were moist and pink, he did appear to be mildly dehydrated per history because the patient states he feels thirsty. Patient states that while in basic training he is forced to drink a number of canteens of water per day. As a result, I feel that that has maintained this patient's fluid levels; otherwise, this patient appears to be in DKA. He has a significant anion gap. His serum ketones are positive. Therefore, in the ED the patient was initially given a 2 liter normal saline IV bolus. Chemistries and labs were drawn with results as above. Upon completion of the 2 liter normal saline bolus, the patient was switched to D5 half normal saline plus 40 of KCl at 200 mL per hour. An insulin drip was started at 2 units per hour. The patient was also given KCl 40 mEq p.o. x1. At that point it was set up to establish a test every hour, alternating between a Chem-7 and a VBG, in order to check the resolution of this patient's acidosis and the normalization of this patient's gap.

Patient felt that he was still having difficulty urinating, and with the mildly distended bladder appreciated on CT scan, it was felt this patient would benefit from a Foley catheter. After discussion with the patient regarding the risks and benefits of the Foley catheter, however, the patient proceeded to produce a significant amount of urine on his own. He states that his symptoms of urinary hesitancy have resolved. The patient is now resting comfortably in bed 5. He continues on his D5 half normal saline drip plus 40 of potassium chloride. In addition, the patient is also receiving 2 units per hour of insulin.

This patient's case was presented to the MICU team, specifically Dr. Patricia Kofos, Intensivist, who arrived in the ED in a prompt and professional fashion. The patient was evaluated, with orders promptly written for admission to the MICU. At this point the patient remains in the ED pending admission to the MICU with diagnoses as follows.

EMERGENCY DEPARTMENT DIAGNOSES
1. Diabetic ketoacidosis.
2. Diabetes mellitus.

DISPOSITION
Admit to MICU.

PLAN
Admit to MICU.

_____

Samuel Ernest, MD
Emergency Room Physician

SE:cks
D:05/28/----
T:05/28/----

c: Patrick Keathley, MD, Endocrinology Service
   Patricia Kofos, MD, Intensivist

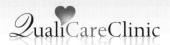

QualiCareClinic

Vascular Surgery Clinic Followup Note

Patient Name: Raul Jaramillo   **PCP:** Ly An Tabor, MD

Date of Exam: 2/3/----   **Age/Sex:** 56/M   **ID#:** M-5

REASON FOR VISIT: First postoperative visit after coronary artery bypass grafting.

HISTORY OF PRESENT ILLNESS: The patient is a 56-year-old gentleman with no prior cardiac history who presented in transfer to the Hillcrest Medical Center emergency department on 1/17/---- after having been transferred from a facility in Texas. Patient was found to have elevated cardiac enzymes consistent with a recent myocardial infarction. He had no pain on presentation but had evidence of an anterolateral infarct on EKG. He was taken to the catheterization laboratory for coronary angiogram, which demonstrated a high-grade proximal LAD stenosis and lesions in his proximal right coronary and circumflex arteries. His ejection fraction was noted to be moderately decreased with hypokinetic to akinetic distal anterior wall and apex. Patient was stabilized and subsequently underwent myocardial perfusion scan, which demonstrated perfusion of the areas of infarct. After several days to allow his Plavix to wear off, patient was taken to the operating room on 1/23/----, at which time he underwent 3-vessel off-pump coronary artery bypass grafting with left internal mammary artery to left anterior descending artery plus saphenous vein graft to obtuse marginal artery and saphenous vein graft to distal right coronary artery. Patient tolerated the procedures well, and he did well postop. He was extubated on the day of surgery and subsequently progressed satisfactorily. He was discharged to home on postop day four, 1/27/----, doing well.

Since being at home, patient states that he has had no problems with anginal symptoms. He is eating well, having regular bowel movements, has no dyspnea, no fevers, no chills.

PHYSICAL EXAMINATION

Temperature 97.0, pulse 72, respirations 18, blood pressure 97/54, height 5 feet 8 inches, weight 165 pounds. CHEST: Clear to auscultation bilaterally. HEART: Regular rate and rhythm. Normal S1, S2 with a 2/6 murmur along his aortic outflow tract at the right upper sternal border. Sternal incision is healing well, and the sternum is stable. He has 3 chest tube sutures remaining, which are removed at this time. Patient has good healing of all his wounds. EXTREMITIES are warm with no cyanosis, clubbing, edema, or tenderness. He has good healing of his saphenous vein harvest sites in his right lower extremity with no significant edema in his leg.

MEDICATIONS
1. Imdur 30 mg daily.
2. Plavix 75 mg daily.
3. Lipitor 40 mg daily.
4. Lisinopril 5 mg daily.
5. Aspirin 81 mg daily.
6. Metoprolol 25 mg b.i.d.
7. Percocet for pain.

(Continued)

ID#: M-5   PAGE 2

IMPRESSION/PLAN
1. Patient doing quite well post 3-vessel off-pump coronary artery bypass grafting.
2. He has been instructed to follow up with his cardiologist in Texas.
3. I will see him back in 4 weeks with a chest x-ray and electrocardiogram.
4. Patient is instructed to call if he has questions or concerns in the meantime.

_____
Ly An Tabor, MD
Vascular Surgery

LAT:cks
D:2/3/----
T:2/5/----

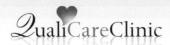

Orthopedic Services Preoperative History and Physical

Patient Name: Christopher R. Burke   **PCP:** David Castillo, MD

Date of Exam: 11/17/----   **Age/Sex:** 32/M   **ID#:** M-6

CHIEF COMPLAINT: Left knee pain.

HISTORY OF PRESENT ILLNESS: Mr. Burke is a 32-year-old male who has a history of left knee pain status post an injury sustained while playing basketball in February of this year. The patient was originally evaluated by Dr. David Castillo. He had an MRI ordered, which was performed in May of this year. The patient was unable to have his surgery as previously scheduled, and he is here in followup for the scheduled operation on his left knee in early December of this year.

The patient states that he has the sensation of instability, as he was told that he had an ACL injury as well as a meniscal injury on exam and MRI. He states that he has no locking or catching but just the instability sensation. He does periodically feel some catching in his left knee, however. He also has some persistent and progressive pain in his left knee. He denies any recent swelling, but with activity, the patient states that he does get some swelling about his left knee.

PAST MEDICAL HISTORY: Negative.

PAST SURGICAL HISTORY: His past surgical history includes an appendectomy. Anterior cruciate ligament repair of the right knee.

FAMILY HISTORY: Significant for diabetes on his grandfather's side.

SOCIAL HISTORY: The patient is a nonsmoker who reports rare alcohol use. He does not chew tobacco or use illicit drugs. He is on active military duty.

ALLERGIES: The patient has no known drug allergies.

MEDICATIONS: He takes no medications.

REVIEW OF SYSTEMS: Multiorgan review of systems is negative other than the present illness.

PHYSICAL EXAMINATION

GENERAL: The patient is alert and oriented x3 and in no acute distress.

HEENT: He is normocephalic, atraumatic. His cranial nerves are grossly intact.

CHEST/LUNGS: The respirations are unlabored, without distress.

CARDIOVASCULAR EXAMINATION: The patient has a regular rate and rhythm. He has intact distal pulses in the lower extremities, which are 2+, and a less-than-2-second capillary refill.

ABDOMEN/GENITALIA/PELVIC/RECTAL: Soft, nontender.

BACK/EXTREMITIES: The left knee range of motion is from 0 to 130 degrees. He has no tenderness to palpation about the medial or lateral joint line. He does have positive lateral McMurray findings on exam.

(Continued)

ID#: M-6   PAGE 2

NEUROLOGIC EXAMINATION: He has intact sensation distally in all dermatomes. He has 5/5 strength in both lower extremities in all motor groups. On stability testing, the patient has no instability noted at 0 varus and valgus. He does have a positive Lachman's at 1+ with no firm end point noted.

SKIN/LYMPHATICS: He has intact skin over his knee and is without signs of erythema or edema.

X-RAY DATA: Review of his magnetic resonance imaging scan shows a chronic anterior cruciate ligament (ACL) tear as well as a left lateral meniscal bucket-handle-type tear.

IMPRESSION
1. Left anterior cruciate ligament tear, chronic.
2. Lateral meniscal injury with history of sensation of instability and occasional catching and pain.

PLAN
The patient will be preop'd today. He will plan on surgery on approximately 12/4/---- with Dr. Rodriguez and team. The patient will follow up sooner should there be any complications or concerns.

_____
Raquel Rodriguez, MD
Orthopedic Surgery

RR:cks
D:11/17/----
T:11/17/----

c: David Castillo, MD, Orthopedic Surgery

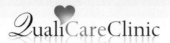

Colorectal Surgery Consult

Patient Name: Michele Bourn   **PCP:** Ronald Reardon, DO

Date of Consultation: 10/6/----   **Age/Sex:** 21/F   **ID#:** M-7

REASON FOR CONSULTATION: Fecal incontinence.

HISTORY OF PRESENT ILLNESS: Patient is a 21-year-old female who had perfect fecal continence until the delivery of her first child approximately 8-1/2 months ago. Patient was informed that she had a fourth-degree perineal laceration following an episiotomy but was not informed at the time what type of episiotomy or what type of repair had been performed. Currently, a lawsuit is pending regarding that case. Patient developed incontinence to liquid stool and gas, but not to solid stool, following this delivery. The frequency and severity of these episodes of incontinence have been worsening over the past several months. Patient reports constipation to solid stool, by which she relates that she has only one bowel movement per week and that the stool is usually hard in consistency. She denies nausea or vomiting. Patient also reports stress urinary incontinence, which is not significantly changed from the amount of urinary incontinence that she had prior to delivery.

PAST MEDICAL HISTORY: None.

PAST SURGICAL HISTORY: Dilation and curettage 3 years ago in December.

MEDICATIONS: None.

ALLERGIES: NKDA.

SOCIAL HISTORY: No tobacco, alcohol, or drugs of abuse.

OBSTETRIC HISTORY: Patient is a G2, P1, A0. Delivery-wise, vaginal at 38 weeks with no complications other than as mentioned above.

REVIEW OF SYSTEMS: Patient does report dyspareunia. Denies cardiac and pulmonary problems. Patient's constipation has not been adequately treated. She is taking no stool softener, fiber, or laxatives. She denies perineal or vaginal splinting for bowel movements.

PHYSICAL EXAMINATION

Temperature 98.2, blood pressure 119/73, pulse 76, respirations 17. In general, patient is in no acute distress. CARDIOVASCULAR: Regular rate and rhythm. No murmur. LUNGS are clear to auscultation bilaterally. ABDOMEN: Minimally tender to palpation in bilateral lower quadrants. No palpable masses. No distention. EXTREMITIES: No cyanosis, clubbing, or edema. RECTAL EXAM: Patient has normal sensation of the perianal area. Obvious decrease of perineal length on visual inspection. Normal sphincter tone. Palpably diminished soft tissue in the perineal body. No internal anal canal masses. Good squeeze tone on internal exam as well. There is thinning of the rectovaginal septum but no rectocele on examination. No obvious cystocele on vaginal examination.

X-RAY DATA: Endoanal ultrasound was performed in the clinic during this same visit. Patient was found to have obvious internal and external anal sphincter defect in the midcanal region. Puborectalis is intact, and the internal anal sphincter is intact superiorly but not inferiorly.

(Continued)

ID#: M-7   PAGE 2

ASSESSMENT

Patient has combined internal and external anal sphincter defect, presumably from a fourth-degree perineal laceration during vaginal delivery. Patient also suffers from constipation to solid stool and incontinence to liquid stool and gas.

PLAN

1. Patient will begin a bowel regimen with twice-daily fiber supplementation and increased hydration in her diet.
2. Surgical plan will be for overlapping sphincteroplasty and possible levatorplasty on 10/24/----. Patient will return for preop visit on 10/23/---- and will undergo bowel prep with a Fleet enema only on the morning of surgery.
3. Patient was counseled on the risks and benefits of surgery to include pain, bleeding, infection, failure of sphincteroplasty repair, and continued incontinence. Patient voiced understanding of these risks and desires to proceed. Her chance of a successful reversal of fecal incontinence at this time should be approximately 70% to 80%.

_____

James A. McClure Jr, MD
Colorectal Surgery

JAM:cks
D:10/7/----
T:10/8/----

cc: Ronald Reardon, DO, Family Practice

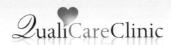

Radiation Oncology Consultation

Patient Name: Kazuo Matsui   **PCP:** Marie Aaron, DO

Date of Consultation: 08/26/----   **Age/Sex:** 22/M   **ID#:** M-9

REASON FOR CONSULTATION: Fracture of the right acetabulum.

HISTORY OF PRESENT ILLNESS: Kazuo Matsui is a 22-year-old man who was involved in a high-speed MVA on 08/21/---- during which he was thrown from his vehicle. Plain radiograph of the right femur done 08/21/---- showed a posterior right hip dislocation with a posterior superior acetabular rim fracture. CT scans of the chest, abdomen, and pelvis done on 08/21/---- showed dependent consolidation of left upper and lower lobes. The mediastinal contents were intact. There was a chip fracture of the posterior superior acetabular rim with an intra-articular fragment displacement. The femoral head had been reduced into the acetabulum. There was subcutaneous edema in the left buttock. CT of the head and spine the same day showed a left frontal, tiny subarachnoid bleed with possible small parenchymal contusions and likely right posterior frontal subdural bleed. The skull was intact. There was a 3 mm foreign body in the soft tissues of the right zygoma. There was no cervical spinal injury.

On 08/25/---- Mr. Matsui underwent open reduction, internal fixation. He now presents to the Radiation Oncology Clinic.

PAST HISTORY: Mostly unremarkable. He has no medical illnesses, no surgeries prior to this admission.

ALLERGIES: No known drug allergies.

MEDICATIONS: Patient is currently on Lovenox, Dilantin, multivitamins, ferrous sulfate, vitamin C, Colace, Vicodin, and morphine sulfate.

FAMILY HISTORY: Not obtained.

SOCIAL HISTORY: He had been using ethanol and cannabinoids.

REVIEW OF SYSTEMS: No anorexia or weight loss. No neurovascular dysfunction.

PHYSICAL EXAMINATION

He is intensely uncomfortable in spite of doses of intravenous morphine. Complains of pain throughout the procedure. He has a Foley catheter in place. He has contusions compatible with his history of trauma. Lungs are clear to auscultation anteriorly. Cardiovascular: Heart with regular rate and rhythm with a normal S1, S2. No murmurs heard. Abdomen: Flat, soft, nontender, with normal bowel sounds. No masses. Extremities: No lower extremity edema. Right lower extremity is wrapped in bandages but is neurovascularly intact with good pulse and capillary refill. Neurologic Exam: Cranial nerves II through XII are intact. Skin is otherwise within normal limits.

IMPRESSION

Kazuo Matsui is a 22-year-old man with a right acetabular fracture following motor vehicle accident. He has had open reduction, internal fixation. According to the radiation oncology literature, the risk of heterotopic ossification in this setting without adjuvant therapy is 60% to 80%. This may be reduced to as low as 5% with application of a single fraction of radiation therapy.

(Continued)

ID#: M-9   PAGE 2

I have reviewed radiation therapy in this setting with Mr. Matsui. I discussed treatment setup and simulation. I discussed side effects during treatment, which would likely include only fatigue and skin reaction. I discussed potential long-term complications of treatment, such as hip stiffness, arthritis, skin changes, neurovascular injury, failure to prevent heterotopic ossification, cancer in the irradiated field, and/or decreased fertility. His testicles are removed from the treatment field and will receive some scattered dose, but I think the actual dose to the testicles will be very low. Patient had a chance to have his questions answered and appeared to be satisfied with the discussion.

PLAN
We will proceed with radiation therapy. I plan to deliver a single fraction of 7 Gy units prescribed to midplane with 6 MV photons. If possible, I am going to place his testicles in a clamshell.

_____
L. (Lonnie) Willem Erwin, MD
Radiation Oncology

LWE:cks
D:08/26/----
T:08/27/----

cc: Marie Aaron, DO, Family Practice

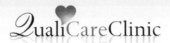

Bone Marrow Transplant Clinic Followup Note

Patient Name: Lance Everett   **PCP:** Solomon T. Fisher, MD

Date of Exam: 06/10/----   **Age/Sex:** 64/M   **ID#:** M-10

INTRODUCTION: Mr. Everett is a 64-year-old gentleman who was recently discharged from the hospital after having been admitted with febrile neutropenia.

HISTORY OF PRESENT ILLNESS: Mr. Everett is currently cycle 1, day 24 status post reduced-dose mitoxantrone and VP-16 for recurrent/ongoing extramedullary leukemia. Patient states that he is feeling pretty well at this time. He denies nausea, vomiting, and diarrhea. Patient denies any chest pain or shortness of breath. Patient states that he is still having some loose stools but not diarrhea. Denies fevers. Patient states that he is eating fairly well.

CURRENT MEDICATIONS

1. Acyclovir 400 mg p.o. q.12 h.
2. G-CSF 480 mcg today.
3. Flagyl 500 mg p.o. t.i.d.
4. Cefepime 2 g IV q.12 h.
5. Hydrocortisone 20 mg in the morning and 10 mg at night.
6. Colace p.r.n.
7. Oxycodone IR p.r.n.
8. Restasis eye drops p.r.n.

PHYSICAL EXAMINATION

VITAL SIGNS: Blood pressure 92/57, temperature 97.2, heart rate 100, pulse oximetry 95% on room air. **GENERAL:** No acute distress. **HEENT:** Normocephalic, atraumatic. Oropharynx is dry without new oral changes. The patient does have changes that are from his chronic graft-vs-host disease. **NECK:** Supple. **LUNGS:** Clear to auscultation bilaterally. **CARDIAC:** Tachycardic with normal S1, S2. **EXTREMITIES:** No cyanosis, clubbing, or edema. **ABDOMEN:** Bowel sounds are hyperactive. Nontender and nondistended.

LABORATORY DATA: White blood cells 0.7, hemoglobin 10.1, hematocrit 29.3, platelets 16,000. Glucose 124, BUN 16, creatinine 0.9, sodium 139, potassium 3.5, chloride 103, bicarbonate 26, calcium 9.4, total protein 6.2, albumin 3.4, alk phosphatase 913, AST 25, total bilirubin 0.5, ALT 41, magnesium 1.9.

IMPRESSION

Mr. Everett is a 64-year-old gentleman who is cycle 1, day 24 status post reduced-dose mitoxantrone with VP-16.

PLAN

1. Patient to get 1 liter normal saline in clinic today.
2. Patient will get 480 mcg of G-CSF in clinic today.
3. Patient did come back *Clostridium difficile*-positive as I was dictating this, so I will continue his Flagyl at 500 mg p.o. t.i.d. for another 10 days.

(Continued)

ID#: M-10   PAGE 2

4. Patient is to return to clinic on 06/13/----.
5. I will order a CBC, renal, magnesium, and LFTs for that visit.

_____
Solomon T. Fisher, MD
Hematology

STF:cks
D:06/10/----
T:06/10/----

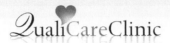

Orthopedic Clinic Consultation

Patient Name: Stephen Landstuhl   **PCP:** Susan McGinnis, MD
Date of Consultation: 11/02/----   **Age/Sex:** 22/M   **ID#:** M-11

REASON FOR VISIT: Nonunion of the right tibia.

HISTORY OF PRESENT ILLNESS: The patient is a 22-year-old Operation Iraqi Freedom veteran who in January was injured by an IED blast in Iraq, and it resulted in an open right tibia fracture. The patient was taken to Baghdad where he was initially débrided. He had fasciotomies and an external fixator placed. He was then transferred to Germany where he underwent intramedullary nailing of his right tibia. Also of note, while he was in Baghdad he apparently suffered a respiratory arrest as well as seizures. He had followup care done in the states, where he underwent multiple I&Ds for his fasciotomies. The patient comes in now, approximately 10 months out from placement of the intramedullary nail, for evaluation and treatment of his nonunion. His only complaint is pain over the fracture site as well as some ankle pain. He denies any knee pain. He states that he has pain basically with ambulation. He does not do any running or any other activity. He is currently unemployed and wants to start school next year. He does note that he has a slight flapping of his foot when he ambulates secondary to a nerve injury, but this has been followed by Neurosurgery. He also notes occasional tingling in his lower extremity in the distributions along the deep and superficial peroneal nerves. It should be noted that in June, when he had followup, it was noted that he had a questionable nonunion as well as a broken screw in the distal part of the nail.

PAST MEDICAL HISTORY: Noncontributory.

PAST SURGICAL HISTORY: Significant only for the operation on his right tibia.

ALLERGIES: He is allergic to MORPHINE and NAPROXEN.

CURRENT MEDICATIONS: His current medications include Ultram.

SOCIAL HISTORY: Negative for smoking. Occasionally he uses alcohol, less than 6 drinks per week.

PHYSICAL EXAMINATION

The patient is alert and oriented x3 and in no acute distress. His vision is intact as are his hearing and speech, and he is without respiratory distress. Evaluation of his right lower extremity shows healing fasciotomy sites that are both medial and lateral, the full length of his lower extremity. He does have a visible deformity to his right lower extremity over the fracture site, that is, where the bone is trying to heal itself. He has full range of motion of his knee. There is no palpable tenderness. He has full range of motion of the ankle with no palpable tenderness. He has decreased sensation in the deep peroneal and superficial nerve distributions. He is intact to the tibial nerve. His strength is 4/5 anterior tib, EHL, and 5/5 for the gastrocnemius.

LABORATORY AND X-RAY DATA: X-rays taken today confirmed the distal screw is broken and that he continues to have a nonunion at the fracture site.

IMPRESSION
Right tibial fracture, nonunion, with an intramedullary nail in place.

PLAN
The patient will be sent upstairs for laboratory evaluation to see if there is an infection. This will include CBC, ESR, CRP, as well as nutrition labs and a Chem-10. He will be given crutches to use to help with the pain he has on ambulation. It was also discussed with him, as well as his father who was present, surgical treatments. At this

(Continued)

ID#: M-11   PAGE 2

time it is recommended that he undergo exchange nail as his first procedure and hopefully the only procedure; however, other procedures were discussed, which included removing the nail and plating the tibia as well as the addition of bone graft to the fracture site after his exchange nail. As stated, though, primarily he will go through an exchange nail.

The tentative date for surgery will be 12/05/---- with a preop date of 11/30/----. By that time he should have all the labs complete. We will also work on a Secretary of the Air Force Package for him so that we can continue his care here, since his benefits through the Army expire in February of next year, and I anticipate that he will need followups after that time period with the possibility of additional surgery if he continues not to heal. The patient had all his questions answered, including the risks of surgery. He has no further questions at this time and neither does his father.

_____
Raquel Rodriguez, MD
Orthopedic Surgery

RR:cks
D:11/02/----
T:11/03/----

c: Susan McGinnis, MD, Family Practice

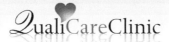

<u>**Vascular Surgery Clinic Followup Note**</u>

Patient Name: Adam L. Berkman   **PCP:** Ly An Tabor, MD

Date of Exam: 10/27/----   **Age/Sex:** 72/M   **ID#:** M-12

HISTORY OF PRESENT ILLNESS: This 72-year-old gentleman was initially seen in the hospital back in October when he was admitted for *Staphylococcus aureus* osteomyelitis of the back, and he was having a workup for his aortic valve disease. At that time CT scan revealed that he had a 3.5 cm infrarenal abdominal aortic aneurysm. He was asymptomatic at that time, and recommendation was for followup at 6 months. This is his first visit back since then.

Patient reports that he has had no problems. He has had no episodes of back pain. He has been asymptomatic otherwise.

SOCIAL HISTORY: He plays golf several times a week, and he is able to walk 18 holes with no significant leg pain. He reports that he smoked 2 to 2-1/2 packs a day for 5 years but stopped over 25 years ago. He is not a diabetic.

PAST MEDICAL HISTORY: He has aortic valve disease, osteomyelitis of his back that is now resolved, history of prostate cancer, hemorrhoids, and cardiac arrhythmia.

PAST SURGICAL HISTORY: Significant for inguinal hernia repair and prostatectomy as well as aortic valve replacement with a bovine valve.

ALLERGIES: No known drug allergies.

MEDICATIONS: Percocet and Lopressor.

PHYSICAL EXAMINATION

Temperature 97.6, blood pressure 142/92 in left arm, blood pressure 142/90 in right arm, pulse rate 60, respirations 16. In general, he is in no acute distress. Alert and oriented x3. HEENT AND NECK: Pupils are equal, round, and reactive to light and accommodation, extraocular movements intact. No lymphadenopathy. No JVD and no tracheal deviation. No bruits noted in his neck. CARDIOVASCULAR: Regular rate and rhythm with no murmur, rub, or gallop noted. LUNGS are clear to auscultation bilaterally. ABDOMEN is soft, nontender, nondistended with positive bowel sounds. He has no bruits over his midline on auscultation. PULSE exam shows 2+ femoral, popliteal, dorsalis pedis, and posterior tibial pulses. He also has a 2+ radial and brachial bilaterally.

ASSESSMENT

Patient is a 72-year-old gentleman who had a 3.5 cm infrarenal abdominal aortic aneurysm found on CT scan done in October during a workup for osteomyelitis and his cardiac valvular disease. He was to follow up in 6 months, which would have put him back in February; however, apparently either no appointment was scheduled or the patient did not follow up.

(Continued)

ID#: M-12   PAGE 2

PLAN is to have patient follow up within 1 month. Since he is not n.p.o. today, he will follow up within 1 month for an ultrasound of his infrarenal AAA. He will follow up again 6 months after that for a repeat ultrasound of his carotids and his AAA.

_____

Ly An Tabor, MD
Vascular Surgery

LAT:cks
D:10/27/----
T:10/27/----

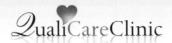
QualiCareClinic

Emergency Department Treatment Record

Patient Name: Mark N. Scott   **PCP:** N/A

Date of Exam: 02/18/----   **Age/Sex:** 18/M   **ID#:** M-13

CONSULTING SERVICE: Internal Medicine Service.

CHIEF COMPLAINT: This is an 18-year-old male who was seen in the ED for generalized myalgias, pain all over, fatigue, and dry mouth.

HISTORY OF PRESENT ILLNESS: Patient presented to the ED at about 1100 hours and was seen shortly thereafter. Initial triage demonstrated that he appeared slightly dehydrated, and he was initially started on intravenous fluid boluses. Laboratory studies were sent and are pending. Patient complained of 1 day of generalized achy pain in his legs, arms, and torso. No swelling, no bleeding, no swollen glands noted. No history of anaphylaxis or immune deficiency. No dysuria or penile discharge. He had no nausea, vomiting, or diarrhea. He had no chest pain, dyspnea on exertion, or palpitations. He denies shortness of breath, cough, wheezing, and pulmonary symptoms. He had no sore throat, ear pain, or congestion. He had no double vision, change in vision, or eye discharge. Denied fever, weight loss, and headache. He did feel some generalized fatigue and weakness all over. He had no suicidal ideation, homicidal ideation, difficulty sleeping, or agitation. Denied focal weakness, numbness, or other neurologic symptoms.

REVIEW OF SYSTEMS: As in History of Present Illness.

PAST MEDICAL HISTORY: Denies any significant past medical history.

PAST SURGICAL HISTORY: He had some right shoulder surgery in the distant past and has had no residual problems with that.

MEDICATIONS: Takes no medications.

ALLERGIES: NKDA.

SOCIAL HISTORY: Denies tobacco, alcohol, or illicit drug use.

FAMILY HISTORY: Denies.

PHYSICAL EXAMINATION

VITAL SIGNS on presentation: Blood pressure 161/85, pulse 68, respirations 16, temperature 98.3, O2 sat. 100%. In general, patient is noted to be uncomfortable but is in no acute distress. He is well nourished and well developed. Pupils are equal, round, and reactive to light and accommodation. Normal conjunctivae. Normal nose and ear inspection. Oropharynx is dry. No exudate, edema, or erythema in his throat. No masses or lymphadenopathy in his neck or supraclavicular regions. Normal thyroid gland. His pulmonary effort is normal bilaterally. Lungs are clear. He has a slightly tender chest wall diffusely. Regular rate and rhythm on his heart exam with no murmurs, rubs, or gallops. Normal pulses. No jugular venous distention and no edema. Abdomen is tender, nondistended. No CVA tenderness. Liver and spleen are normal to exam. He has no rashes, lesions, or skin ulcers. No induration noted. Has an antalgic gait. He has no gait abnormality; however, he moves very gingerly as he claims that he hurts all over when he moves. Equal strength in bilateral upper and lower extremities. Normal tone, no cyanosis noted. Cranial nerves II through XII are intact. He has a normal cerebellar exam. Mood and affect are normal. He is alert and oriented to person, place, time, and situation.

(Continued)

ID#: M-13   PAGE 2

EMERGENCY DEPARTMENT COURSE/MEDICAL DECISION MAKING: This is a young male who appears to be slightly dehydrated and who was started on some fluids. Initial laboratory values showed that he was slightly acidotic with bicarbonate of 21. His anion gap was 22. He had a creatinine of 6.1, and eventually I discovered that his total CK was greater than 92,000. Patient continued to be fluid hydrated.

Internal Medicine was consulted, and patient will be admitted to the intensive care unit under their service. He remained in stable condition in the ED. A bicarbonate drip was ordered, but per the admitting team at the time of dictation, we are awaiting final results on a urine pH before administering a bicarb drip. The rest of his laboratory values were reviewed by me. He had a white count of 17,000 and other laboratory studies as in the computer.

EMERGENCY DEPARTMENT DIAGNOSIS
Pending. Dr. Wells was present and participated in all aspects of this patient's exam and medical decision making.

_____
Samuel Ernest, MD
Emergency Room Physician

SE:cks
D:02/18/----
T:02/18/----

c: A. Leigh Wells, MD, Internal Medicine

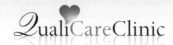

QualiCareClinic

Pediatrics Consultation

Patient Name: Roy Michaels   **PCP:** Ronald Reardon, DO

Date of Consultation: 5/11/----   **Age/Sex:** 11/M   **ID#:** M-14

REASON FOR CONSULTATION: Patient presents today for evaluation of his dog bites to bilateral upper extremities.

HISTORY OF PRESENT ILLNESS: Roy is an 11-year-old male who was bitten by a bullmastiff on the left hand and right forearm and hand on 5/10/----. He was initially seen in the Hillcrest Medical Center Emergency Department, evaluated by the emergency medicine physicians as well as an orthopedic surgeon, and patient was found to have most significant bites—one on the volar ulnar aspect of his midforearm of the right upper extremity and also another puncture-type wound with some erythema, induration, and edema on the thenar eminence volarly of his left hand. The patient received one dose of intravenous Zosyn while at Hillcrest and was discharged at 5 o'clock on 5/11/----. Orthopedics in the emergency department at Hillcrest had intended on getting him oral Augmentin; however, it was inadvertently prescribed at the outpatient clinic, which was closed at the time of the patient's discharge. The mother went back to the ER Help Desk and was told to just pick up her son's antibiotics when she had a followup visit at 2 p.m. on that same day.

The patient followed up with Orthopedics at 1400 hours on 5/11/---- and was found to be not significantly improved. He was subsequently referred to Forrest General Hospital for admission if deemed necessary by our service. The patient has no fevers. He has been doing reasonably well at home with no significant change in his overall pain status.

The background on the dog is that it was a stray dog that had been taken from an animal shelter, as the patient's mother is doing work with these types of animals. The child had been playing in the back yard with the animal, unsupervised, and apparently in somewhat of a playful but not exactly provoked manner the dog bit the child on the right wrist and forearm and the left hand, as previously described. The dog has since been euthanized and decapitated for cranial analysis for rabies. All appropriate forms have been filled out by the shelter from whence the dog came and also from the ED at Hillcrest.

MEDICATIONS: None. Previous antibiotics received include Unasyn IV at Hillcrest. None at Forrest General.

PAST MEDICAL HISTORY: None.

PAST SURGICAL HISTORY
1. Pressure equalization tubes x2.
2. Arteriovenous malformation in the antecubital fossa in the right upper arm, which was corrected surgically.
3. Left tympanoplasty.
4. Right neck biopsy of benign tissue.

SOCIAL HISTORY: Patient lives at home with his mother only.

PHYSICAL EXAMINATION

Weight is 30.5 kg, vital signs are stable. No fevers are noted. Exam of patient's upper extremities reveals full strength with strength 5/5 in bilateral deltoids, biceps, triceps, brachioradialis, wrist flexors, wrist extensors, finger flexors, finger extensors, and interossei. Overall light touch sensation is intact in both upper extremities along the median, ulnar, and radial dermal distribution. Distal neurologic status shows a 5/5 strength in and along the anterior interosseous and posterior interosseous as well as ulnar nerve distribution. Capillary refill is less than 2 seconds in all fingers. Radial pulse is easily palpated and is 2+ in nature bilaterally. Specific attention to the skin

(Continued)

ID#: M-14   PAGE 2

findings shows multiple very small and shallow puncture/abrasions on the volar and dorsal aspects of the forearm of the right upper extremity and also on the palm and dorsum of the left hand. None of these are deep and each has a very scant coagulated scab present. No fluid is expressible from any of these sites. The only ones that have mild erythema associated with them include one on the volar ulnar aspect of the midforearm in the right upper extremity and also the hypothenar eminence of the left hand, which has a fair amount of erythema; however, no induration and no fluctuance is noted. The thenar eminence is soft, and the patient tolerates palpation of the area without difficulty. Passive finger extension and flexion is unimpeded and pain-free. No fluid or pus is expressed from any of these lesions.

LABORATORY AND X-RAY DATA: Patient's WBC count is 8.3, ESR is 14, CRP is 0.8.

X-ray studies on May 10 from Hillcrest Medical Center show a right forearm and left hand with no foreign objects, no fractures noted. There is some subcutaneous air noted along the volar aspect of the radius in the right forearm. The left hand shows some soft tissue swelling over the thenar eminence but no fractures, foreign objects, or subcutaneous emphysema.

X-rays done on May 11 of the right forearm and hand: The left hand shows no interval changes. Still with some subcutaneous air in the volaris back to the distal radius on the right. Forearm series: There are again no dislocations, fractures, and no foreign objects noted. Bilateral hands and forearms show no significant degree of soft tissue swelling at this time.

ASSESSMENT

This is an 11-year-old male with bilateral hand and forearm dog bites with cellulitis over left thenar eminence and over the volar ulnar midforearm of the right hand without evidence of abscess at this time.

PLAN

1. I plan to have the patient admitted overnight to the pediatric service at Forrest General Hospital for intravenous antibiotics for the next 12 to 24 hours.
2. I plan to have the patient start Zosyn 2.4 g intravenously q.8 h., which is 80 mg/kg/8 h.
3. Patient will take Tylenol for pain control.
4. Will follow closely in the morning with laboratory evaluation as well as repeat examination of his wounds. Patient will be n.p.o. past midnight tonight; however, he can eat dinner this evening.
5. I plan to place the patient in a small pancake volar splint for the left hand for soft tissue rest and reevaluate in the morning as previously described.

_____

Danila R. Fry, MD
Plastic Surgery

DRF:cks
D:5/12/----
T:5/13/----

cc: Ronald Reardon, DO, Family Practice

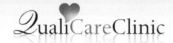

Radiation Oncology Clinic Followup Note

Patient Name: Joel Flores   **PCP:** Sherman Loyd, MD

Date of Exam: 08/29/----   **Age/Sex:** 57/M   **ID#:** M-15

DIAGNOSIS: Squamous cell carcinoma of the floor of mouth, stage IVA (T4aN2M0).

RADIATION THERAPY: Following resection and bilateral neck dissection, Mr. Flores was irradiated to his floor of mouth, receiving a total dose to the tumor bed of 64.4 cGy units delivered in 35 fractions over 51 elapsed treatment days, completed on December 29 of last year.

INTERVAL HISTORY: Mr. Flores is continuing to improve. He has a feeding tube but drinks all his nutrition orally. He is able to swallow. He will eat liquefied beef stew that his wife makes, for example. His sense of taste is continuing to improve, but he has continuous oral dryness. He has no complaints of pain. His most recent CT of neck on May 31 of this year showed extensive postoperative changes from his right hemimandibulectomy and reconstruction as well as 2 nonspecific enhancing nodules in the right submandibular space. A CT of the chest, abdomen, and pelvis on July 25 of this year showed no evidence of metastatic disease. In general he feels well and is quite cheerful. This was the first time he has been able to come to an appointment in a long time. He is walking with his wife's assistance without the use of a wheelchair or similar device.

PHYSICAL EXAMINATION

He is not acutely ill. He is visually impaired, wearing sunglasses. His weight is 174 pounds (175 pounds on March 17 of this year). His blood pressure is 162/94, heart rate 78, temperature 98.1. There is no scleral icterus. The neck has no adenopathy. He has obvious changes from his hemimandibulectomy and previous radiation therapy. Examination of the oral cavity and oropharynx reveals no visible tumor. He has thickened, tenacious mucus. There is no palpable tumor in the tongue, the accessible areas in the floor of mouth, or the tonsillar bed or base of tongue. Endoscopy to the right nasion shows no evidence of tumor, but he does have thick, tenacious mucus. There is normal adduction of the vocal cords with phonation. His lungs are clear to auscultation. Cardiovascular exam shows a regular rate and rhythm without murmurs. His abdomen is benign. The extremities have no edema. He has intact cranial nerves II through XII, mentation, and gait.

IMPRESSION

Mr. Flores is a 57-year-old male with stage IVA (T4aN2M0) squamous cell carcinoma of the floor of mouth. Currently he has no evidence of disease. He feels quite well and is continuing to recuperate from his radiation therapy.

DISCUSSION/PLAN

1. He will return for followup in our clinic in 3 months, at which time we will repeat CT scan of the neck.
2. He will continue to follow up with the ENT Clinic, and at the next visit we will also begin checking TSH on an annual basis.

L. (Lonnie) Willem Erwin, MD
Radiation Oncology

LWE:cks
D:08/30/----
T:09/01/----

c: Sherman Loyd, MD, Internal Medicine

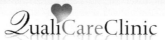

Vascular Surgery Followup Note

Patient Name: Arthur T. Richeson   **PCP:** Ronald Reardon, DO

Date of Exam: 02/03/----   **Age/Sex:** 76/M   **ID#:** M-16

HISTORY: Mr. Richeson is a 76-year-old male who underwent bilateral common iliac artery stenting in November of last year. Since that time, his half-block claudication in the bilateral calves has now gone to no claudication. He does complain of both his legs feeling numb if he sits too long, especially in the morning, such as when he is watching the news. He also complains of 1 episode of dizziness. He has had this before and had a pacer placed for this reason. Patient is going to get his pacer interrogated next week. Denies chest pain, denies amaurosis fugax, unilateral weakness, numbness, and/or clumsiness.

PHYSICAL EXAMINATION

Temperature 96.7, blood pressure 116/70 on the left, 109/65 on the right, pulse 71, respirations 16.

HEENT EXAM: The patient is normocephalic with multiple what appear to be seborrheic or actinic keratoses on the face. He has a ruddy complexion. His face is symmetric. NECK: Supple with no adenopathy. Normal carotid pulsations. There are no carotid bruits. HEART is regular with no murmurs. LUNGS: Clear to auscultation bilaterally. ABDOMEN: Soft, nontender, nondistended, no pulsatile abdominal mass. EXTREMITIES: Patient has very mildly diminished, easily palpable bilateral femoral, popliteal, and dorsalis pedis artery pulses.

X-RAY DATA: Noninvasive vascular imaging ABIs performed in clinic today reveal an ABI of 1.29 on the right, 1.05 on the left. Screening carotid duplex reveals bilateral, mild, 16% to 49% internal carotid stenoses with left vertebral artery occlusion. The right vertebral artery is antegrade. The aortoiliac duplex performed on February 1 of this year revealed widely patent bilateral common iliac artery stents. There appears to be a mild external iliac artery stenosis on the right by velocity criteria with a velocity ratio of just over 2.

ASSESSMENT

1. Widely patent bilateral common artery stents with no residual claudication and normal ankle-brachial indices bilaterally. Will follow the patient in 6 months with repeat aortoiliac duplex.
2. Mild carotid disease picked up bilaterally on screening, with an occluded left vertebral artery. We will follow this in 1 month with repeat carotid duplex, as the patient remains asymptomatic on aspirin.

_____

Ly An Tabor, MD
Vascular Surgery

LAT:cks
D:02/03/----
T:02/04/----

cc: Ronald Reardon, DO, Family Practice

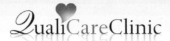

QualiCareClinic

Vascular and Neurovascular Surgery Followup Note

Patient Name: James E. Stotler   **PCP:** Chris Salem, DO

Date of Exam: 08/03/----   **Age/Sex:** 79/M   **ID#:** M-17

CHIEF COMPLAINT: Bilateral lower extremity pain with ambulation.

HISTORY: The patient is a 79-year-old Caucasian gentleman who is currently being evaluated for a diarrheal illness for the last year. He states that over the last several years his walking has become incrementally worse based upon pain in his calves with walking. Started mostly on the left but does involve both relatively equally. The pain is consistent at about 5 to 6 blocks currently. When it initially started, it was mostly at longer distances. He does state that if he pushes it, it starts to move up into his thighs. If he really, really "goes after it," the pain may come up into his buttocks. He denies postprandial pain. Denies TIAs or stroke-like symptoms. His cardiovascular risk factors include coronary artery disease. He has hypertension and hyperlipidemia, for which he is medically controlled. He denies having diabetes, and he quit smoking in 1998 after a 40-pack-year history. He does have a history of mild congestive heart failure, although he has never had a heart attack. He denies having any active chest, left shoulder, or jaw pain.

Medications currently include niacin, metoprolol, lisinopril, cilostazol, simvastatin, and pantoprazole.

ALLERGIES: No known drug allergies.

PHYSICAL EXAMINATION

VITAL SIGNS: Temperature 97, left arm pressure is 113/56, right arm pressure is 109/80, pulse is 88, respirations 19. He has easily palpable normal upper extremity pulses with easily palpable subclavian arteries bilaterally. No supraclavicular bruits. He has 2+ carotid pulses bilaterally with good upstroke and bilateral bruits. He has easily palpable superficial temporal pulses. He has no epigastric pulsation, no epigastric or flank bruits. He has diminished femoral pulses bilaterally, but they are palpable, and he has had no palpable pulses below this bilaterally. He has stigmata of peripheral vascular disease at his distal leg and foot level; however, he has no tissue breakdown.

DIAGNOSTIC DATA: Imaging and noninvasive vascular laboratory data: He underwent lower extremity segmental pressures and PVRs on July 19 of this year, which revealed evidence of multilevel occlusive disease bilaterally. This is moderate to severe in nature with a right ABI of 0.5 and a left ABI of 0.7. On the left it does appear the majority of his disease is actually in the SFA/popliteal region, and his right-sided disease is multifactorial with both aortoiliac and superficial femoral popliteal disease. His toe pressure on the right is 49. His toe pressure on the left is 44. His PVRs do reveal a bit of blunting and some latency, suggesting multilevel disease bilaterally.

IMPRESSION/PLAN

Overall, Mr. Stotler states that this is not greatly limiting him. I discussed with him a structured walking program and that he should again start to walk. There is no danger with this.

After claudication education and a discussion of intermittent claudication, I discussed with him that he needs, as well, an aortic screening and a carotid duplex. Based upon his segmental pressures, we will see him again in 6 months with an aortoiliac duplex and ABIs to evaluate for progression.

(Continued)

ID#: M-17   PAGE 2

He understands this and will begin his structured walking program. I believe that from a medical standpoint, he appears to be overall well controlled. He is on a beta blocker, an ACE inhibitor, and a statin medication. Further, he is already taking 100 mg b.i.d. of cilostazol. I gave him my card and said that he can follow up with us sooner if need be.

_____

Ly An Tabor, MD
Vascular Surgery

LAT:cks
D:08/04/----
T:08/04/----

c: Chris Salem, DO, Family Practice

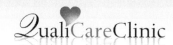

Hematology/Oncology Bone Marrow Transplant Note

Patient Name: Richard J. Fisher   **PCP:** David H. Cohen, MD

Date of Exam: 03/01/----   **Age/Sex:** 47/M   **ID#:** M-18

INTRODUCTION: Richard Fisher is a 47-year-old African American gentleman with a history of lymphoplasmacytic lymphoma who is status post high-dose melphalan and autologous stem cell support in June of last year. He presents today for possible collection of autologous cells.

HISTORY OF PRESENT ILLNESS: Patient was referred from his primary oncologist for possible collection of autologous cells. In December of last year, the patient collected 1.8 x 10⁶ over a 2-day period. At that time, patient did not want to pursue a collection of further stem cells. Since that time, he has had slow progression of his disease. His primary oncologist has discussed with the patient starting Velcade, and he felt that we should collect autologous cells before any further stem cell toxic therapy.

Mr. Fisher is actually a patient of Dr. David Cohen. Dr. Cohen had discussed with the patient allogenic stem cell transplant from a sibling. As it turns out, he does have a brother who is a 6/6 HLA match. Patient states that he is considering either an autologous stem cell transplant or a nonmyeloablative allogenic transplant at this time.

Since patient's last collection, he has had no significant change in his past medical history. He has not traveled outside of the state since his last collection.

PHYSICAL EXAMINATION

VITAL SIGNS: Blood pressure 126/81, temperature 98.3, pulse 89, respirations 16, weight 93.7 kg. GENERAL: Middle-aged male, awake, alert, and oriented x3 in no acute distress. HEENT: Sclerae nonicteric. Conjunctivae pink. Oral mucosa clear. LYMPH NODES: No cervical, supraclavicular, axillary, or inguinal adenopathy. LUNGS have slightly decreased breath sounds at the bases, otherwise clear. ABDOMEN is soft and nontender. EXTREMITIES are without edema.

LABORATORY AND X-RAY DATA: Kappa free light chains 4134 mg/dL from February 15 of this year. This is increased from 2078 in October 2 years ago and 1834 in August of last year. Kappa-free light chains preautologous transplant in June of last year were 48,724.

On February 15 of last year his beta-2 microglobulin was 5.4 and creatinine 2. White blood cells 4, hemoglobin 12.3, and platelets 144,000.

IMPRESSION

This is a 47-year-old black male with lymphoplasmacytic lymphoma with progressive disease post autologous stem cell transplant. I think it is reasonable to complete stem cell collection at this time. With collection of his last stem cells, this was done at 15 mcg/kg. I suspect patient should be able to complete collection in 2 to 3 days. I did discuss with patient, however, that this would be only temporizing for his disease and that he had evidence of progression of disease within 4 months of his autologous transplant. I think his only chance of disease-free survival is with an allogenic stem cell transplant, although this does carry the risk of mortality up front.

(Continued)

ID#: M-18   PAGE 2

PLAN

1. Will begin high-dose G-CSF at 15 mcg/kg on March 22. Will begin stem cell collection on March 26.
2. Patient will follow up with me on day of collection, March 26. After this, I will refer patient back to his primary transplant doctor, Dr. Cohen.

_____
Solomon T. Fisher, MD
Hematology/Oncology

STF:cks
D:03/01/----
T:03/02/----

cc: David H. Cohen, MD, Hematology/Oncology

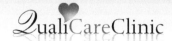

<u>**Internal Medicine Clinic Note**</u>

Patient Name: Jack T. Lampe, PhD   **PCP:** Sherman Loyd, MD
Date of Exam: 09/30/----   **Age/Sex:** 76/M   **ID#:** M-19

CHIEF COMPLAINT: This 76-year-old white male is here for followup medical care.

HISTORY: The patient describes being Dr. Ramirez's patient, describes appreciation for his thoroughness. He goes on to note that he needs no medications renewed but has had a hard time getting into our clinic and hopes that in the next few months he would be able to reestablish care.

PAST MEDICAL HISTORY
1. Dyslipidemia.
2. Once a smoker, discontinued 3 years ago.
3. Sensorineural hearing loss.
4. Chronic ischemic heart disease, apparently.
5. Symptomatic bradycardia. He had a pacemaker placed 8 years ago.
6. Chronic atrial fibrillation.
7. Anticoagulation, chronic, and this for #6 above.
8. Slow urinary stream.
9. Pulmonary tuberculosis, left kidney focus. This was found when he presented with recurrent urinary tract infections. Multiple urinary samples done at different medical facilities found the culprit organism, with diagnosis eventually made.
10. Cataracts, both eyes. There is a question as to whether or not amiodarone is involved. (The stromal deposits are called verticillata.)

PAST SURGICAL HISTORY
1. He had a coronary arteriogram and a permanent pacer placed 8 years ago in January.
2. Left kidney revision by a Dr. Green in the remote past.
3. Rectal melanoma excision 10 years ago.
4. Tympanoplasty and mastoidectomy 20 years ago.
5. Right cataract surgery 7 years ago.

ALLERGIES: STREPTOMYCIN and ALDOMET. Manifestations unknown.

MEDICATIONS (mg p.o. daily unless otherwise noted)
1. Warfarin 223 as of today.
2. Tamsulosin 0.4 mg b.i.d.
3. Simvastatin 20.
4. Potassium chloride 10.
5. Omeprazole 20.
6. Metoprolol 200.
7. Lisinopril 40.
8. Hydrochlorothiazide 25.
9. Finasteride 5.

FAMILY HISTORY: Patient describes his mother dying of tuberculosis 8 to 9 months after he was born. A sister succumbed to cancer as an adult. He thinks it was lymphoma.

(Continued)

ID#: M-19   PAGE 2

SOCIAL HISTORY: Patient lives locally with his wife. He has been seeking medical care from Quali-Care Internal Medicine Clinic for some time. He once smoked and he rarely drinks. History of being a pipe smoker.

REVIEW OF SYSTEMS

CONSTITUTIONAL: Patient has gained approximately 8 pounds in the last year. There has been no weakness.

NEUROLOGIC: Denies headaches, seizures. There have been no falls.

HEENT: Denies description of sore throat, vision, or hearing change. He admits to being hard of hearing.

ENDOCRINE: He has had no diabetes or thyroid problems. He has had hypertension.

CARDIAC: There has been no heart attack or heart failure. He has had no rapid heart rates.

PULMONARY: No known pulmonary disease. He has no cough or wheeze. There has been no pulmonary embolism.

GASTROINTESTINAL: He denies description of odynophagia, dysphagia, bleeding ulcers, or epigastric pain. He describes an empty feeling that led him to seek medical attention. A diagnosis of what sounds like GERD was made. Prilosec started. His chief complaint was 100% resolved. He has had no liver disease. No change in stool color, caliber, or consistency. He thinks his last colonoscopy was 3 years ago in our facility.

RENAL: He has had the renal disease as described above. His kidneys are now functional from his point of view. Denies dysuria or kidney stones.

HEMATOLOGIC: No bleeding or clotting abnormalities. No transfusions.

SKIN: No skin color changes. No new lumps or bumps.

RHEUMATOLOGIC: Denies muscle pains or joint aches.

PHYSICAL EXAMINATION

VITALS show blood pressure 129/86, pulse 91, respirations 16, temperature 98.7, height 5 feet 10 inches, weight 171 pounds. Generally, he is a white male of medium build, very careful with his speech, in no apparent respiratory distress. Has minimal upper body segment obesity.

HEENT: No dominant skin lesions. Mouth and nose clear. Eyes without arcus senilis. No injection. Ears clear bilaterally.

NECK is without cervical lymphadenopathy, thyromegaly, or nodules. There are no carotid bruits or murmurs.

PULMONARY: Lungs are clear to auscultation.

HEART: Regular. S1 and S2 are normal.

ABDOMEN: Soft, nontender, with bowel sounds present.

EXTREMITIES are without cyanosis, clubbing, or edema.

ANCILLARY DATA

Cardiac catheterization from 8 years ago showed normal coronaries with ejection fraction of 45%. Eight years ago his pulmonary function tests showed FEV1 of 86% of predicted, FVC 106%, DLCO (an adjusted value, namely D/VA) 103% of predicted. Plethysmography showed vital capacity 81% of predicted. Spirometry showed normal inspiratory and expiratory flow volume loops. Three years ago he had a transthoracic echo that showed an ejection fraction of 60% and normal left ventricular size and function. Valves were unremarkable. Last January

(Continued)

ID#: M-19   PAGE 3

(9 months ago) his LDL and HDL were within normal limits. Creatinine was 1.3 and slowly increasing, when viewing the trend. Total bilirubin increased and decreased.

ASSESSMENT

1. Hypertension, controlled on medical therapy.
2. Extrapulmonary tuberculosis, eventuating in an undocumented surgery.
3. Symptomatic bradycardia, now with pacer in place. Normal left ventricular function.
4. Vacillating total bilirubin.
5. Chronic atrial fibrillation, now anticoagulated.
6. Slow creatinine rise, etiology unclear. Patient clinically stable.

PLAN

1. I have reviewed patient's medical record, which dates back approximately 8 years. I see no evidence of colonoscopy.
2. I would like to see him back in 6 months.
3. Patient clinically stable. No medications to renew.

_____

Jean W. Mooney, PA
Internal Medicine

JWM:cks
T:09/30/----
D:10/01/----

c: Sherman Loyd, MD, Pulmonology
   Saul Thompson, MD, Cardiology

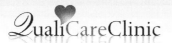

Emergency Department Treatment Record

Patient Name: Tristan R. Leher   **PCP:** Linda L. Kingston, DO
Date of Exam: 07/08/----   **Age/Sex:** 19/M   **ID#:** M-20

CONSULTING SERVICE: Genitourinary Service.

CHIEF COMPLAINT: Penile discharge.

HISTORY OF PRESENT ILLNESS: This is a 19-year-old male who states that approximately 2 or 3 days ago he was masturbating and noticed a brownish discoloration to his ejaculate. Patient states that this was not painful, and he knows of no history of prior incidences of this; however, he does state that in late April or early May he was diagnosed with Chlamydia and was given azithromycin for that. Patient states that he was given no other antibiotics to include no other antibiotic injections and no other medications at that time. He completed his course of azithromycin and had no followup. Patient states that he has had no dysuria, hematuria, abdominal pain, testicular pain, and no penile discharge with the exception of that noted above. No back pain, fevers, chills, or rashes. Patient states he has been sexually active in the past, but he has not been sexually active since April or May of this year.

REVIEW OF SYSTEMS: As in HPI.

PAST MEDICAL HISTORY: Negative.

PAST SURGICAL HISTORY: Negative.

MEDICATIONS: None.

ALLERGIES: No known drug allergies.

SOCIAL HISTORY: Patient was sexually active 2 months ago. No alcohol use, no smoking, no illicit drugs.

PHYSICAL EXAMINATION

VITAL SIGNS on presentation: Pulse 74, blood pressure 118/67, respiratory rate 18, temperature 98.5, saturating 98% on room air. In general, the patient is alert and oriented, in no apparent distress. HEENT: Atraumatic. Extraocular movements intact. Pupils are equal, round, and reactive to light and accommodation bilaterally. Oropharynx and nasopharynx clear. NECK: Supple, no adenopathy. No jugular venous distention. CARDIOVASCULAR: Heart rate and rhythm regular. No murmurs, gallops, or rubs. PULMONARY: No respiratory distress. Lungs are clear to auscultation in all fields bilaterally. ABDOMEN: Nondistended, nontender to palpation. No masses or hepatosplenomegaly, no costovertebral angle tenderness. INGUINAL REGION: No adenopathy. GENITOURINARY: Testicles nontender, both descended. No masses. Penis is uncircumcised. Foreskin is retracted. There is no discharge. No lesions. Penis is nontender. EXTREMITIES: No cyanosis, clubbing, or edema. Pulses 2+ in upper and lower extremities bilaterally. SKIN: No rashes, no lesions.

(Continued)

ID#: M-20   PAGE 2

EMERGENCY DEPARTMENT COURSE/MEDICAL DECISION MAKING: This is a 19-year-old male with a history of urethritis, which, per the patient, was treated with only a single week of azithromycin. He states that he was given no further medications for this, was given no other antibiotics, was given no injections during this time, and he now has this discharge with his ejaculate. It is therefore possible that this patient still has a urethritis, possibly gonococcal, since he apparently was not treated for gonococcal infection. He is nontoxic here in the ED, has no signs of infection, is afebrile, and his physical exam was completely benign. I think it is possible that he has urethritis, perhaps gonococcal, at this time. Cultures were taken from the penile region and the urethra. I suspect no epididymitis since the patient's testicles are nontender. He has no inguinal adenopathy, so I suspect no significant spread of disease. His skin is otherwise without lesions, and he has no history of medical problems. He has not been sexually active for 1 to 2 months.

EMERGENCY DEPARTMENT DIAGNOSIS
Urethritis, possible gonorrheal versus chlamydial.

DISPOSITION
I will treat him with a 7-day course of doxycycline 100 mg b.i.d., ceftriaxone 1 g IM x1 here in the ED. Cultures were sent. Consult to be arranged for patient's followup with Dr. Mendesz in the urology clinic for results of the culture and any further treatment necessary at that time.

_____
Samuel Ernest, MD
Emergency Room Physician

SE:cks
D:07/08/----
T:07/08/----

cc: Charles Mendesz, MD, Urology
     Linda L. Kingston, DO, Family Practice

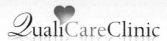

QualiCareClinic

Bone Marrow Clinic History and Physical Examination

Patient Name: Miguel Trujillo   **PCP:** Jean W. Mooney, PA

Date of Admission: October 7, ----   **Age/Sex:** 36/M   **ID#:** M-21

CHIEF COMPLAINT: The patient is a 36-year-old male with refractory Hodgkin lymphoma who will be admitted today with progressive hypoxia.

HISTORY OF PRESENT ILLNESS: Patient has known parenchymal Hodgkin lymphoma. In addition, he has bilateral pleural effusions, left effusion large, right effusion small. His left effusion is known to be a chylous effusion. This was tapped several weeks ago at the pulmonary clinic. It has reaccumulated and has been stable over the past several weeks. In addition, on September 20 he had a pulmonary embolism, which was small, on the right. He has been on Lovenox anticoagulation. His pulmonary embolism resulted in oxygen requirement. Two days ago in clinic his oxygen saturation at rest was 95% on room air. Yesterday he presented to clinic and was saturating in the 70s on 2 liters with exertion. He denied having increased symptoms of shortness of breath. CT angiogram was obtained, which was unable to be compared with previous CTs; however, it was reviewed by pulmonary staff, who felt that the pleural effusion was stable in size as well as his lymphomatous involvement. He demonstrated no new PE. There were no areas of consolidation to suggest pneumonia; however, he does have bilateral compressive atelectasis, left greater than right, and we cannot exclude pneumonia in these areas. Patient was afebrile in clinic yesterday, his oxygenation improved on 4 liters' oxygen, and he was sent home. When patient returned to clinic today, he was 87% on 5 liters, which improved to 99% on a nonrebreather. He had no new complaints overnight; however, he was febrile in clinic this morning at 101.5. He has a chronic dry cough that has increased in frequency over the past several days.

Patient's Hodgkin lymphoma most recently recurred in July three years ago. He underwent 2 cycles of "mini bine" with progressive disease. He is currently on cycle 1 of salvage gemcitabine, Navelbine, and Doxil. He will be due for cycle 2 on October 11. He is currently undergoing growth factor stimulation for stem cell collection. He is to begin his stem cell collection today.

Patient currently has a pruritic rash over his back. This is being treated with triamcinolone and Atarax.

PAST MEDICAL HISTORY
1. Chemo-refractory Hodgkin lymphoma.
2. Depression.
3. Herpes zoster.

PAST SURGICAL HISTORY: None.

FAMILY HISTORY: Noncontributory. He has 1 full sister.

SOCIAL HISTORY: No tobacco or alcohol. He currently lives locally with his wife.

ALLERGIES: No known drug allergies.

MEDICATIONS
1. Zoloft 75 mg daily.
2. Lovenox 100 mg subcutaneously daily.
3. Acyclovir 800 mg p.o. b.i.d.
4. Aranesp 300 mg subcutaneously weekly.
5. Neupogen 960 mcg subcutaneously daily.
6. Atarax 25 mg every 8 hours p.r.n. pruritus.
7. Triamcinolone cream 0.1% to back b.i.d.
8. Hydromorphone 2 mg every 4 hours p.r.n. cough.

(Continued)

REVIEW OF SYSTEMS: Per HPI. In addition, patient has had drenching night sweats over the past several weeks. He has pruritus. Denies nausea, vomiting, diarrhea, melena, or dysuria.

PHYSICAL EXAMINATION

VITALS: Temperature 101.5, blood pressure 95/58, pulse rate 121, respirations 32, 87% on 5 liters, improved to 99% on nonrebreather, with decrease in pulse rate to 111.

GENERAL: Young, cachectic Hispanic male in no acute distress.

HEENT: Sclerae nonicteric. Conjunctivae pink. Oral mucosa clear.

LYMPH NODES: No cervical, supraclavicular, or infraclavicular adenopathy palpable. There are multiple, small, right axillary lymph nodes.

LUNGS: Decreased breath sounds bilaterally at the bases; left is to the midlung field.

HEART is tachycardic.

ABDOMEN is soft and nontender.

EXTREMITIES are without edema.

LABORATORY DATA: CBC, CMP pending.

IMPRESSION

This is a 36-year-old male with refractory Hodgkin lymphoma, bilateral pleural effusions, left greater than right, recent pulmonary embolism, worsening hypoxia, and increasing cough. With no significant change on CT scan, the etiology for patient's worsening hypoxia is unclear. It is possible, with his fever, that he has pneumonia in the areas of atelectasis.

PLAN

1. We will start double gram-negative coverage with Levaquin 750 mg daily and cefepime 2 g every 12 hours.
2. Obtain blood cultures x2, urinalysis, urine culture, and chest x-ray.
3. Continue Neupogen through stem cell collection. Goal is to collect enough stem cells for 2 transplants. It is not ideal to collect patient while he is febrile; however, patient has received multiple chemotherapy regimens and concern is we will be unable to collect patient at a future date. Patient may need to receive antibiotics when stem cells are reinfused.
4. Hold Lovenox for now. Will consult Pulmonary regarding possible thoracentesis of the left effusion. I do not think this is the cause of the patient's acute hypoxia, as the effusion has been stable; however, this may improve his hypoxia by giving him increased lung volume. Because this is a chylous effusion, and we have not fixed the leak, it will reaccumulate rapidly, and this will be just a temporary fix.
5. Oxygen to maintain O_2 sats greater than 93%.
6. Admit to inpatient BMT Unit.

_____

Solomon T. Fisher, MD
Hematology

STF:cks
D:10/07/----
T:10/07/----

cc: Jean W. Mooney, PA, Internal Medicine
    Joshua Stephen Gatlin, MD, Pulmonology

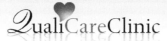

Internal Medicine Followup Note

Patient Name: Daniel J. Tremblay   **PCP:** Anne Basswood, MD

Date of Exam: 2/17/----   **Age/Sex:** 35/M   **ID#:** M-23

REASON FOR VISIT: Routine followup.

HISTORY OF PRESENT ILLNESS: Mr. Tremblay is a pleasant 35-year-old gentleman with a past medical history significant for severe closed-head injury with resulting cerebral palsy, B12 deficiency, seborrheic dermatitis, nonalcoholic fatty liver disease, history of seizure disorder, wheelchair dependence, and lower extremity spasticity treated with baclofen pump. Per his mother's report, who is also his caregiver, the patient has been doing okay. He has been in desperate need of a new wheelchair with a stander. Because of his decreased standing, he has had worsening compaction and worsening lower extremity spasticity. Mr. Tremblay is unable to ambulate without use of his wheelchair in his home. He cannot stand independently. Patient is able to communicate appropriately with short, 1- to 3-word answers; however, he cannot use the phone, read, or participate otherwise in his own ADLs. His mother is his around-the-clock caregiver.

Mr. Tremblay was recently evaluated and was found to be able to use a power wheelchair independently to some extent as well as with the assistance of his caregiver. His limitations cannot be corrected with the use of just a cane or a walker. His home has been adapted for the use of a wheelchair. He has the appropriate ramps into the home as well as widened doorways and other access as appropriate. His mobility cannot be completely resolved with a manual wheelchair, as he cannot propel himself in a manual wheelchair. Due to patient's limited upper extremity strength as well as his spasticity, a scooter would not be appropriate. Patient needs the proper positioning and pressure relief provided only by a power wheelchair. Given patient's history of significant spasticity that is treated to some extent with a baclofen pump, he needs the capability to be able to be put into a standing position. Standing and stretching has significantly improved his spasticity in the past.

Patient recently has had significant irritation of his left eye. He has a condition known as filamentitis. He is being followed by the cornea specialist in the ophthalmology clinic. He is able to open his eye today, which is somewhat improved from our last encounter. At that time patient could not open his left eye. His caregiver agrees that it has improved, but it has not yet resolved.

CURRENT MEDICATIONS
1. B12 injections, 1000 mcg monthly.
2. Lamictal 100 mg b.i.d.
3. Tegretol 200 mg b.i.d.
4. Potassium chloride 20 mEq daily.
5. Prilosec solution 10 mL b.i.d.
6. Claritin 10 mg daily.
7. Restasis eye drops daily.
8. BenzaClin gel p.r.n.
9. Selenium sulfate shampoo daily.
10. Tube feeds nightly.
11. Intrathecal baclofen pump.

PHYSICAL EXAMINATION

VITALS: Blood pressure 106/68, pulse 89, respirations 16. Height was previously 5 feet 8 inches.

GENERAL: Alert and awake. He answers simple questions appropriately.

HEENT: Pupils equal, round, and reactive to light and accommodation. Extraocular motions intact. No significant conjunctival injection; however, the left eye is tearing. The patient squints with that eye.

(Continued)

ID#: M-23   PAGE 2

NECK: Supple without bruits.

CARDIOVASCULAR: Regular rate and rhythm. Normal Sl, S2, no S3 or S4, no murmurs.

CHEST is clear to auscultation bilaterally.

EXTREMITIES: Lower extremities with no clubbing, cyanosis, or edema.

LABORATORY AND X-RAY DATA: None.

ASSESSMENT
This 35-year-old gentleman with past medical history as listed above is doing okay at this time but would significantly benefit from a new power wheelchair with standing capability secondary to increased compaction of the spine as well as increased lower extremity spasticity.

PLAN
1. Mobility impaired, as above: Recommend that patient receive a new power wheelchair with standing capability. He has been seen by the physical medicine and rehabilitation physician in the past, and a prescription for the correctly fitting chair has been acquired.
2. Seizure disorder: Patient has been without seizures for many, many years. He is followed in the neurology clinic. He is to continue his Lamictal and Tegretol at their current doses.
3. Corneal filamentitis: Patient is to follow up in the ophthalmology clinic as previously instructed.
4. Healthcare maintenance: Patient is up to date.

DISPOSITION: Follow up with me in 3 to 4 months, sooner as needed.

_____

Jean W. Mooney, PA
Internal Medicine

JWM:cks
D:2/17/----
T:2/18/----

c: Anne Basswood, MD, Neurology

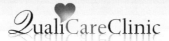

Hematology/Oncology Clinic Outpatient Progress Note

Patient Name: Otto Rentz   **PCP:** A. Leigh Wells, MD

Date of Exam: 7/31/----   **Age/Sex:** 61/M   **ID#:** M-24

HISTORY OF PRESENT ILLNESS: Mr. Rentz is a 61-year-old gentleman who presents to the hematology clinic for followup of myelodysplastic syndrome with a 5q- mutation. He is currently treated with every-other-week Aranesp. His last dose was last Wednesday, the 26th of July. Since our last visit, the patient has been seen by Nephrology here at Quali-Care Clinic as well as initial and followup care with his primary care doctor in internal medicine. He has had medication changed to include the discontinuation of Lasix and spironolactone for acute on chronic kidney failure. However, his Lasix was recently restarted due to increasing lower extremity edema and hyperkalemia. The patient states that overall he is feeling well. He states that his energy level is improved since our last visit. He continues to be limited in his physical activity by pain secondary to his gout. The pain is most pronounced in his bilateral knees, right greater than left, as well as bilateral feet. He was scheduled to undergo knee corticosteroid injection last week; however, there was limited evidence of inflammation at that time and the injection was canceled.

MEDICATIONS: Except as above, there have been no medication changes since his last visit.

SOCIAL HISTORY: He was prescribed Zyban for tobacco cessation, states that he has not noticed much of a difference in his cravings. However, he is still interested in smoking cessation.

PHYSICAL EXAMINATION

VITAL SIGNS are 104/62, heart rate of 80, temperature 98.1, weight 130.6 pounds, which is an improvement from his weight on our last visit, which was 128 pounds.

LABORATORY AND X-RAY DATA: CBC shows a hemoglobin of 11.1, which is improved from his previous value. Patient underwent CT of his chest last week to follow up on abnormal PET scan results. The CT chest showed significant mediastinal lymphadenopathy. However, there were no lung parenchymal findings to correlate with the CT results.

ASSESSMENT AND PLAN

This is a 61-year-old gentleman with a complicated medical history to include myelodysplastic syndrome with a 5q- mutation. He is currently responding well to Aranesp. I will continue Aranesp 300 mcg every other week, and I will follow up with another CBC in 1 month. If he does not continue to respond, I will consider a course of Revlimid, given his improving performance status, and follow up in the medical system. The remainder of his medical problems are stable and are well managed by his PCP.

_____

Solomon T. Fisher, MD
Hematology

STF:cks
D:7/31/----
T:7/31/----

c: A. Leigh Wells, MD, Internal Medicine
    Trevor Jordan, MD, Nephrology

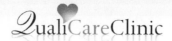

QualiCareClinic

Physical Medicine and Rehabilitation Consultation

Patient Name: Dawn T. Peterson   **PCP:** A. Leigh Wells, MD

Date of Consultation: 08/10/----   **Age/Sex:** 63/F   **ID#:** M-25

REASON FOR CONSULT: Low back pain and left greater than right radiating thigh pain.

HISTORY OF PRESENT ILLNESS: Ms. Peterson is a 63-year-old female who is referred to me by Dr. Wells of internal medicine for evaluation of this patient's chronic intermittent low back pain for almost 15 years, although this pain particularly worsened 4 years ago when she subsequently began to have radiating, left greater than right anterior thigh pain. She states this pain is particularly aggravated with activities, especially with standing and walking, and she is limited to less than 200 feet before needing to sit down after the onset following that duration and distance. She has some improvement with leaning forward, such as pushing a cart, as well as when she initially lies down on her back. Nevertheless, she still has pain at night when she sleeps in one position for a prolonged period. She states the majority of her pain is across her back, but she also has this radiating, left greater than right anterior thigh pain. The pain severity ranges from 0/10 to 7/10.

REVIEW OF SYSTEMS: Neurologic review of systems is remarkable for the left greater than right radiating anterior thigh pain that is generally in an L3 to, less likely, L4 distribution. There are some associated numbness and paresthesias on that left thigh. There is also some weakness in the left thigh, particularly noted when attempting to climb stairs. She occasionally will have some falls and stumbling on that left leg due to such weakness. She has some mild bilateral numbness and tingling in her feet related to her diabetes mellitus. Denies bowel/bladder changes or incontinence. Constitutional review of systems is unremarkable for fevers, chills, progressive night pain, although she has some pain at night. She denies any malignancy, history of malaise, or recent infection.

Treatment for this back pain has consisted of physical therapy as well as some injections in the distant past. She does continue to do some exercises on a regular basis.

PAST MEDICAL HISTORY: Hyperlipidemia, hypertension, IDDM with associated polyneuropathy and retinopathy, TIA, GERD, essential tremor, knee osteoarthritis.

PAST SURGICAL HISTORY: CABG, tonsillectomy, hysterectomy, C-section, laser eye surgery, carpal tunnel release.

SOCIAL HISTORY: Denies tobacco or alcohol beverage consumption.

MEDICATIONS: Her only analgesic is Tylenol up to 1 g t.i.d., but she rarely uses that much. Other meds include insulin, lisinopril, Pletal, Protonix, primidone, aspirin, and Zocor.

ALLERGIES: ERYTHROMYCIN, AUGMENTIN, MACRODANTIN, and SEPTRA/SULFA.

RADIOLOGY: Lumbosacral spine MRI in April two years ago was remarkable for severe acquired degenerative central canal stenosis at L3-4 plus the left foraminal stenosis related to a broad, diffuse disk protrusion, facet hypertrophy, and ligamentum flavum thickening.

PHYSICAL EXAMINATION

GENERAL APPEARANCE: Well-nourished, well-developed female, A&O x3, appropriate mood and affect, pleasant, and in no acute distress.

(Continued)

ID#: M-25   PAGE 2

SPINE: Posture: Mildly increased thoracic kyphosis and slight loss of lumbosacral lordosis. Lumbopelvic

AROM: Moderate aggravation of the left greater than right lumbosacral area back pain with quadrant loading as well as with extension and some relief with flexion. Unable to reproduce any of the radiating left anterior thigh pain. Palpation: Mild tenderness in the lower lumbar spinous/paraspinous region.

NEUROLOGIC: Gait: There is diminished heel walking as well as tandem walking, although she is better able to do some toe walking. Motor: The lower extremity muscle groups are as follows: Iliopsoas and quadriceps are 5/5. Anterior tibialis −5/5. EHL 4+/5, peroneal 4+/5, and gastrocsoleus 5−/4 or 5. Fairly symmetric. Sensory: There is some decrease in a stocking distribution on her bilateral legs below the midportion of the lower leg. The proximal regions are intact to both light touch and pinprick. Reflexes: Right patella is 1− and the left is 1+. Achilles is absent. No response from Babinski testing. Nerve tension signs: There is a left femoral nerve stretch test on the nerve tension signs, and the right is normal as well as having a negative straight-leg raise for the right and left.

EXTREMITIES/VASCULAR: Normal temperature and coloration of distal legs and feet, with palpable dorsalis pedis pulses 2+ and symmetric and without cyanosis or edema.

ASSESSMENT

1. L3-4 canal and left L3-4 foraminal stenosis with secondary low back pain as well as left greater than right L3 greater than L4 neurogenic/radicular leg pain.
2. Insulin-dependent diabetes mellitus with distal sensory polyneuropathy.

PLAN

1. Left L3-4 and L4-5 transforaminal epidural steroid injection is scheduled after discussion of risks and benefits.
2. Extensively discussed her limitations, particularly to avoid prolonged standing and walking due to likely aggravation of her neurogenic leg pain.
3. Would recommend use of a stationary bicycle or a pool/aquatic exercises.
4. Also will request a multibreaking rolling walker to assist her for ambulation outside the home.
5. She will continue with her Tylenol up to 1 g q.i.d. at her request for her analgesic needs.

_____

Jean W. Mooney, PA
Physical Medicine and Rehabilitation

JWM:cks
D:08/10/----
T:08/11/----

cc: A. Leigh Wells, MD, Internal Medicine

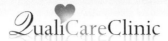

Emergency Room Treatment Record

Patient Name: Gayle Ann Moss   **PCP:** Jean W. Mooney, PA

Date of Exam: 02/18/----   **Age/Sex:** 27/F   **ID#:** M-26

CONSULTING SERVICE: Internal Medicine.

CHIEF COMPLAINT: Assault.

HISTORY OF PRESENT ILLNESS: This is a 27-year-old white female with no significant past medical history who presents today for medical evaluation after an encounter with another physician. She says she is a reservist who was getting her yearly physical done and was seen this morning by a Dr. Smolz. She said that during the course of the evaluation she told the doctor about some mild persistent wrist pain. He performed the exam and diagnosed early carpal tunnel syndrome. He then asked her if she had ever had acupuncture before. She replied she had not, and then the patient states that he instructed her to remove her socks and shoes. He then withdrew a solid copper needle from a pouch, a plastic pouch, which had been contained in one of the pockets of his flight suit. He then inserted the needle into various surfaces of her forearm and wrist and bilateral lower extremities— between 5 and 10 times on each extremity. The patient states that at no point was she asked if she would like to undergo acupuncture. There was no explanation, and no consent was obtained. The therapeutic risks and benefits were not explained to her.

Furthermore, patient states that her skin was not prepared and that Dr. Smolz did not wash his hands. She also reports that the physician requested that she "not tattle," as he has apparently been counseled on performing acupuncture by a general officer prior to this date. She then proceeded to go to lunch. She noticed some transient red rash and some minor aches and pains, most especially on her right foot, with some bruising over the top of the right midfoot. As time went on, she thought more about the episode and began to feel that she had been victimized. The patient relates a history of sexual abuse at age 8, and she said she felt a return to that victimized state. She felt strongly that she had been taken advantage of, and she then proceeded to discuss the situation with her friends and colleagues. They advised her to get checked out.

REVIEW OF SYSTEMS: Reviewed 9 of 12 systems; all are unremarkable except for the HPI.

PAST MEDICAL HISTORY: As noted above.

PAST SURGICAL HISTORY: Wisdom teeth extraction.

FAMILY HISTORY: Noncontributory.

SOCIAL HISTORY: No alcohol, illicit drugs, or tobacco.

MEDICATIONS: Birth control pills.

ALLERGIES: No known drug allergies.

IMMUNIZATIONS: Up to date.

PHYSICAL EXAMINATION

VITAL SIGNS on presentation: Temperature 99, pulse 96, respirations 18, blood pressure 135/83, pulse oximetry is 99%. In general, this is a well-developed, well-nourished white female in no acute distress.
HEENT: Normocephalic, atraumatic. Pupils are equal, round, and reactive to light and accommodation. Extraocular movements intact. No scleral icterus or injection. Nares clear. Oropharynx unremarkable.
NECK: No lymphadenopathy. CHEST: Regular rate and rhythm with no murmur, rub, or gallop.

(Continued)

ID#: M-26   PAGE 2

LUNGS: Clear to auscultation bilaterally. ABDOMEN: Soft, nontender, nondistended with normoactive bowel sounds. EXTREMITIES: are warm, well perfused. SKIN: There are a few scattered areas of mild erythema over the dorsal surfaces of the bilateral forearms. There is also a 2 x 3 cm area of mild ecchymosis over the dorsal midfoot of the right lower extremity. Scattered, punctate, erythematous lesions are seen consistent with needle insertion sites about the dorsal surfaces of the distal 4 extremities. Pulses are 2+ and symmetric x4. Full range of motion of all joints of the upper and lower extremities. No significant edema or erythema and no tracking.

EMERGENCY DEPARTMENT COURSE/MEDICAL DECISION MAKING: This is a 27-year-old white female who presents for evaluation after apparently undergoing acupuncture in another physician's office earlier this morning. She feels very strongly that she was victimized by this physician and has presented for further evaluation. At this time Security Police have been notified as well as the patient's chain of command, and her supervisor and first sergeant are present at the bedside. In addition to law enforcement, we have notified Family Advocacy and Medical Photo is present and will take photographs to document the physical findings.

At this time there are a few medical issues that I have counseled the patient on:

1. Long-term wrist pain, which I feel needs no further investigation during this visit to the ED.
2. Any risk of disease transmission with multiple punctures with a solid bore needle. I advised her that even if the needle was not sterile and her skin was not prepared, the chances of significant disease transmission, to include hepatitis and HIV, is vanishingly small. I would recommend that the patient undergo no prophylactic antimicrobial therapy at this time. There is always a risk of infection or bleeding whenever the skin is pierced; however, there is no apparent evidence of bleeding, and I am unconcerned by the ecchymosis on the right foot. It is too early to diagnose any possible skin infection at this time. She was given strict precautions to return for fever, swelling, redness, heat, pain, or any kind of discharge from the needle puncture sites.
3. In addition, especially given the patient's prior history of sexual abuse, I have counseled her that should she feel the need to speak with a physician again, if this episode should trigger any depression or anxiety, the ED is always available to her. She can come back and be reevaluated at any time. She now feels well enough to proceed home without further psychological or psychiatric intervention.

EMERGENCY DEPARTMENT DIAGNOSIS: Multiple needle punctures to all 4 extremities.

DISPOSITION: At this time I am going to complete my documentation and discharge the patient to home. From my standpoint at this time, the case is closed from a medical standpoint. It is pending further investigation by law enforcement.

DISCHARGE INSTRUCTIONS: Close return precautions.

_____

Samuel Ernest, MD
Emergency Room Physician

SE:cks
D:02/18/----
T:02/18/----

c: Jean W. Mooney, PA, Internal Medicine

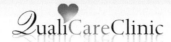

Orthopedic Clinic Consultation

Patient Name: Lisa Marie Jones   **PCP:** Reed Phillips, MD

Date of Exam: 09/30/----   **Age/Sex:** 3 months/F   **ID#:** M-27

REASON FOR CONSULTATION: Right arm pain.

HISTORY OF PRESENT ILLNESS: Lisa Marie is a 3-month-old female infant who was brought to the Hillcrest ED by her parents after the father noted that Lisa Marie was not moving her right upper extremity. He states that he went into the bedroom to check on her in the evening and that she was extremely fussy. She cried even worse with the movement of her right upper extremity. The parents brought her to the ED for evaluation. X-rays performed in the ED showed a right displaced humeral shaft fracture. The orthopedics service was subsequently consulted for evaluation of this fracture.

ALLERGIES: The patient has no known drug allergies.

MEDICATIONS: She is on no medications.

PAST MEDICAL/SURGICAL HISTORY: There is no past medical or surgical history.

PERINATAL HISTORY: The patient was the term product of a normal spontaneous vaginal delivery. She had no birth complications.

FAMILY HISTORY: Not significant.

PHYSICAL EXAMINATION

The right upper extremity shows a swelling over the right brachium. She moves her fingers spontaneously. She has a 2+ radial pulse. Capillary refill is less than 2 seconds. There are no areas of ecchymoses, swelling, or tenderness in her lower extremities, back, or left upper extremity.

X-RAY DATA: The right humerus shows a spiral mid to distal third humeral shaft fracture. A skeletal survey performed the day after the initial ED evaluation showed a right posterior rib fracture as well as a periosteal reaction at the right distal femur and left distal humerus.

ASSESSMENT
1. This is a 3-month-old female with right mid to distal spiral humeral shaft fracture.
2. Periosteal reaction on the right distal femoral metaphysis and left distal humerus, concerning for nonaccidental trauma.

PLAN
1. A well-fitting splint was placed on the right upper extremity to immobilize the humeral shaft fracture. X-rays following this showed an acceptable alignment.
2. Patient was admitted to the pediatric service. Child Protective Services was consulted to evaluate the concerns of nonaccidental trauma.
3. A full genetic workup and pediatric workup will be performed while an inpatient.

(Continued)

ID#: M-27   PAGE 2

4. We will follow Lisa Marie as an outpatient in 2 weeks. At that point we will repeat the x-rays on her right upper extremity to ensure that there is still proper alignment. We anticipate a total of approximately 4 weeks of immobilization for this fracture. Further nonaccidental trauma evaluation, workup, and planning will be performed by the pediatric service as well as by Child Protective Services.

_____

Raquel Rodriguez, MD
Orthopedic Surgery

RR:cks
D:09/30/----
T:10/01/----

cc: Reed Phillips, MD, Pediatrics

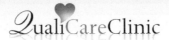

Bone Marrow Transplant Clinic Followup Note

Patient Name: Rodolfo Garcia **PCP:** Solomon T. Fisher, MD
Date of Exam: 07/10/---- **Age/Sex:** 25/M **ID#:** M-28

INTRODUCTION: Rodolfo Garcia is a 25-year-old Hispanic male, who is day +4 status post a reduced-intensity, matched, related transplant for non-Hodgkin lymphoma, who is seen today in followup.

HISTORY: Patient is doing well overall. He denies nausea, vomiting, diarrhea, and rash. He is eating and drinking well.

REVIEW OF SYSTEMS: Patient denies fevers, sore throat, mucositis, shortness of breath, chest pain, abdominal pain, dysuria, hematuria, hematochezia, epistaxis, and chills.

MEDICATIONS
1. Coumadin 8 mg daily.
2. AcipHex 20 mg daily p.r.n.
3. Fluconazole 400 mg daily.
4. Acyclovir 800 mg b.i.d.
5. Magnesium 400 mg b.i.d.
6. Tacrolimus 2 mg b.i.d.
7. Actigall 600 mg a.m. and 300 mg p.m.
8. Levaquin 500 mg daily.

PHYSICAL EXAMINATION

Temperature 96.9, blood pressure 119/80, pulse 85, respirations 20, weight 67.1 kg, oxygen saturation 98% on room air. GENERAL: No acute distress. HEENT: Sclerae nonicteric. Sinuses are nontender. Oral mucosa is clear. Lungs are clear to auscultation bilaterally. HEART: Regular rate and rhythm without murmurs, rubs, or gallops. Extremities are without edema. Skin is without rash. PICC line is without erythema, tenderness, or discharge.

LABORATORY DATA: White blood cells 0.7, hemoglobin 13.2, platelets 92,000. Creatinine 0.8, magnesium 1.2, potassium 4.5.

IMPRESSION
This is a 25-year-old male, day +4 post a reduced-intensity, matched, related transplant. Overall he is doing well.

PLAN
Patient will follow up with me in clinic tomorrow. Will stop Coumadin when platelet count is greater than 80,000.

_____
Solomon T. Fisher, MD
Hematology

SCG:cks
D:07/11/----
T:07/12/----

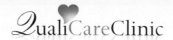

Internal Medicine Clinic Followup Note

Patient Name: Nicholas Berry   **PCP:** A. Leigh Wells, MD

Date of Exam: 01/05/----   **Age/Sex:** 58/M   **ID#:** M-29

REASON FOR VISIT: Routine followup.

HISTORY OF PRESENT ILLNESS: Mr. Berry is a pleasant 58-year-old gentleman with a past medical history significant for hypertension, hyperlipidemia, degenerative disk disease of the lumbar spine, osteoarthritis of the knees, lower extremity discomfort (likely secondary to peripheral neuropathy), as well as erectile dysfunction and continued tobacco use.

Patient reports that he was seen in Neurology for evaluation of his lower extremity discomfort. He states that they also felt this was secondary to neuropathy. He had further laboratory evaluation that revealed no clear etiology. However, he states that the discomfort that he has at night has significantly improved with reinitiating nortriptyline 25 mg at night. He is doing this and sleeping well. He has had no progression of symptoms. He has had no weakness in his lower extremities and no other symptoms.

Patient also reports that he was back to Orthopedics for evaluation of his right knee pain. It was felt that he has had no worsening of his meniscal injury, and the pain is likely secondary to osteoarthritis. He received a therapeutic injection and had significant benefit with that. He continues to take Mobic on a regular basis with fair relief of pain. He will follow up with Orthopedics if his knee continues to be bothersome.

Patient also reports that he used Levitra one time. He states that he did have good results with it; however, he developed a significant headache after using it. He has not used it since that time. He is questioning whether it is okay for him to try using it once again.

REVIEW OF SYSTEMS: Denies visual changes. No chest pain, orthopnea, paroxysmal nocturnal dyspnea, or lower extremity edema. He has had no fevers, chills, night sweats, or weight loss. Denies nausea, vomiting, or abdominal pain. Denies bright red blood per rectum or melena. Has no difficulty emptying his bladder. No significant nocturia. Mood is good. He is otherwise doing well.

CURRENT MEDICATIONS
1. Lipitor 20 mg daily.
2. Lisinopril 10 mg daily.
3. Mobic 7.5 mg daily.
4. Nortriptyline 25 mg at bedtime.
5. Levitra 20 mg p.r.n.
6. B12 1000 mcg intramuscularly monthly.

PHYSICAL EXAMINATION

Blood pressure 133/81, pulse 97, respirations 18, temperature 97, height 5 feet 11 inches, weight 194 pounds. He reports 4/10 pain in his knee. In general, he is a well-nourished, well-developed male in no acute distress. HEENT: Unremarkable. NECK: Supple without bruits. CARDIOVASCULAR EXAM: Regular rate and rhythm with normal S1, S2. No S3 or S4. No murmurs. CHEST is clear to auscultation bilaterally. ABDOMEN is soft, nontender. LOWER EXTREMITIES: No clubbing, cyanosis, or edema. He has dorsalis pedis pulses bilaterally. NEUROLOGIC exam is nonfocal. He has a normal gait without assistive device.

(Continued)

ID#: M-29   PAGE 2

LABORATORY DATA: No new laboratory studies.

ASSESSMENT
This is a 58-year-old gentleman with past medical history as listed above who is doing well at this time with improvement in symptoms in his lower extremity discomfort and cramping at night with use of nortriptyline. Patient with continued right knee pain secondary to osteoarthritis, fairly well controlled on Mobic 7.5 mg daily.

PLAN
1. Right knee osteoarthritis: Patient is to continue Mobic 7.5 mg daily or Tylenol p.r.n. pain. He will follow up in the orthopedic clinic if he wishes to pursue further injection or knee replacement.
2. Idiopathic peripheral neuropathy: Patient has had a thorough metabolic workup and neurologic evaluation. He is doing quite well with his symptoms and has had no progression of symptoms at this time. He is to continue nortriptyline 25 mg at bedtime.
3. Hypertension: Good control on lisinopril 10 mg daily. Will continue this at the current dose.
4. Hyperlipidemia: Patient was at goal when lipids were checked in July of last year. He is having no significant myalgias on Lipitor 20 mg daily. He will continue this at the current dose.
5. Erectile dysfunction: Patient had a good response from Levitra other than the associated headache. He has had no associated lightheadedness, dizziness, chest pain, or other symptoms. He was advised to try the Levitra once again. He is to notify me if he has similar side effects. We will consider a change to Cialis or back to Viagra as needed.
6. Healthcare maintenance: Patient received an influenza vaccine this season. He had a colonoscopy at age 50. He is otherwise up to date.

DISPOSITION: Patient is to follow up with me in 4 to 5 months, sooner as needed.

Jean W. Mooney, PA
Internal Medicine

JWM:cks
D:01/05/----
T:01/05/----

cc: Anne Basswood, MD, Neurology
    David Castillo, MD, Orthopedic Surgery
    A. Leigh Wells, MD, Internal Medicine

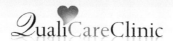

Physical Medicine and Rehabilitation Followup Note

Patient Name: Lorena Mae Oppenheimer **PCP:** Kenneth Shaker, MD

Date of Exam: 04/05/---- **Age/Sex:** 75/F **ID#:** M-30

CHIEF COMPLAINT: Chronic low back pain.

HISTORY: Ms. Oppenheimer is a 75-year-old female whom I have been following for the last couple of years for her mechanical low back pain, which is attributed to L4-5 facet osteoarthritis with some mechanical back pain as well as some previous mild neurogenic/radicular leg pain, which has since resolved. She presents stating that her back pain continues to be aggravated with standing, less so with walking, and only generally then with walking long distances. She also has aggravation of that mechanical low back pain when she comes from a sitting to a standing position. She generally has minimal discomfort or actually some relief with walking at a slower or comfortable pace. She states the back pain is generally a dull aching pain, and she occasionally has a stabbing sensation.

Patient states she also has some mild discomfort in the right lateral hip region, which is noted when she lies on that side, as well as when she is sitting in a soft chair. The patient's pain generally ranges from a 4/10 to a 7/10.

REVIEW OF SYSTEMS: Neurologic review of systems is unremarkable for any type of sciatica or for radicular/ neurogenic leg pain. She denies numbness, paresthesias, or weakness of her lower extremities. She denies bowel or bladder changes or incontinence. Constitutional review of systems is unremarkable for fevers, chills, progressive night pain, malaise, weight loss, history of malignancy, or recent infection.

PAST MEDICAL HISTORY: Hypertension, asthma, seasonal allergies.

PAST SURGICAL HISTORY: Total abdominal hysterectomy and cataract resection.

MEDICATIONS: Her analgesic medication regimen is Mobic 7.5 mg 1 tab q.day. Other medications include Zestril, Premarin, and Atarax.

ALLERGIES: No known drug allergies.

PHYSICAL EXAMINATION

GENERAL APPEARANCE: A very well nourished, well-developed female, younger than her chronologic age in appearance. She is alert and oriented x3 and in no acute distress.

Spine

- Posture: Mildly increased thoracic kyphosis, otherwise with a good lumbosacral lordosis and without scoliosis.
- Lumbopelvic AROM: Aggravation of the low back pain with buttock pain when she extends or when she undergoes quadrant loading positions, particularly to the ipsilateral side. She has some relief with forward flexion.

Palpation: Mild tenderness noted at the lumbosacral junction on both right and left.

Neurologic

Gait: Normal heel-toe and tandem walk.

Motor: Five out of 5 in all muscle groups of the lower extremities.

(Continued)

ID#: M-30   PAGE 2

Sensory: Normal to light touch in the lower extremity dermatomes.

- Reflexes: Two-plus and symmetric at the patella; 1+ and symmetric at the Achilles with a normal flexion response on Babinski testing.

Nerve tension signs: Negative right and left straight-leg raise.

Lower Extremity/Vascular

- Hip: Passive range of motion of the hips is symmetric without discomfort and with the following values: Forward flexion 110 degrees and symmetric; flexion and external rotation: right 70 degrees and left 60 degrees; flexion and internal rotation: right 30 degrees and left 25 degrees. Palpation of the hips demonstrates focal tenderness on the right superior-posterior aspect of the greater trochanteric region consistent with the greater trochanteric bursa.
- Vascular: Normal temperature and coloration of the distal legs and feet with palpable dorsalis pedis pulses and without cyanosis or edema.

ASSESSMENT

1. L4-5 disk protrusion with facet osteoarthritis with predominantly facet-related mechanical low back pain.
2. Right greater trochanteric bursitis.

PROCEDURE: A right greater trochanteric bursa injection is performed after discussion of risks and benefits. The patient's right greater trochanteric lateral hip area was prepped and draped in the usual sterile fashion. Utilizing a "no touch" technique, a 25-gauge, 2-inch needle was inserted down to the greater trochanteric bursa region. After contact with the os, the needle was slightly withdrawn, and injection of 3 mL of 1% lidocaine plus 3 mL of 0.5% Marcaine plus 2 mL of Depo-Medrol 40 mg/mL was performed without difficulty. The needle was removed. The patient's hip area was cleansed. The patient indicated about 50% relief of discomfort in that area.

PLAN

1. Right greater trochanteric bursa injection, as described above.
2. Updated x-rays will be obtained today to assess for further evidence of facet arthropathy, particularly at the L4-5 level.
3. Demonstrated appropriate stretches for her lumbosacral and hip abductors.
4. Nuclear medicine bone scan will be requested to further affirm the level of her facet arthropathy that is most likely to be symptomatic.
5. Will provide a trial of increasing the Mobic from 7.5 to 15 mg per day.
6. Recommend stationary bicycling for cardiovascular exercises.
7. The patient will return to clinic in a few weeks after completion of a nuclear medicine bone scan.

Jean W. Mooney, PA
Physical Medicine and Rehabilitation

JWM:cks
D:04/05/----
T:04/05/----

cc: Kenneth Shaker, MD, Internal Medicine

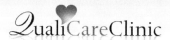

Colorectal Surgery Consultation

Patient Name: Leonard C. Thomas   **PCP:** Chris Salem, DO

Date of Exam: 03/02/----   **Age/Sex:** 41/M   **ID#:** M-31

REASON FOR CONSULT: Perirectal bleeding and drainage.

HISTORY OF PRESENT ILLNESS: This is a 41-year-old male with a 1-month history of persistent purulent blood drainage from his perianal area. He reports, just before this happened, having a large bowel movement accompanied by some pain and bleeding. Since then he has had some bloody drainage and discharge in the area. He has had hemorrhoids banded previously x2 and previous perianal fistulae that have resolved spontaneously.

PAST MEDICAL HISTORY: Significant for hemorrhoid banding, genital herpes, basal cell carcinoma, and eczema.

PAST SURGICAL HISTORY: Tonsillectomy, colonoscopy, and basal cell excision.

MEDICATIONS include acyclovir, hydrocortisone suppositories.

ALLERGIES: No known drug allergies.

SOCIAL HISTORY: He denies alcohol and tobacco use.

FAMILY HISTORY is significant for colon cancer in some distant relatives.

REVIEW OF SYSTEMS: Unremarkable. Specifically, he denies nausea, vomiting, constipation, fever, chills, and shortness of breath.

PHYSICAL EXAMINATION

He is a well-developed man in no acute distress. Temperature is 97.8. LUNGS are clear. HEART has regular rate and rhythm. On DIGITAL RECTAL EXAM he has a posterior midline fissure with scant amount of purulent drainage. He has normal rectal tone.

IMPRESSION

By exam patient has a posterior midline fissure, but by history this is likely a ruptured abscess without fistula formation.

PLAN

This area will likely heal without intervention. He is to keep his stool soft, the area clean, and is to follow up with me in 6 weeks if this persists.

_____

James A. McClure Jr, MD
Colorectal Surgery

JAM:cks
D:03/02/----
T:03/02/----

cc: Chris Salem, DO, Family Practice

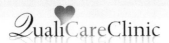

<u>**Vascular Surgery Consultation**</u>

Patient Name: Gloria C. Santivanez   **PCP:** Marie Aaron, DO
Date of Exam: 04/09/----   **Age/Sex:** 60/F   **ID#:** M-32

REASON FOR REFERRAL: This is a 60-year-old Hispanic female with stage 4 chronic kidney disease from diabetic nephropathy, here now for evaluation of AV fistula placement.

HISTORY OF PRESENT ILLNESS: Ms. Santivanez is a delightful female who has had a creatinine of 2.3, although I ordered it today, and it is 2.5. She has a creatinine clearance that is roughly 30 to 50, and she has stage 4 chronic kidney disease. She actually says that she, herself, is currently not interested in hemodialysis. However, I did sit down and talk with her, and it sounds like she would undergo hemodialysis if it meant staying alive. We sat and had a long discussion about hemodialysis and arteriovenous fistulae and access, and she seems to understand. I am not sure she understands all the intricate details, however.

PAST HISTORY: Diabetes, gastroesophageal reflux disease, hyperlipidemia, coronary artery disease, and hypertension.

MEDICATIONS include NovoLog, Avapro, hydrochlorothiazide, AcipHex, Plavix, aspirin, nifedipine, Zocor, Lasix, estriol, Lopressor, and iron sulfate.

PHYSICAL EXAMINATION

PE today reveals a well-developed, well-nourished, mildly obese female in no acute distress.

VITAL SIGNS show temperature 97.0, blood pressure 132/63, pulse 77, respirations 18.

HEENT exam is normocephalic, atraumatic.

NECK: She has 2+ carotid upstrokes. LUNGS are clear. HEART is regular.

ABDOMEN is soft and nontender.

EXTREMITIES show 2+ radial pulses and 2+ femoral pulses bilaterally.

X-RAY DATA: Her venous duplex examination revealed cephalic vein in the upper arm to be adequate for a fistula. The lower arm was small on the left side, and she is right-side dominant. The basilic vein appeared adequate along the entire arm for fistula placement.

ASSESSMENT: Ms. Santivanez is a delightful female with mild to moderate renal insufficiency, stage 3 to 4. She is going to see her nephrologist again in the near future, and I have told her that we ought to have her talk with him again and see if she should have a fistula placed sooner or later.

PLAN

I am going to have patient follow up with me in 1 to 2 months. I have told her that we would be willing to place a fistula if she is willing to let us; however, she has to be willing to undergo this procedure. I think she understands the risks, benefits, and alternatives to the procedure, although, again, I am not 100% sure she understands all the intricate details.

Her daughter was with her today, and I think that she can help make that decision for her.

_____
Ly An Tabor, MD, Vascular Surgery

LAT:cks
D:04/10/----
T:04/11/----

cc: Marie Aaron, DO, Family Practice
    Trevor Jordan, MD, Nephrology

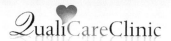

Orthopedic Surgery Followup Note

Patient Name: Jennifer Ann Adcock   **PCP:** Martha C. Eaton, MD

Date of Exam: 08/09/----   **Age/Sex:** 47/F   **ID#:** M-34

HISTORY: This 47-year-old patient is here in followup. She was last seen on July 18 when she was started on physical therapy for range of motion, as her range of motion at her last appointment was 5 to 110 degrees. She states that she had some difficulty getting her insurance company to set her up with physical therapy in a timely fashion. She has had only a couple of appointments since we saw her last. She has some chronic pain along the lateral side of her right knee, and it is noted that she is status post patellectomy. She states that her complaints are unchanged compared to before. She also states that she has had a 10- to 15-pound weight loss since her total knee arthroplasty was performed and that she has been somewhat sluggish. We had her see her internist, who was concerned with her anemia, and sent her for fecal occult studies as well as setting her up for a flexible sigmoidoscopy in the future.

REVIEW OF SYSTEMS: She denies fevers, chills, or sweats.

PHYSICAL EXAMINATION

RIGHT KNEE EXAMINATION: Active range of motion is from 10 to 115 degrees. Passive range of motion is from 5 to 115 degrees. She has diminished quad girth on the right compared to the left, which is 1 cm at all portions of the quadriceps. She has tenderness to palpation overlying the iliotibial band in the region of her femoral component. She has a 5 mm superficial abrasion overlying the distal portion of her incision, roughly 2 cm from the distal-most end of her incision. She states that she stumbled or fell in the parking lot over the weekend. She states that there has been no pus and no fluid draining from that abrasion. Today there is no pus, no expressible fluid, no purulent drainage noted on her bandage or from her wound. The knee is without signs of superficial or deep infection at present. She has 5/5 strength in the EHL, FHL, gastrocnemius/soleus complex, tibialis anterior, and the peroneals. She has intact light touch sensation grossly below the ankle in the deep peroneal, superficial peroneal, and sural distributions. She has palpable dorsalis pedis pulse and less than a 2-second capillary refill in all digits.

IMPRESSION

She is status post right total knee arthroplasty with early take-back for acute infection on polyethylene exchange. She appears at this time to have some component of capsular tightness as well as iliotibial band friction syndrome, given that she is post patellectomy and has had minimal physical therapy postoperatively.

PLAN

The plan for Ms. Adcock is to continue with aggressive physical therapy for range of motion as well as a massage over the region of her discomfort at the iliotibial band. It is very concerning that the patient has had pronounced weight loss postoperatively. We will obtain a number of nutrition labs as well as an iron study, CBC, Chem-10, and CEA. If any of those values are abnormal, we will consult the appropriate service for her to be seen and evaluated further.

She is to follow up with orthopedic clinic in a couple of weeks to see how she is doing with her physical therapy and to review her laboratory results. Alternatively, she may page me. I gave her my pager number, and I can give her her laboratory results.

_____

Raquel Rodriguez, MD
Orthopedic Surgery

RR:cks
D:08/09/----
T:08/10/----

cc: Martha C. Eaton, MD, Internal Medicine

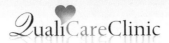

Orthopedic Followup Note

Patient Name: Kelsi Shaffer   **PCP:** Reed Phillips, MD

Date of Exam: 03/09/----   **Age/Sex:** 11/F   **ID#:** M-36

HISTORY: Patient is a spastic, quadriplegic 11-year-old child with cerebral palsy status post unit rod scoliosis instrumentation 2 months ago. Patient has been doing well. They have been trying to get her to stand with physical therapy. There is a concern about her left leg internally rotating during this. Patient has been in a wheelchair otherwise, doing well, no complaints, afebrile.

PHYSICAL EXAMINATION

Exam reveals a spastic, diplegic female with symmetric abduction. She has slight increased internal rotation of her left leg compared to her right leg. Incision is clean, dry, intact, and well healed. One small area at the distal third, about a 1 mm area, has a stitch extrusion. No erythema, warmth, or significant drainage. There is slight prominence to the unit rod proximally.

X-RAY DATA: X-ray evaluation shows no change in alignment. Sitting balance is stable with slight prominence of the proximal unit rod.

ASSESSMENT

Spastic, diplegic female, 5 weeks status post scoliosis deformity unit rod correction. Doing well.

PLAN

Patient is able to participate in aquatic therapy. She is to do no lifting and no significant bending. She is to wear a Band-Aid over her stitch extrusion area.

She is to follow up sooner for any signs or symptoms of infection; otherwise, she is to follow up in May with preclinic x-rays, seated scoliosis films.

_____

Gilbert M. Fields, MD
Orthopedic Surgery

GMF:cks
D:03/09/----
T:03/10/----

c: Reed Phillips, MD, Pediatrics

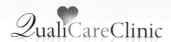

QualiCareClinic

Emergency Room Treatment Record

Patient Name: Briggs Jackson   **PCP:** N/A

Date of Exam: 07/24/----   **Age/Sex:** 60/M   **ID#:** M-37

CONSULTING SERVICE: Ophthalmology.

CHIEF COMPLAINT: Eye irritation.

MODE OF ARRIVAL: Privately owned vehicle.

HISTORY OF PRESENT ILLNESS: This 60-year-old male has a history of herpes keratopathy and presents with right eye irritation and the sensation that he has when he has had glaucoma in the past. He has a history of multiple ocular surgeries, including penetrating keratoplasty, trabeculectomy, cataract extraction with intraocular lens implantation, glaucoma drainage, implant insertion, and cyclophotocoagulation. He has had several episodes of glaucoma in the past related to his herpes infection. He is not having much pain in that way, but he says when he palpates his globes, the right eye feels a little firmer than the left eye. He is therefore concerned that he is having glaucoma attack. Patient cannot see at all from his right eye and is legally blind in his right eye. He is generally able only to count fingers at 1-1/2 feet.

REVIEW OF SYSTEMS: Negative for fevers, chills, weight loss, weight gain, sinus congestion, sore throat pain, neck pain, neck stiffness, shortness of breath, cough, wheezing, chest pain, palpitations, abdominal pain, nausea, vomiting, diarrhea, hematochezia, hematemesis, melena, dysuria, urgency, frequency, myalgias, arthralgias, easy bruising or bleeding, hot or cold intolerance, rash, seizure, numbness, or tingling in the extremities.

PAST MEDICAL HISTORY: Hypercholesterolemia, gastroesophageal reflux disease.

PAST SURGICAL HISTORY: See HPI.

MEDICATIONS: Viroptic, Zocor, Prevacid.

ALLERGIES: No known drug allergies.

SOCIAL HISTORY: Denies smoking, drinking, and using illicit drugs.

FAMILY HISTORY: Noncontributory.

PHYSICAL EXAMINATION

VITAL SIGNS on presentation: BP 149/98, P 70, R 18, T 98.5, saturating at 97% on room air. In general, patient is in no acute distress. PULMONARY exam: Clear to auscultation bilaterally. No wheezes, crackles, rhonchi. CARDIOVASCULAR exam: Regular rate and rhythm with no murmurs, rubs, or gallops. ABDOMEN: Soft, nontender, nondistended. Normal bowel sounds. No rebound, guarding, or hepatosplenomegaly. EYE exam: Extraocular muscles intact bilaterally. Pupils are equal, round, and reactive to light bilaterally. The ocular pressure, right eye, is 18. Ocular pressure, left eye, is 11. No signs of foreign body. Patient's vision at 1.5 feet: He cannot count numbers. He can count numbers at 1 foot. Before fluorescein staining of the eye could take place, Ophthalmology had arrived. They took the patient to the ophthalmology clinic for further examination of his eye.

(Continued)

ID#: M-37   PAGE 2

EMERGENCY DEPARTMENT COURSE

No tests were done on this patient. Patient was seen and evaluated and taken to the ophthalmology clinic for further examination.

MEDICAL DECISION MAKING

This patient had a possible eye irritation secondary to herpes keratopathy. I do not think the patient had glaucoma, as he has normal pressure in the right eye. Treatment will be based on recommendations from Ophthalmology, which are pending at the time of this dictation. Their recommendations will be recorded in the chart.

EMERGENCY DEPARTMENT DIAGNOSIS

Viral keratitis.

DISPOSITION

Discharge to home. Follow up with Ophthalmology as needed. Return for signs and symptoms of glaucoma or any other concerns. Patient voiced complete understanding and was discharged from the ED in good condition.

_____

Samuel Ernest, MD
Emergency Room Physician

SE:cks
D:07/24/----
T:07/24/----

cc: Midori Okano, MD, Ophthalmology

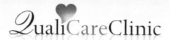

Hematology/Oncology Followup Note

Patient Name: Gene Dale
Date of Exam: 02/21/---
        Age/Sex: 47-year-old male
        PCP: Lynne Andrew, MD
        ID#: M-38

DIAGNOSES
1. Carcinoid of distal ileum diagnosed 10 years ago.
2. Recurrent carcinoid 7 years ago.

TREATMENT
Resection of lesions at both diagnosis and recurrence.

HISTORY: Patient is a 47-year-old male here today in routine followup. Since our last visit patient has done well. He is currently without complaints. Denies diarrhea, flushing, and new abdominal pain. He denies weight loss, and his appetite is good.

PHYSICAL EXAMINATION

VITAL SIGNS: Vitals show blood pressure 138/80, pulse 73, temperature 96.7, height 72 inches, weight 206 pounds.

GENERAL: Middle-aged male in no acute distress.

HEENT: Within normal limits.

LYMPH NODES: No cervical, supraclavicular, axillary, or inguinal adenopathy. LUNGS are clear to auscultation bilaterally without wheezing.

HEART is regular rate and rhythm without murmurs, rubs, or gallops.

ABDOMEN: Soft, nontender without hepatosplenomegaly. Normally active bowel sounds.

EXTREMITIES: Without edema.

X-RAY DATA: An octreotide scan last month was indeterminate in appearance of the liver on SPECT imaging. A new focus of activity in the abdomen on planar images only. A 3-phase CT of the liver and pelvis is recommended for further evaluation.

IMPRESSION
This is a 47-year-old male with a history of carcinoid. Patient is now 7 years out from recurrence of disease with questionable new activity on octreotide scan.

PLAN
1. Obtain 3-phase CT of the liver and pelvis.
2. Check chromogranin and 24-hour urine 5-HIAA.

_____

Solomon T. Fisher, MD
Hematology/Oncology

STF:cks
D:02/21/----
T:02/22/----

cc: Lynne Andrew, MD, Internal Medicine

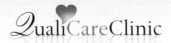

Vascular Surgery Followup Note

Patient Name: Frieda Kasanjian	**PCP:** A. Leigh Wells, MD
Date of Exam: 08/04/---- **Age/Sex:** 70/F	**ID#:** M-39

HISTORY: Ms. Kasanjian is a 70-year-old female, well known to our service. She has had multiple failed dialysis accesses in the left arm. She underwent an attempt at a right Cimino fistula, which failed. She then had a right forearm loop graft placed with ligation of the AV fistula. Since that time she has had problems with significant arm swelling and pain, with chronic wounds at each of her incision sites. These have crusted over with eschar. She returns today complaining that one of the crusted eschars has split her skin. No complaints of fever. The dialysis unit took her off vancomycin again, even though she has had 2 recent nasal cultures that showed her to be MRSA positive.

PHYSICAL EXAMINATION

Temperature 97.6, blood pressure 136/71 on the left, pulse 75, respirations 22. Right upper extremity exam reveals a good thrill in the fistula. There is still some rubor and induration to the forearm, although the woody edema that was present for many weeks postoperatively is gone. There is a crusted eschar above the incision, just below the antecubital fossa. There is a crusted eschar at the distal incision for the loop graft. Several sutures were removed from the distal incision, and some of the eschar was removed, with healthy skin underneath. Some of the eschar was removed from the more proximal incision with some sutures removed. There is some healing, early granulation tissue underneath this eschar. There is no overt pus. There is a fissure in the skin where the eschar has pulled away from the skin.

ASSESSMENT/PLAN

1. Chronically poorly healing wounds with significant devitalized tissue still present. I think she will need to go to the operating room for debridement and washout and to see if there is any way we can improve these wounds. Perhaps put a wound V.A.C. on the proximal wound.
2. The patient will be called on Monday, and we will plan surgery early on Tuesday. I feel this is not definitely infected, although it certainly could be, given her methicillin-resistant *Staphylococcus aureus* (MRSA) history.
3. Patient knows that if she has any problems, she is to go to the Hillcrest Medical Center emergency department immediately. She states that overall her arm feels like it is improving rather than getting worse. She is just worried about this fissure in her skin.

Ly An Tabor, MD
LAT:cks

D:08/04/----
T:08/05/----

c: A. Leigh Wells, MD, Internal Medicine
Trevor Jordan, MD, Nephrology

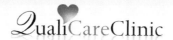

QualiCareClinic

<u>**Orthopedic Surgery History and Physical Examination**</u>

Patient Name: Jennifer Day   **PCP:** Reed Phillips, MD

Date of Exam: 04/13/----   **Age/Sex:** 12/F   **ID#:** M-40

CHIEF COMPLAINT: Bilateral hip pain, left greater than right.

HISTORY OF PRESENT ILLNESS: Jennifer Day is a 12-year-old female who has recently moved here from Alaska with a history of bilateral developmental dysplasia of the hip, diagnosed in infancy. As a child she was treated with triple diapers until 3 months. At age 3 months, treatment with a Pavlik harness was started. She was treated with this through the age of 10 months. At 10 months she was noted to have bilateral dislocated hips; therefore, she was treated in traction followed by closed reduction and a spica cast placement for 6 weeks at the age of 13 months. She later had imaging that showed bilateral dislocated hips again. She was treated with open reduction and casting of the right hip at 15 months with open reduction of the left hip at 17 months. Subsequently, Jennifer had few difficulties during childhood and into adolescence through elementary school. She had no problems playing at recess, playing with her friends; however, she has started in the sixth grade and has been more active in PE, playing some volleyball and other activities. She has noted increased pain, worse in the left hip than in the right hip. She states that she has pain that is increased with activities and is relieved with rest. She does have occasional night pain, typically when she has had a more active day prior.

According to her records from prior providers, she has been known to have residual dysplasia of the hips, more significant on the left than on the right. This has been followed conservatively until now.

Also of concern is a small "cyst" in the left acetabulum that warrants further evaluation. The patient was referred to me for evaluation of both her bilateral hip pain and this left acetabular "cyst." When the patient is asked where her pain is, she points bilaterally, more to her iliac crests than to her hips. She denies any pain deep in her groin areas bilaterally.

PAST MEDICAL HISTORY is insignificant other than the bilateral hip dysplasia.

PAST SURGICAL HISTORY is as above.

SOCIAL HISTORY: The patient is an A/B student and is now in the sixth grade.

MEDICATIONS: The patient is prescribed narcotics for her pain, but she has not been taking them.

PHYSICAL EXAMINATION

The patient stands with a level pelvis, level shoulders without apparent limb length discrepancy. She has tenderness to palpation bilaterally over the iliac crests and the proximal origins of the abductors. She has no groin tenderness, no greater trochanteric tenderness on exam. The right hip has active flexion to 100 degrees, 60 degrees of internal rotation, and 10 degrees of external rotation. The left hip has 120 degrees of active flexion, 50 degrees of internal rotation, and 20 degrees of external rotation. She has increased deep hip pain on the left at the ends of the internal/external rotation. The strength is 5/5 throughout. The sensation is normal. She is vascularly intact bilaterally. Her gait is within normal limits.

X-RAY DATA: AP and frog-leg views of the pelvis 2 months ago are reviewed. There is no residual acetabular deformity on the right. She does have some mild dysplasia of the femoral head on the right; however, there are no degenerative changes, and she has good alignment on the right. The left hip, however, does have increased acetabular index significant for acetabular dysplasia. The femoral head shows no significant dysplasia. There is a small, approximately 1.5 x 1.5 cm, well-defined, well-marginated lytic lesion in the superior aspect of the acetabulum that does not disrupt any of the cortices or expand the bone. CT images of this same lesion were obtained and are consistent with a lucent process without cortical destruction. MRI of the same lesion shows a well-defined, heterogeneous low signal on T1 and some increased signal on T2.

(Continued)

ID#: M-40

ASSESSMENT

1. Bilateral developmental dysplasia of the hips with normal-appearing right hip and increased acetabular index on the left.
2. Bilateral iliac crest/abductor pain.
3. Left acetabulum lytic lesion that appears benign, geode versus chondroblastoma.

PLAN

I counseled the patient and her father extensively on the treatment for developmental dysplasia of the hip at her age. The only surgical procedure I would recommend at this point would be a Ganz periacetabular osteotomy. I did counsel them, however, that it would take far more symptoms to sway me toward that route. Given the minimal degree of actual hip symptoms at this time, I would not consider that. Secondly, I would need to refer her to someone who performs Ganz periacetabular osteotomy, as I do not perform this procedure.

In regard to this lucent lesion in her acetabulum, I will take this MRI to the musculoskeletal radiologist at Forrest General Hospital for review. It is my opinion that this lesion is benign; however, I would like to get an opinion on its appearance and see if it warrants further imaging. The question is whether or not this lesion is contributing to her symptoms. Chondroblastomas have been known to appear in the triradial cartilage and typically cause pain in the adjacent joints, so this is a possibility. This could be a degenerative cyst, as well, however.

I will have the MRI reviewed and will contact the patient's father for further recommendations and followup.

_____

Raquel Rodriguez, MD
Orthopedic Surgery

RR:cks
D:04/13/----
T:04/13/----

cc: Reed Phillips, MD, Pediatrics

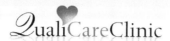

Colorectal Surgery Consultation

Patient Name: Sheena Ferruzzi   **PCP:** Ronald Reardon, DO
Date of Exam: 08/10/----   **Age/Sex:** 44/M   **ID#:** M-41

REASON FOR CONSULT: Anorectal pain.

HISTORY OF PRESENT ILLNESS: This is a 44-year-old Middle-Eastern male with a 5-year history of rectal tenderness and muscle spasm. This begins as a dull pain and increases to a sharp 10/10 pain. This occurs once every 1-1/2 to 2 weeks and will occasionally wake him up from sleep. Episodes last from 30 seconds to 30 minutes. He also reports some crampy, right lower quadrant and left lower quadrant abdominal pain, relieved with loose bowel movement.

PAST HISTORY: Significant for hypoglycemia.

PAST SURGERIES have included bilateral knee surgeries. He had a prior colonoscopy when his 3 polyps were removed.

MEDICATIONS: Gemfibrozil.

ALLERGIES: SULFA drugs.

SOCIAL HISTORY: He has rare alcohol use. No smoking. No other tobacco or illicit drug use. No prostitute contact, no homosexual contact, no STDs.

REVIEW OF SYSTEMS: Unremarkable. Specifically, he denies constipation, nausea, vomiting, abdominal pain, shortness of breath, chest pain.

PHYSICAL EXAMINATION

Normal male in no acute distress. Temperature is 97.1, blood pressure 127/86, pulse 58, respirations 16. HEENT exam is within normal limits. LUNGS are clear. HEART has regular rate and rhythm. ABDOMEN is soft, nontender with normoactive bowel sounds. ANAL EXAM is normal to inspection. On DIGITAL RECTAL EXAM he has taut levator tendons, right greater than left. Palpation of these reproduces his pelvic floor symptoms.

IMPRESSION
Levator ani syndrome.

PLAN
Will prescribe the patient Flexeril for amelioration of acute attacks and refer to Dr. Jesus Mayoral at Hillcrest Medical Center for consideration of pelvic floor biofeedback.

_____

James A. McClure Jr, MD
Colorectal Surgery

JAM:cks
D:08/10/----
T:08/11/----

c: Jesus Mayoral, MD, Colorectal Surgery/Pelvic Floor Medicine
   Ronald Reardon, DO, Family Practice

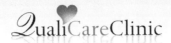

$\mathcal{Q}$ualiCareClinic

Emergency Room Treatment Record

Patient Name: Don Q. Fogarty   **PCP:** Nancy Lawrence, MD

Date of Exam: 06/18/----   **Age/Sex:** 68/M   **ID#:** M-42

CONSULTING SERVICE: Internal Medicine.

CHIEF COMPLAINT: Nausea and vomiting.

HISTORY OF PRESENT ILLNESS: This 68-year-old Caucasian male has a history of a nephrectomy, status post isolated renal cell carcinoma, and has had a protracted history of nausea and vomiting along with p.o. intolerance for approximately 1 week. The patient was seen in another emergency room on Monday. He had a workup, and everything was apparently normal at that time, so he was subsequently discharged. The patient came in today because he has since become diffusely weak, and his nausea, vomiting, and abdominal pain have persisted. The patient states that before all this happened in the Sunday/Monday time frame, he was completely in his baseline physical condition. The patient's wife has been eating the same foods that he has, and she has none of these symptoms. No one around him, in fact, has been sick.

REVIEW OF SYSTEMS: Positive chills, nausea, vomiting, abdominal pain. No headache, loss of consciousness, or vision changes. Positive generalized weakness. No paralysis. No chest pain, shortness of breath, dyspnea on exertion, orthopnea, dysuria, hematuria, diarrhea, or constipation. States his bowel movements have been normal. He had one earlier today, which was unremarkable and normal.

PAST MEDICAL HISTORY: Stroke, myocardial infarction, renal cell carcinoma.

PAST SURGICAL HISTORY: Nephrectomy, aortobifemoral bypass, aortic valve replacement.

MEDICATIONS: Aspirin, Norvasc, folic acid, lisinopril, atenolol, Lipitor.

ALLERGIES: MORPHINE, MOTRIN.

SOCIAL HISTORY: Does not drink, smoke, or use illicit drugs. Denies recent medication changes, denies any known sick contacts, denies any known toxic ingestion or unusual foods.

PHYSICAL EXAMINATION

VITAL SIGNS on presentation: Pulse 89, blood pressure 74/30, respirations 24, temperature 97.5 rectally, O_2 saturation 92% on room air. In general, the patient is a cachectic, decompensated, emaciated 68-year-old Caucasian male who is in mild distress secondary to weakness; however, he is otherwise alert and oriented x4. HEENT: Atraumatic. Extraocular muscles intact. Pupils are equal, round, and reactive to light and accommodation bilaterally. Oropharynx and nasopharynx clear. Mucous membranes are tacky. NECK: No nuchal rigidity. Supple, no adenopathy. No jugular venous distension. CARDIOVASCULAR: Heart rate and rhythm regular. No murmurs, gallops, or rubs. PULMONARY: No respiratory distress. Lungs are clear to auscultation bilaterally in all fields. ABDOMEN: Nondistended. Diffusely tender to palpation. There is a midline surgical scar, well healed. No costovertebral angle tenderness, no mass or hepatosplenomegaly. EXTREMITIES: No cyanosis, clubbing, or edema. Pulses 2+ in upper and lower extremities bilaterally. Strength 5/5 in upper and lower extremities bilaterally. GU exam: No lesions, no discharge. RECTAL exam: Good rectal tone. Guaiac-negative. SKIN: No rashes, no lesions.

(Continued)

ID#: M-42   PAGE 2

LAB AND X-RAY: Bedside ultrasound showed no evidence of gallbladder pathology, no presence of AAA. Chest x-ray and flat plate abdomen: Normal. No acute process. CBC: White blood cells 6, hemoglobin 16, hematocrit 47, platelets 228,000. Sodium 147, potassium 3.7, chloride 91, bicarb 38, BUN 60, creatinine 3.3, glucose 138, calcium 9.5, phosphorus 8.4, anion gap of 18, lactate of 5.2. PT 12.6, PTT 29, INR 0.95. Urinalysis: No glucose, no ketones, no blood, no nitrites, no leukocyte esterase. AST 16, ALT 13, alk phos 87, total bilirubin 0.4, direct bilirubin less than 0.1, amylase 20. Urine creatinine is 140, urine sodium 30 with a FENa of 0.46%. A serum creatinine was drawn 5 days ago, which was 1 at that time.

EMERGENCY DEPARTMENT COURSE: The patient was given an initial bolus of 1 L of fluid, and his blood pressure came up to the 90s/40s. He was given a repeat bolus, after which his pressure went up to the mid-90s/50s to 60s. After a third liter of fluid bolus, his blood pressure increased to the one-teens to the 120s/70s. Following those fluid boluses, the patient stated he felt significantly better and did not feel as weak. Electrocardiogram was normal sinus rhythm in the 60s with normal intervals, normal axis. No ST-T wave changes, no pathologic Q waves, good R-wave progression. Patient was given 4 mg Zofran x2 for his abdominal pain and nausea. He was then started on a maintenance dose of normal saline at 120 mL per hour. Foley was placed to ensure adequate urine output.

MEDICAL DECISION MAKING: This is a 68-year-old Caucasian male with a history of nephrectomy secondary to renal cell carcinoma, not believed to be metastatic, who comes in today for protracted nausea and vomiting. He was found to have a creatinine of 3.3. A creatinine done 5 days previously was 1. His urine electrolytes show a FENa of 0.46%, indicating that this is a prerenal renal failure, likely secondary to his nausea and vomiting.

It is unclear, but it is possible that he may have had a renal insult to his kidney that could have caused the azotemia and subsequent nausea and vomiting to ensue. The patient, although he does have a lactate of 5, is afebrile, has no elevated white count, and has no obvious source of infection on physical examination or on radiographic films. Therefore, I do not suspect that he is septic at this time. His blood pressure has continued to improve on fluids alone, not requiring pressors, and his abdomen following the interventions is actually benign. It is nontender and soft with no masses. All of his belly labs and his lipase along with the LFTs are within normal limits. Therefore, I suspect no significant intra-abdominal pathology. He has no right upper quadrant pain, seemed to have no evidence of gallbladder pathology on bedside ultrasound; therefore, I suspect no cholelithiasis or cholecystitis or ascending cholangitis.

I suspect this is quite possibly prerenal renal failure secondary to decreased p.o. intake, which could be secondary to a gastritis, which may be improving by now per physical examination. Either way, the patient will require admission to close his gap to ensure that his lactic acidosis resolves and that his renal failure is appropriately treated. I suspect it is possible, as this patient has a history of aortobifemoral bypass and coronary artery disease, that he is likely a vasculopath. Therefore, even mild changes in his blood pressure, even mild hypotensive periods, would tend to cause an anaerobic metabolism in all peripheral tissues. Therefore, it is quite possible that the lactate is secondary to anaerobic metabolism in any of his peripheral organs. He will continue to be monitored, and if he does spike a temp or shows any localizing sources of infection, he will be treated with antibiotics as appropriate; otherwise, I suspect no infectious etiology at this time.

EMERGENCY DEPARTMENT DIAGNOSES
1. Acute renal failure.
2. Nausea and vomiting.

(Continued)

ID#: M-42

PLAN

1. Continue judicious fluid infusion as the patient is cardiovascularly able to tolerate.
2. Control the nausea and vomiting.
3. Admit to Internal Medicine.

_____

Samuel Ernest, MD
Emergency Room Physician

SE:cks
D:06/18/----
T:06/18/----

c: Nancy Lawrence, MD, Internal Medicine
    Trevor Jordan, MD, Nephrology
    Saul Thompson, MD, Cardiology

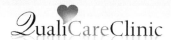

Radiation Oncology Followup Note

Patient Name: Joel Flores   **PCP:** Sherman Loyd, MD

Date of Exam: 11/16/----   **Age/Sex:** 57/M   **ID#:** M-43

DIAGNOSIS: Squamous cell carcinoma, floor of mouth, stage IVA (T4aN2M0).

INTERVAL HISTORY: Compared to his last visit 4 months ago there has been no change. Mr. Flores continues to feel well. He is able to swallow liquefied foods. Dysgeusia continues to resolve but oral dryness persists.

PHYSICAL EXAMINATION

He looks well. Weight is 179 pounds (increased from 174 pounds on his last visit), blood pressure 170/90, heart rate 72, and temperature 96.9. HEENT AND NECK: Patient is blind. No scleral icterus. No adenopathy in the neck or clavicular region. There are obvious persistent defects from his hemimandibulectomy and previous radiation therapy. He has evidence of a partial glossectomy and graft. Thickened, tenacious mucus is present. There is no palpable tumor in the oral tongue, floor of mouth, tonsillar bed, or base of tongue. Endoscopy to the right nasion: No evidence of tumor in the nasopharynx, base of tongue, vallecula, supraglottic or glottic larynx. Vocal folds adduct normally with phonation. LUNGS: Clear to auscultation. CARDIOVASCULAR: Regular rate and rhythm without murmurs. ABDOMEN: No masses. EXTREMITIES: No edema. NEUROLOGIC: Cranial nerves intact, as are mentation and motor power.

IMPRESSION

The patient is a 57-year-old blind man with stage IVA (T4aN2M0) squamous cell carcinoma of the floor of the mouth, who currently has no evidence of disease. He has persistent sequelae of his therapy and his cancer, but he is doing quite well.

PLAN

He will return to the radiation oncology clinic in 3 months for followup evaluation, and he will also follow up in the ENT clinic. I have ordered a TSH as well as CT of the head and neck in routine followup.

_____

L. (Lonnie) Willem Erwin, MD
Radiation Oncology

LWE:cks
D:11/16/----
T:11/17/----

cc: Leah Pittfield, MD, Otorhinolaryngology
    Sherman Loyd, MD, Internal Medicine

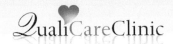

Emergency Department Treatment Record

Patient Name: Roberto Ruenes   **PCP:** Unknown

Date of Exam: 03/26/----   **Age/Sex:** 47/M   **ID#:** M-44

CONSULTING SERVICE: Trauma Surgery.

CHIEF COMPLAINT: Subdural bleed.

MODE OF ARRIVAL: EMS, Code 3 transfer.

PREHOSPITAL SUMMARY: This is a 47-year-old Mexican male brought Code 3 trauma via EMS with the chief complaint of a fall with a resultant right subdural hemorrhage and a left frontal subdural hemorrhage. Vital signs in the field: Blood pressure 150/80, pulse 87, respirations 16, temperature 99 rectal, pulse oximetry 100%.

INTERVENTIONS IN THE FIELD: This patient had been put into a C-collar on a long board. He had a cardiac monitor. He had already been intubated with a size 8-French endotracheal tube and was receiving 750 mL tidal volume at a rate of 16 per minute, 100% FiO_2 with a PEEP of 5, with a propofol drip hanging at 8 mg per hour. Foley catheter placed.

AMPLE History as reported included **A**, no drug allergies; **M**, no medications known; **P**, no past medical history or surgical history known; **L**, last meal unknown; and **E**, event was that he apparently fell from standing. He was seen at an outside hospital and diagnosed with a subdural bleed and transferred to the emergency room.

PRIMARY SURVEY

Vital signs on arrival showed blood pressure 146/86, heart rate 84, respirations 16, saturating at 100% on a ventilator. Sedated GCS for this patient was 3T.

A. Airway: Had the ET tube in good position. End-tidal CO_2 detector picked up good respirations.

B. Breathing: His lungs were bilaterally expanding. Trachea is midline.

C. Circulation: No flail chest, no subcu air circulation. Palpable pulses in all extremities.

D. Disability: Pelvis stable. C-spine precautions. C-spine immobilization maintained at all times with C-collar in place. Deficits: Glasgow coma score was 3T, but he was sedated on a propofol drip and intubated at the time. He is moving. He did not move any extremities spontaneously.

E. Exposure: He was fully exposed, log-rolled off the long board with C-spine immobilization maintained.

PRIMARY INTERVENTIONS

Basic safety net was applied. Cardiac monitor. Patient was transferred over to the vent and off the portable vent. He had three IV lines already in place: an 18-gauge in the right antecubital, an 18-gauge in left hand, and a 16-gauge in the left hand. He had pulse oximeter and noninvasive blood pressure cuffs in place.

A. Airway: Patient had a portable chest x-ray that showed the tube to be approximately 2 cm too high, so it was lowered 2 cm. Still had good breath sounds at that time. Still saturating at 100%. The patient had the propofol drip turned up to keep him sedated.

B. Breathing: He was given oxygen through the ventilator, 100% FiO_2. Pulse oximeter in place.

C. Circulation: Cardiac monitor placed. Noninvasive blood pressure. No more intravenous access was placed other than that prior to arrival.

INTRAVENOUS FLUIDS: He had 1 L normal saline run in.

(Continued)

ID#: M-44   PAGE 2

SECONDARY SURVEY

REPEAT VITAL SIGNS: Blood pressure 144/75, heart rate 80, respirations 16, saturating 100% on the vent. HEENT: Moist oral mucosa without active bleeding. He did seem to have some chipped teeth, but had no midface instability. Had a right hemotympanum with blood behind the tympanic membrane and also in the external auditory canal. Also had what appeared to be hematoma on the back left occiput. There was also wet blood, but a laceration was not visualized. He had no step-offs or palpable deformities in his C-spine. No Battle sign or raccoon eyes. No conjunctival hemorrhage. No subcutaneous emphysema. CARDIOVASCULAR: Regular rate and rhythm. Palpable distal pulses in all extremities. No jugular venous distension, no pedal edema. LUNGS: Bilaterally clear to auscultation. CHEST: Symmetric expansion. No clavicular chest wall tenderness to palpation, no contusions, laceration, hematomas, or crepitus. ABDOMEN: Soft, nondistended belly. He did have a small area of healing hematoma in his midaxillary line, approximately the T6-8 space. No other contusions, lacerations, or hematomas noted. BACK: No T- or L-spine step-offs or bony deformities. No contusions, lacerations, hematomas. GU: No blood at the meatus. Foley catheter in place prior to arrival. No scrotal hematoma, no perineal lacerations or contusions. RECTAL: No gross blood from his rectum. EXTREMITIES: No obvious deformities. No contusions or lacerations.

SECONDARY INTERVENTIONS: He had a portable chest x-ray that showed his ET tube initially to be about 2 cm too high. It was placed lower. Complete laboratory work, including ABG, done with results pending at the time of his discharge. The trauma surgery team will follow these results. FAST exam was negative. No additional IV access. He had a Foley placed prior to arrival. No CPAP or BiPAP was needed. Patient was just put on a vent with the setting at 750 on assist control, 750 mL of tidal volume, along with a respiratory rate of 18, with 100% FiO2 and a PEEP of 5. No tetanus was given. No antibiotics or pain meds given. One liter total normal saline IV fluids were given. He was on a Diprivan drip for sedation.

ASSESSMENT
This is a 47-year-old male status post fall, intubated, with a right subdural and a left frontal bleed seen at CT scan at outside facility.

DISPOSITION
Trauma Surgery Team took him to CT scanner for more tests, evaluation, and treatment. He will be transferred to the surgical intensive care unit for further evaluation. There they will follow up on all labs. Patient was in stable condition when he left the ED.

_____

Samuel Ernest, MD
Emergency Room Physician

SE:cks
D:03/26/----
T:03/26/----

cc: Mack Stolga, MD, Trauma Surgery

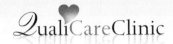

<u>**Bone Marrow Followup Note**</u>

Patient Name: Curtis L. Johnson

Date of Exam: 01/01/----

Age/Sex: 32/M

PCP: Lynne Andrew, MD

ID#: M-45

IDENTIFICATION: The patient is a 32-year-old African American male with chemorefractory Hodgkin lymphoma with a large mediastinal mass who is now day +113 post matched-related donor, allogenic peripheral blood stem cell transplantation.

HISTORY: Patient is most recently status post a hospital admission with a flare of acute graft-versus-host disease manifesting as nausea and vomiting, diarrhea, and a fever. During his hospital course 1 blood culture was also positive for nonanthrax species bacillus, and his stool specimen was positive for *Clostridium difficile* colitis 2 days ago. Patient remains on treatment with Flagyl p.o. as well as Tequin systemic antibiotic therapy. As part of his hospital course, he has also experienced a bout of pancytopenia, and at the time of discharge yesterday his white blood cell count was 0.9, with platelets of 20,000. Both of these counts are stable to slightly decreased from the day before with the CBC showing a white count of 1.6 and platelets of 24,000.

Because of improvement in his GI symptoms, he was discharged to an outpatient status. Solu-Medrol IV is continued at 1 mg/kg IV every morning, Tequin IV is given in the clinic, and Flagyl p.o. is continued for treatment of *C. difficile* colitis.

Overnight, the patient continues to do very well in terms of GI symptoms. He has had no further nausea and vomiting and is taking his pills without complaint. He has had some semiformed stool but no frankly watery stools and has 2 to 3 pudding-like stools per day. Patient's biggest complaint is increased bilateral lower extremity swelling, which started yesterday. He feels he has had an excessive amount of fluid retention.

PHYSICAL EXAMINATION

Blood pressure 115/75, pulse 92, respirations 16, temperature 97.5, weight 76.6 kg, which is up from 73 kg upon discharge. His baseline weight in the clinic was 71.4 kg approximately 6 weeks ago. GENERAL: Well-developed, well-nourished, pleasant black male in no apparent distress. Looks well, alert and oriented x4. HEENT: Pupils are equal, round, and reactive to light and accommodation. Oropharynx is clear. LUNGS: Clear to auscultation with no basilar rales. Saturating 96% on room air. CARDIOVASCULAR: Normal S1, S2. Regular with no murmur. ABDOMEN: Soft, nontender, nondistended. EXTREMITIES: Plus-two pedal edema, bilateral and symmetrical.

CURRENT MEDICATIONS
1. Solu-Medrol 70 mg IV every morning.
2. Tequin 400 mg IV every morning.
3. Flagyl 500 mg p.o. q.6 h.
4. Norvasc 5 mg p.o. daily.
5. Dapsone 100 mg p.o. daily.
6. Fluconazole 200 mg p.o. b.i.d.
7. Aranesp 200 mg subcutaneously every week.
8. G-CSF 480 mcg subcutaneously daily.
9. Kytril 1 mg p.o. every morning.
10. Compazine p.r.n.
11. Cyclosporin 100 mg p.o. q.12 h.
12. Acyclovir 200 mg p.o. b.i.d.

(Continued)

ID#: M-45 PAGE 2

LABORATORIES FROM TODAY: CBC, Chem-10, LFTs, and cyclosporin level are currently pending.

IMPRESSION

This is a 32-year-old African American male with chemorefractory Hodgkin disease who is status post allogenic peripheral blood stem cell transplant and is now status post mediastinal radiation therapy, which was completed approximately 3 weeks ago, for treatment of progressive disease after allogenic transplant. Patient was admitted with a flare of graft-versus-host disease involving predominantly the GI tract. This has now improved with systemic glucocorticoid therapy. He has no evidence of active infection, although he continues to have pancytopenia, but no temperatures greater than 101 degrees. He does have evidence of fluid retention.

His inpatient course was remarkable for an increased creatinine to 1.3 two days ago, although yesterday his creatinine decreased to 1. The etiology of the fluid retention may be multifactorial at this point, and in any event, he is in no respiratory distress.

CURRENT PLAN

1. Hematology: Await the results of his CBC and continue with daily G-CSF therapy.
2. Graft-versus-host disease: Continue with cyclosporin 100 mg p.o. b.i.d. Will plan to check a cyclosporin level today. The patient's most recent cyclosporin done yesterday was 209 ng/mL.
3. Infectious disease: Continue Flagyl p.o. and Tequin IV for the time being.
4. Gastrointestinal: Patient's GI symptoms are under control, and he is taking p.o. medications well.
5. Fluid, electrolytes, and nutrition: I will reevaluate the patient tomorrow morning. If he has gained further weight, I will plan to start him on Lasix diuresis as long as his creatinine remains stable. Additionally, we will await the results of his chem panel from today.

_____

Solomon T. Fisher, MD
Hematology

STF:cks
D:01/01/----
T:01/01/----

cc: Lynne Andrew, MD, Internal Medicine

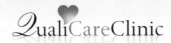

Emergency Room Treatment Record

Patient Name: Marian Parry   **PCP:** N/A

Date of Exam: 11/13/----   **Age/Sex:** 64/F   **ID#:** M-46

CONSULTING SERVICE: Ophthalmology.

CHIEF COMPLAINT: Blurred vision.

MODE OF ARRIVAL: Privately owned vehicle.

HISTORY OF PRESENT ILLNESS: This 64-year-old female presents to the ED complaining of blurred vision in her right eye. She states that 2 to 3 days ago she had blinking lights in the periphery of her right vision that has persisted off and on. In addition, patient complains of floaters behind her right eye. Patient states that yesterday she experienced the sensation of having a sharp dark ribbon down the right side of her eye that resolved spontaneously. Patient denies any type of pain in her eye, denies any type of trauma.

REVIEW OF SYSTEMS: Positive in the ED for floaters in the patient's right vision and diplopia. ROS is otherwise negative for the following: Headache, change in hearing, dysphagia, nausea, vomiting, diarrhea, fever, chills, chest pain, shortness of breath, abdominal pain, dysuria.

PAST MEDICAL HISTORY: Hypothyroid, depression.

PAST SURGICAL HISTORY: Hysterectomy.

MEDICATIONS: Synthroid and Effexor.

ALLERGIES: No known drug allergies.

SOCIAL HISTORY: Denies tobacco use.

PHYSICAL EXAMINATION

VITAL SIGNS on presentation: Pulse 78, BP 156/81, respirations 16, temperature 96.7, O_2 sat. 98% on room air. GENERAL APPEARANCE: Awake, alert, oriented x3, in no acute distress. EYE exam consists of the following: Visual acuity is 20/25 bilaterally with correction. Pupils full and round reactively from 5 mm to 3 mm with normal reflexes. Extraocular muscles intact. No deficits in her movements. No pain with movements. Visual fields, right eye, are full to confrontation in that the patient could see shapes; however, she complained of blurriness to the midline and to the medial aspect. Visual fields, left eye, are full to confrontation. Intraocular pressures: Right eye 15, left eye 13. Patient's external exam is negative for ecchymoses, crepitus, or numbness. No changes in the skin. Slit lamp exam: Corneas are normal. Anterior chambers are deep and quiet bilaterally. Irides are normal bilaterally. Lenses are normal bilaterally. Floaters are appreciated in the patient's right eye in the posterior chamber. Lids, lashes, and lacrima are all within normal limits. Conjunctivae are normal.

TEST RESULTS WITH INTERPRETATION: None.

EMERGENCY DEPARTMENT COURSE/MEDICAL DECISION MAKING: The patient was seen and examined. She received a full physical exam with examination of her eyes with a slit lamp and Tono-Pen. This patient appears stable with normal vital signs; however, I cannot exclude a small retinal detachment or vitreous hemorrhage. Dr. Okano of ophthalmology was consulted at 1345 hours. Dr. Okano requested the patient be discharged to her clinic, and she is on her way to the hospital at this time to evaluate the patient. The patient is stable for discharge to the care of Ophthalmology, and the patient need not return to the ED for further evaluation. She was given strict return precautions, however, regarding worsening of symptoms. She was cautioned against driving a motor vehicle if there is impairment of her vision. Patient verbalized full understanding of these discharge instructions and indicated that she would comply as directed.

(Continued)

ID#: M-46   PAGE 2

EMERGENCY DEPARTMENT DIAGNOSIS
Diplopia.

DISPOSITION
Discharge to ophthalmology clinic.

PLAN
Discharge to ophthalmology clinic. Return with any questions or problems. Do not drive a motor vehicle until cleared by Ophthalmology.

_____
Samuel Ernest, MD
Emergency Room Physician

SE:cks
D:11/13/----
T:11/13/----

cc: Midori Okano, MD, Ophthalmology

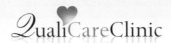

Orthopedic Surgery Followup Note

Patient Name: Robert M. Sager   **PCP:** Susan McGinnis, MD

Date of Exam: 08/10/----   **Age/Sex:** 43/M   **ID#:** M-47

HISTORY: Patient is a 43-year-old gentleman who is well known to our clinic. He presents today for his Euflexxa injections #3 bilaterally. Patient has done well in the last week since his previous injections with some notable aching knees, which were similar to his previous series of Euflexxa injections. Patient denies fevers, chills, nausea, vomiting, and has no complaints otherwise.

PHYSICAL EXAMINATION

Patient is in no acute distress today. He is alert and oriented x3. Examination was limited to his musculoskeletal system. He has mild varus angulation of both knees. Patient's range of motion is from 5 degrees to 125 degrees, with some crepitus. Very little varus and valgus angulation on stress testing at 0 and 30 degrees of flexion.

ASSESSMENT/PLAN

Patient is a 43-year-old male with bilateral knee osteoarthritis. The plan is to perform the Euflexxa injection #3 bilaterally.

After prepping both knees with Betadine, inferolateral portals were used to inject the correct dose of Euflexxa into each knee. The injections were carried out under sterile technique. Patient tolerated the procedure well with no complications.

The patient will follow up with us as needed in the orthopedic clinic.

_____
Gilbert M. Fields, MD
Orthopedic Surgery

GMF:cks
D:08/10/----
T:08/11/---

cc: Susan McGinnis, MD, Family Practice

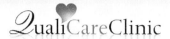
QualiCareClinic

<u>**Vascular Surgery Consultation**</u>

Patient Name: Hamilton Jones   **PCP:** Kenneth Shaker, MD
Date of Exam: 03/16/----   **Age/Sex:** 78/M   **ID#:** M-48

REASON FOR REFERRAL: Abdominal aortic aneurysm, juxtarenal/infrarenal, with relatively rapid growth.

HISTORY OF PRESENT ILLNESS: Mr. Jones, a 78-year-old male, is well known to our clinic. He had a history of a small aneurysm that has grown recently. He has had significant enlargement of the size of the aneurysm with the aneurysm now being 5.7 cm to 6 cm, depending on measurement axis. This is a significant increase since 6 months ago, at which time it measured 5.3 x 4.7 cm. One year prior to that it measured less than 5 cm, at around 4.6 to 4.7 cm. He has basically an infrarenal aneurysm except the left renal artery has a fairly low takeoff. It is about 1 to 1.5 cm lower than the right renal artery. Just distal to that, it has some ectasia of the infrarenal aorta just distal to the left renal artery. He presents today for operative discussion, planning, and options.

PHYSICAL EXAMINATION

His physical examination today is unchanged from previous. VITALS: His temperature is 96.6, blood pressure 144/85, pulse 61, respirations 20. His focal exam reveals a moderately obese male in no acute distress. ABDOMEN: Soft, nontender. Cannot palpate this aneurysm secondary to its size. He has 2+ femoral pulses.

X-RAY DATA: CT scan was reviewed with the patient. Again, he does have a neck adequate for endografting below his right renal artery that is roughly 1.5 cm long. However, the left renal artery comes off approximately 1 cm lower than the right renal artery and about 5 mm above the infrarenal neck. The patient has a large 5.7 mm, by radiology read, but 6 to 6.1 cm maximal diameter aneurysm below that. Normal, widely patent iliac arteries.

ASSESSMENT AND PLAN
The patient is a delightful gentleman with an enlarging aneurysm, now roughly 6 cm in size. He really requires repair of this at 6 cm. Even at 78 years of age, he is relatively healthy. He has a mild heart history, having had a stent placed 2 years ago. Postoperative to that he has had a stress test, during which he was said to have had some minor symptoms; however, the stress test was relatively negative. The patient is currently asymptomatic from the heart standpoint and is relatively active as well. He desires surgery for intervention.

We discussed the options of (1) open surgery versus (2) an attempt at a fenestrated endograft with (3) possible open surgery and/or (4) possible left renal artery bypass graft if we inadvertently cover that left renal artery or (5) leaving the renal artery covered and letting the kidney die, as he has normal kidney function, at least by creatinine standards, currently. Patient understands all these options, and we will plan to perform a fenestrated endograft of this aneurysm with possible left renal artery bypass versus possible open aneurysm repair. He understands all these options, the indications, and the risks. He desires to proceed.

We are going to admit him the day before surgery to hydrate him. We will perform the surgery in 6 weeks and will have him get a preop evaluation by Anesthesia in 2 weeks.

_____
Ly An Tabor, MD
Vascular Surgery

LAT:cks
D:03/16/----
T:03/16/----

c: Kenneth Shaker, MD, Internal Medicine

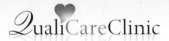

QualiCareClinic

Emergency Department Treatment Record

Patient Name: Roy T. Holloday **PCP:** Unknown

Date of Exam: 11/11/---- **Age/Sex:** 14/M **ID#:** M-50

CONSULTING SERVICE: Neurosurgery.

CHIEF COMPLAINT: Status post motor vehicle collision with head injury.

MODE OF ARRIVAL: Code 3, EMS.

HISTORY OF PRESENT ILLNESS: This is a 14-year-old male who was involved in an MVC. It was a vehicle versus tree. The patient was a nonrestrained passenger. The patient came in after suffering a large blow to the right side of the head. EMS picked up the patient, put the patient in a C-collar, provided C-spine support, started him on some oxygen, and transferred him to the Hillcrest Medical Center emergency room, Code 3. The patient presented with a GCS of 4 and was posturing.

PRIMARY SURVEY

A. Airway: The patient had no spontaneous breaths.
B. Breathing: Lungs sounds were clear to auscultation with bag-valve-mask.
C. Circulation: Distal pulses were 2+ in all extremities.
D. Disability: The patient had decerebrate posturing and, other than posturing, did not spontaneously move extremities. GCS was 4 upon arrival.

PRIMARY INTERVENTIONS: Secondary IV access was obtained. The patient was placed on 100% oxygen with a bag-valve-mask and given breaths. He was placed on a monitor. The patient was prepared for intubation. He was hyperventilated with the bag-valve-mask. Patient was given 20 of etomidate and 100 of succinylcholine. The patient was intubated with RSI technique while holding C-spine precautions. A Mac 3 blade was inserted into the oropharynx. Suction was used to get out blood and debris. The vocal cords were visualized, and a 7.0 tube was passed and visualized through the vocal cords. After the tube was passed, tube placement was confirmed with bilateral breath sounds and positive color change on 6 breaths using end-tidal CO_2.

SECONDARY SURVEY

GENERAL: The patient was now GCS of 3T. His vital signs were stable. His blood pressure was 150/98 with heart rate of 100 and sinus tachycardia. He had no spontaneous breaths. Temperature was 97.1, and he was saturating 100% on monitor. He was 3T and unresponsive. HEENT: The patient had a large, 5 cm gaping laceration to the right temporoparietal area. Also in the same region, the patient had a depressed skull fracture. He had a small laceration on his chin. Patient had no hemotympanum. No septal hematoma, and his midface was stable. HEART: Regular rate and rhythm. Normal S1, S2. No murmurs, gallops, or rubs. LUNGS: Clear to auscultation bilaterally. ABDOMEN: Soft and nondistended. He had a stable chest and stable pelvis. EXTREMITIES: Two-plus pulses in all extremities. No other cyanosis, clubbing, or edema. He had no other evidence of trauma, other than trauma to the head. SKIN: No petechiae, purpura, or rashes.

(Continued)

ID#: M-50   PAGE 2

SECONDARY INTERVENTION: The patient was given 2 mg of Versed and was given 50 g of mannitol. He had an additional 2 repeat boluses of Versed. He was given 30 mg of rocuronium and another 2 mg of Versed. He was given a gram of Ancef. He was given Cerebyx 1 g.

An OG tube was placed. Placement was confirmed, and the patient's stomach was decompressed. A trauma panel was drawn and sent, and the patient was turned over to Trauma Surgery to take to the CT scanner. Also, portable chest x-ray was obtained, which showed no pneumothorax, normal mediastinum, and good tube placement.

EMERGENCY DEPARTMENT COURSE: The patient remained hemodynamically stable while in the emergency department. Patient was given therapy to help with suspected increased intracranial pressure to include mannitol and fosphenytoin. Patient was taken to CT scanner by Trauma Surgery.

IMPRESSION/MEDICAL DECISION MAKING: This is a 14-year-old male who presents Code 3 by EMS, who has a depressed skull fracture and a large gash to his right head consistent with an open skull fracture. The patient presented with a GCS of 4, was intubated, and it was 3T upon discharge from the ER to Trauma Surgery. The patient was given 1 g Ancef to cover antibiotic-wise. I suspect the patient had increased ICP based on posturing in the emergency department. He was intubated and stabilized in the ED prior to being transferred to Trauma Surgery. The blood results and CT scan to be followed by Trauma Surgery.

DISPOSITION
Admission to the SICU in critical condition.

EMERGENCY DEPARTMENT DIAGNOSES
1. Depressed skull fracture.
2. Blunt head injury.
3. Status post motor vehicle collision.

PROGNOSIS
Guarded.

_____

Samuel Ernest, MD
Emergency Room Physician

SE:cks
D:11/11/----
T:11/11/----

c: Arnold R. Youngblood, MD, Neurosurgery
    Mack Stolga, MD, Trauma Surgery

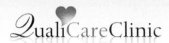

Orthopedic Clinic Consultation

Patient Name: Christopher Lee   **PCP:** Marie Aaron, DO

Date of Exam: 16 Feb ----   **Age/Sex:** 17-year-old male   **ID#:** M-51

REASON FOR CONSULTATION: Right ankle instability.

HISTORY OF PRESENT ILLNESS: Christopher is a 17-year-old semiprofessional skateboarder who presents today with a history of numerous ankle sprains. These ankle sprains are worrisome and bothersome enough that they prevent him from competing at a higher professional level. He desires today to undergo a surgical reconstruction for added stability of the right ankle to pursue a professional career in skateboarding. He has the sensation of right ankle instability with the usual sport bike activities but most specifically with skateboarding.

PAST MEDICAL HISTORY: He has a past medical history of asthma and allergic rhinitis.

PAST SURGICAL HISTORY: There is no past surgical history.

CURRENT MEDICATIONS: Advair 500/50 mg inhaled twice a day, Singulair 10 mg p.o. once a day, Zyrtec-D once a day, Maxair every other day, and albuterol 1 to 2 puffs as needed.

SOCIAL HISTORY: He denies tobacco use, he denies alcohol use, and he denies illicit drug use. He is an eleventh grader in high school.

ALLERGIES: The patient has no known drug allergies.

REVIEW OF SYSTEMS: The review of systems completed today is noted to be positive for right ankle instability and pain. All other systems are negative.

PHYSICAL EXAMINATION

The physical examination reveals a well-developed, well-nourished 17-year-old male whose height is 5 feet 10 inches and weight is 130 pounds. HEENT examination reveals normal teeth, normal gums, normal lips, and a normal buccal mucosa. NECK: There is no evidence of adenopathy, thyromegaly, or carotid bruit. LUNGS are clear to auscultation bilaterally. CARDIOVASCULAR exam is notable for a regular rate and rhythm without murmur. BACK is nontender to palpation. GASTROINTESTINAL examination reveals a nontender, nondistended abdomen. No hepatosplenomegaly, no masses, no aortic or renal bruits. NEUROLOGIC examination is grossly intact. Right ankle: His range of motion is full to passive and active range of motion. There is no instability with examination, although the patient subjectively feels unstable with inversion of the ankle and foot, pain also experienced in the lateral aspect of the ankle joint. Motor examination reveals extensor hallucis longus, gastrocnemius/soleus, anterior tibialis, and peroneals are 5/5. There is a negative anterior drawer test. The sensation is intact to light touch in the deep peroneal, superficial peroneal, saphenous, sural, and tibialis nerve distributions. Vascular examination reveals normal coloration of the skin. There are palpable pulses in the dorsalis pedis and posterior tibialis with capillary refill less than 2 seconds.

IMPRESSION

This is a 17-year-old semiprofessional skateboarder who presents today with a history of right ankle instability.

(Continued)

ID#: M-51   PAGE 2

PLAN
The plan is to take the patient to the operating room on 22 February----for right ankle ligamentous reconstruction. The indications for, details of, alternatives to, as well as known associated risks versus expected benefits to the above-named procedure were discussed with the patient and his mother today. All questions were answered to their satisfaction. They verbalized understanding and gave informed consent to proceed.

_____
Raquel Rodriguez, MD
Orthopedic Surgery

RR:pai
D:2/16/----
T:2/16/----

c: Marie Aaron, DO, Family Practice

QualiCareClinic

Emergency Department Treatment Record

Patient Name: Paula K. Lockhart   **PCP:** Linda L. Kingston, DO

Date of Exam: 21 Oct ----   **Age/Sex:** 68-year-old female   **ID#:** M-52

CHIEF COMPLAINT: Left forearm pain and deformity after a fall.

MODE OF ARRIVAL: The patient arrived by privately-owned vehicle.

CONSULTING SERVICE: Orthopedic Surgery.

HISTORY OF PRESENT ILLNESS: The patient is a 68-year-old female who presents to the emergency department, accompanied by her daughter, after falling and sustaining an injury to her left arm. The patient as well as the daughter who was present at the time state that she was standing, bending over on an uneven surface, slipped, and fell backward. She placed her arms up behind her to stop her and thus sustained injury. There is clearly no history of loss of consciousness either before or after the fall. No dizziness, headaches, weakness, numbness, chest pain, difficulty breathing, or other complaints at this time. She does complain that the arm is mildly tender to palpation. She seems to have minimal pain when the arm is not being manipulated. She does not complain of a headache or pain to her cervical spine, thoracic spine, or lumbar spine. There is no pain in her coccyx.

REVIEW OF SYSTEMS: The patient has a chronic cough. Her review of systems is otherwise negative, except for the History of Present Illness.

PAST MEDICAL HISTORY includes a history of hypertension.

MEDICATIONS: Please see the handwritten chart for a list of the medications.

SOCIAL HISTORY: Please see the handwritten chart for the social history.

PHYSICAL EXAMINATION

The VITAL SIGNS on presentation include a temperature of 100.2 degrees, a pulse of 88, respirations 20, blood pressure 170/85, oxygen saturation 94% on room air. GENERAL APPEARANCE is that of a well-developed, well-nourished white female in no acute distress. HEENT EXAMINATION: The pupils are equal, round, and reactive to light. Conjunctivae are normal. The sclerae are anicteric. The oropharynx is clear, moist, and symmetric. The nose is normal. NECK EXAM: The neck is supple without masses. The thyroid is normal. RESPIRATORY EXAM: The lungs are clear to auscultation bilaterally. The CHEST WALL EXAM is nontender. CARDIOVASCULAR EXAM: S1 and S2 are normal. There are no murmurs noted. There is no peripheral edema. GASTROINTESTINAL EXAM: Abdomen is soft and nontender. No hepatosplenomegaly is noted. INTEGUMENTARY EXAM: There are no rashes, lesions, ulcers, or induration. NEUROLOGIC EXAM: The patient is alert and appropriate. The speech is clear. The gait is stable. EXTREMITIES: There is some deformity over the ulnar aspect of the forearm on the left side. There is ecchymosis noted as well. Minimal tenderness to palpation. The anatomic snuffbox is completely nontender. The thumb and indeed the entire forearm are totally nontender with axial loading. She is neurovascularly intact. She does have some pain with extension of the wrist against resistance.

(Continued)

ID#: M-52   PAGE 2

ANCILLARY STUDIES: The x-ray shows a slightly impacted but otherwise nondisplaced intraarticular distal radius fracture.

MEDICAL DECISION-MAKING PROCESS: There is an isolated distal radius fracture in an elderly female. She has very minimal pain. She is tolerating the injury quite well. Neurovascularly she is intact. Orthopedics was called down and, with some minimal intravenous narcotics, they were able to reduce and cast the fracture with the assistance of the finger traps. The patient tolerated this well.

EMERGENCY DEPARTMENT DIAGNOSIS
Distal radius fracture.

CONDITION: Stable.

DISPOSITION: The patient was discharged from the emergency department to home.

DISCHARGE INSTRUCTIONS: The patient has been discharged with clear return instructions as well as instructions to follow up at the orthopedic clinic as directed by the orthopedic team.

_____
Raquel Rodriguez, MD
Orthopedic Surgery

RR:pai
D:10/21/----
T:10/21/----

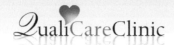

Oromaxillofacial Surgery Consultation

Patient Name: Juan Gutierrez **PCP:** Chris Salem, DO

Date of Exam: 2 Sept ---- **Age/Sex:** 23-year-old male **ID#:** M-54

REASON FOR CONSULTATION: Facial trauma during assault.

HISTORY OF PRESENT ILLNESS: Mr. Gutierrez is a 23-year-old male who was assaulted at approximately 2 a.m. on 2 Sept ----. The patient states that he was assaulted by approximately 7 men when he was leaving a downtown bar. One of these men punched him in the face and also bit off a portion of his right ear. Patient was transported by EMS to Quali-Care, from which he was transported as Code 3 Trauma to Hillcrest Medical Center ED. Upon evaluation by the trauma service, Oromaxillofacial Surgery was consulted to evaluate the patient's facial trauma injuries.

PAST HISTORY: Noncontributory. Patient has had no previous surgery.

ALLERGIES: NKDA.

MEDICATIONS: Patient has been on penicillin for the past week for recent root canal therapy to tooth #31.

SOCIAL HISTORY: Patient admits to using tobacco products infrequently, mainly cigarettes. Patient also admits to drinking alcohol the previous evening. Denies illicit drug use.

PHYSICAL EXAMINATION

Patient is examined in his room at approximately 0620 hours on 2 Sept ----. Vital signs show heart rate of 86, blood pressure of 141/74, oxygen saturation is 99% on room air, and respirations 18. Patient is alert and oriented x3, in no acute distress, with a Glasgow coma scale of 15.

INITIAL HEENT EXAM: Complains of pain on his ear with swelling on his face. Pain is 5/10. Soft tissue exam shows scalp is within normal limits. No axillary abrasions are noted. No major contusions. Patient has no evidence of Battle sign. Has significant periorbital edema on both eyes, more significant supraorbital edema over his left eye. Infraorbital edema over his right eye. There is an 8 mm laceration under his right eye, approximately 1 cm below the lower lid.

CRANIAL BONE EXAM: Bones are all intact. No major facial fractures noted. Eyes show his pupils are equal, round, and reactive to light and accommodation. Subconjunctival heme over the right eye at the lateral portion. Visual acuity is grossly intact. Patient is 20/20 in both eyes on examination with a near card. There is no diplopia on forward gaze or any excursive movements.

EARS show his external auditory canals to be patent bilaterally. There is no hemotympanum. Left ear has no evidence of trauma. Right ear shows complete avulsion of the helix from the right helical tubercle down to the superior portion of the lobule. The avulsed portion has been placed in a bag of ice and is present with the patient at bedside.

NASAL EXAM shows no evidence of septal hematoma, nasal fracture, or septal deviation.

ORAL EXAM: Maxilla is grossly intact. No mobility, no occlusal discrepancies, no soft tissue damage. Mandibles are grossly intact. Multiple carious teeth. No limitation of tongue movement. His occlusion is stable and repeatable.

NEUROLOGIC EXAM shows cranial nerves II through XII grossly intact. No paresthesias.

LABORATORY AND X-RAY DATA: CT exam of his face shows possible bilateral infraorbital floor fractures that are minimally displaced. No other fractures are noted on CT exam. Significant labs include a white count of 14.9. Blood alcohol level at 0445 hours today of 0.64.

(Continued)

ID#: M-54   PAGE 2

ASSESSMENT

This 23-year-old male sustained facial trauma with (1) significant avulsion of a portion of his right ear, (2) bilateral minimally displaced orbital floor fractures, and (3) one minor facial laceration on his right infraorbital region. Ophthalmologic exam is stable.

PLAN/RECOMMENDATIONS

1. After examination of the patient and the avulsed portion of his ear, it was determined that we would attempt to reattach this portion of the ear primarily. It is unknown, however, how much time has elapsed since the actual traumatic incident prior to the patient being evaluated at Quali-Care. The patient was counseled on the possible treatment options and elected to proceed with a primary repair of his ear by reattaching the avulsed portion. However, he was given an extremely guarded prognosis as to the survivability of the portion to be reattached. The patient was subsequently escorted down to the oral surgery clinic with staff present for the procedure to be done.
2. General Surgery indicated that they will consult ophthalmology services concerning the orbital floor fractures. The patient shows no signs of ophthalmologic injury that would require emergent treatment.
   We will continue to follow the patient's eye exam to determine if he will require further treatment.
3. Patient was taken to our clinic for repair of his ear. The dictation will be noted in the patient's record separately.

_____

Leela Pivari, MD
Oromaxillofacial Surgery

LP:pai
D:9/2/----
T:9/2/----

c: Chris Salem, DO, Family Practice

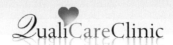

Discharge Summary

Patient Name: Melissa Baker   **PCP:** Susan McGinnis, MD

Date of Admission: 30 Jan ----   **Date of Discharge:** 4 Feb ----   **Age/Sex:** 56-year-old female   **ID#:** M-55

IDENTIFICATION: Ms. Baker is a 56-year-old female with a history of chemorefractory, diffuse, large B-cell, non-Hodgkin lymphoma originally treated with 8 cycles of CHOP and Rituxan therapy, completed in September four years ago. Patient was treated with a splenectomy on 15 Nov last year, and now she has had 2 cycles of CCE and Rituxan therapy with cycle 2 given on 6 Jan ----. Repeat PET scan staging on 24 Jan revealed resolution of the previously visualized right hilar lymphadenopathy and substantial reduction in the anterior abdominal wall of standardized uptake value (SUV) activity. It now is 16 mm in size and has an SUV value of 4.4, having a previous SUV value of 8.2. This is consistent with a partial response from CCE.

For full details, please see the accompanying initial Bone Marrow Transplant Evaluation Note from 1 Nov last year, the Family Conference Note of 26 Jan ----, and the admission H&P dictated by Dr. Lopez on 30 Jan ----.

HOSPITAL COURSE: Patient was admitted to undergo high-dose chemotherapy with Cytoxan, BCNU, and VP-16. This was successfully accomplished over an approximately 96-hour period of time. She was dosed according to an adjusted ideal body weight of 55.8 kg with a height of 59 inches with a dosing body surface area (BSA) of 1.50 m^2. On this she received 1500/m^2 of Cytoxan IV daily for 4 days, BCNU 200 mg/m^2 IV daily for 2 days, and VP-16 at 250 mg/m^2 IV b.i.d. for 4 days for a total of 8 doses. She received this as an inpatient with intravenous fluids with subsequent Lasix to obtain an even fluid balance. Patient also received mesna to prevent hemorrhagic cystitis, and she had no evidence of hemorrhage or hematuria at the time of discharge.

At the time of discharge, patient felt well with minimal nausea and no shortness of breath.

PLAN
Discharge to home today with followup on 6 Feb ---- for peripheral blood stem cell reinfusion. Patient will follow up sooner if she develops increasing nausea over the weekend, hematuria, or other pain symptoms.

DISCHARGE MEDICATIONS
1. Tequin 400 mg p.o. daily.
2. Fluconazole 200 mg p.o. daily.
3. Acyclovir 800 mg p.o. b.i.d.
4. Magnesium oxide 400 mg p.o. b.i.d.
5. Potassium phosphate 250 mg p.o. b.i.d.
6. Atenolol 50 mg p.o. daily.
7. Lisinopril 10 mg p.o. daily.
8. Premarin 0.625 mg p.o. daily.
9. Zofran 8 mg p.o. b.i.d. from 5 to 7 Feb ----.
10. Compazine p.r.n.
11. Colace 100 mg p.o. b.i.d.
12. Actigall 300 mg b.i.d.
13. Allopurinol 300 mg p.o. daily through 5 Feb ----.
14. AcipHex 20 mg p.o. daily.
15. Restoril 15 mg p.o. q.h.s. p.r.n.

(Continued)

ID#: M-55   PAGE 2

    16. Oxycodone p.r.n.
    17. Dapsone 100 mg p.o. daily through 5 Feb ----.
    18. Norvasc 5 mg p.o. daily.

_____
Solomon T. Fisher, MD
Hematology/Oncology

STF:pai
D:2/5/----
T:2/6/----

c: Susan McGinnis, MD, Family Practice

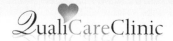
QualiCareClinic

Preop History and Physical Examination

Patient Name: Jerry Graham   **PCP:** Ronald Reardon, DO

Date of Exam: 5 Feb ----   **Age/Sex:** 57-year-old male   **ID#:** M-56

DIAGNOSIS
There is a left upper extremity amputation at the elbow status post reimplantation.

HISTORY OF PRESENT ILLNESS: The patient is a 57-year-old male who was in a motor vehicle accident in August of last year. He had a head-on collision with a guardrail and had his left upper extremity severed at the elbow joint. He underwent reimplantation back in August of last year. He is here today for preop for a left total elbow reconstruction. He is doing well at this time. He denies fevers, chills, nausea, or vomiting. He is otherwise healthy, and he has no complaints at this time.

PAST MEDICAL HISTORY: There is none other than that mentioned in HPI.

PAST SURGICAL HISTORY: Reimplantation of his upper extremity and removal of an external fixator.

SOCIAL HISTORY: The patient works as a custodian. He is married with 3 children and has a good support system.

ALLERGIES: There are no known drug allergies.

PHYSICAL EXAMINATION

GENERAL: On physical examination, the patient is a well-developed, well-nourished 57-year-old white male in no acute distress.

HEENT/NECK: Normocephalic and atraumatic. The neck exam shows no lymphadenopathy.

CHEST/LUNGS: His lungs are clear to auscultation bilaterally, and there are no chest lesions.

CARDIOVASCULAR EXAMINATION: The heart has regular rate and rhythm.

ABDOMEN/GENITALIA/PELVIC/RECTAL: There is a soft, nontender, nondistended abdomen. He has normal male genitalia.

BACK/EXTREMITIES: The patient's left upper extremity shows well-healing wounds. There is an intact dermal layer over all his wounds. The patient has no sensation below the elbow. He has some paresthesias and tingling in the mid aspect of his elbow. The patient has minimal wrist flexion and some long finger flexion. The patient has brisk capillary refill to all of his digits. The patient has no motion at the elbow joint.

DIAGNOSTIC DATA: The patient's plain films today show no changes from previous.

(Continued)

ID#: M-56   PAGE 2

IMPRESSION AND PLAN
Left upper extremity amputation at the elbow status post reimplantation.

The patient is here for his preop for total elbow arthroplasty. The risks, benefits, and adverse effects were discussed with the patient at length, and the patient agrees to undergo the surgery. Outcome expectations were also discussed with the patient at length. The patient expressed understanding of the postoperative outcome goals. There were no barriers to communication.

_____
Raquel Rodriguez, MD
Orthopedic Surgeon

RR:pai
D:2/5/----
T:2/6/----

c: Ronald Reardon, DO, Family Practice

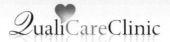

QualiCareClinic

Emergency Department Treatment Record

Patient Name: Ahmed Saleh   **PCP:** Unknown

Date of Exam: 26 March ----   **Age/Sex:** 18-year-old male   **ID#:** M-57

MODE OF ARRIVAL: EMS, ambulatory.

CONSULTING SERVICE: Psychology.

HISTORY OF PRESENT ILLNESS: This 18-year-old male states that he is from Yemen, and while he was in Yemen he wanted to go to college and learn things; however, you need "high scores." He says that there is a lot of pressure to do well, but in his country they sort of assign you your scores, and his were in the 60s, so he could not attend college. He felt that coming to America would allow him to go to college, so he struck a bargain with his father. His father said that he would buy a plane ticket for Ahmed to come to America if Ahmed got married. So the patient is married, for which he takes a lot of responsibility. He says he needs to provide for his wife and family. When he came to America, he states, he was very nervous about providing for the family. He had to get a job in order to pay for an apartment for the family.

Ahmed felt that he could never go to college because of having to work at a job. Upon seeing an advertisement for the Army, he felt that he wanted to do something for this country, for his family, and for himself. He felt that the Army would be a good option because he could be an Arabic translator, which the Army needs, and do a good thing for the country while he earned money for college and obtained some education. He felt this was a great idea, and he joined the US Army. He went to 1 week's basic training prior to being sent to Defense Language Institute (DLI) training to learn English fully. Ahmed states that he really enjoyed his time in basic training. People helped him out. However, once he transferred to DLI training, he said that it became a struggle because he is a perfectionist and wants to do everything right. He tries his hardest to obey his drill instructors; however, he does not understand how the other people in his platoon do so poorly. He does not understand why they are here if they do not want to work hard to learn their jobs. Patient is concerned because when one of them messes up, the entire platoon gets punished. He feels that this is unfair when he has been working so hard. Patient strictly denies suicidal and homicidal ideations, quoting religious reasons, but he states that he really does not get along with the people in his platoon because he does not understand why they are not working hard enough. This afternoon he sort of "had enough" where he walked outside from his barracks to get away from the other people in his platoon. His Drill Instructor (DI) asked Ahmed why he was outside, and he felt that Ahmed was a little bit slow in replying. Patient remarked that he just wanted to get away from the other people.

The DI replied, "Maybe I should just move your cot outside." The patient remarked that he would be fine with that. He said, "Yes, please move me outside to get me away from these people." The DI felt that this was an inappropriate response, said that he needed to talk to a "nervous" doctor over in the ED. The DI promptly sent the patient over to the ED. Patient remarks that he has, again, no complaints at this time other than being just a little bit anxious about going back.

REVIEW OF SYSTEMS: As above, otherwise negative.

PAST MEDICAL HISTORY: Noncontributory.

PAST SURGICAL HISTORY: None.

MEDICATIONS: None.

ALLERGIES: No known drug allergies.

IMMUNIZATIONS: Up to date.

SOCIAL HISTORY: No smoking, no alcohol, no illicit drugs, no herbal medications.

FAMILY HISTORY: Noncontributory except as mentioned above.

(Continued)

ID#: M-57   PAGE 2

PHYSICAL EXAMINATION

VITAL SIGNS on presentation: P 81, BP 130/68, R 15, T 98.0, O2 saturation 96% on room air. In general: Alert and oriented x3 in no apparent distress. Pleasant male who appears his stated age. HEENT: Normocephalic, atraumatic. Pupils are equal, round, and reactive to light and accommodation. Extraocular movements intact. Oropharynx clear with moist mucous membranes. NECK: Supple with no lymphadenopathy or jugular venous distention. CARDIAC: Regular rate and rhythm with no murmurs, rubs, or gallops. LUNGS: Clear to auscultation bilaterally. ABDOMEN: Soft, nontender, nondistended with positive bowel sounds. EXTREMITIES: Pulses +2 x4. No clubbing, cyanosis, clots, or edema. NEURO: Cranial nerves II through XII grossly intact. Patient is ambulatory.

EMERGENCY DEPARTMENT COURSE/ASSESSMENT/PLAN: I spoke to Dr. Stella Rose Dickinson, who is on call. I described the patient's symptoms and how I felt that this soldier is actually a benefit to the Army and that we should try to keep the soldier in the Army. The soldier, in fact, wants to stay in the Army. However, he does not understand and is somewhat stressed out about his training situation at this time. I feel that this patient has no suicidal ideations and no homicidal ideations. I feel that maybe, if he just had someone to talk to, to describe these things to him—maybe due to an ethnic gap or a language barrier, he may not understand exactly what his role is here. Again, I spoke with Stella Rose Dickinson of Psychology, who stated that he would be an appropriate patient for the Walk-In Life Skills Clinic in 24 to 48 hours. He will walk in on Monday morning at 0800 hours to the fourth floor Life Skills Clinic. I will give him a consult to carry with him, and I will fax this narrative to the appropriate number.

EMERGENCY DEPARTMENT DIAGNOSIS
  Anxiety disorder.

PLAN
1. Maintain good oral intake.
2. Follow up with PCP as needed.
3. Follow up with Life Skills Walk-In Clinic at 0800 hours on 28 March, which is 48 hours from now.
4. This plan was discussed with the patient, who expressed understanding and willingness to comply. On reevaluation, patient is asymptomatic with stable vital signs and in no acute distress.
5. Patient ambulated out of the ED under his own power. He was given aftercare instructions on anxiety.

DISPOSITION
Condition stable. Disposition is to home, then to Life Skills Walk-In Clinic in 48 hours.

_____
Samuel Ernest, MD
Emergency Room Physician

SE:pai
D:3/26/----
T:3/26/----

c: Stella Rose Dickinson, PhD, Psychology

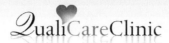

Internal Medicine Clinic Followup Note

Patient Name: Rooster O'Brien   **PCP:** Martha C. Eaton, MD

Date of Exam: 10 Aug ----   **Age/Sex:** 89-year-old male   **ID#:** M-59

CHIEF COMPLAINT
Mr. O'Brien presents in followup to discuss memory

HISTORY OF PRESENT ILLNESS
1. Memory problems: Our last visit was on 12 July ----. He was recently moved home from the hospital after rehab following an inpatient stay for urinary tract infection. I asked his wife if she would bring him in for an appointment today to evaluate his memory and decreased degree of function. I requested today, specifically, to give him a sufficient interval between his acute hospitalization and his return home to ensure he was back to his functional level of baseline.

   Mrs. O'Brien said Rooster spends most of his days watching television but watches intellectually challenging shows, such as the History channel, the National Geographic channel, and the news on PBS. From time to time he walks outdoors and has a ramp from his house down to the street level, so he can ambulate with his Rolator. He has significant nocturia and spends much of his time during the day napping because of sleep deprivation overnight.

   He still needs significant assistance from his wife with his ADLs, but she challenges him as much as possible. She specifically asked him what he did last evening, what they watched on television. He was able to remember that they watched a Dallas Cowboys game. He knew the Cowboys won but was unable to tell me what team they played.

2. Ischemic cardiomyopathy, for which he is followed in Cardiology: He was recently seen in Cardiology to discuss nocturia. Evaluation by the cardiologist includes that she doubts congestive heart failure is an etiology in his significant nocturia. She notes no definitive evidence of significant volume overload by exam. She feels his ischemic cardiomyopathy is adequately compensated.

3. Benign prostatic hypertrophy: He is followed regularly in Urology. They have discontinued Uroxatral and substituted Ditropan. He has been taking Ditropan for only 4 nights, and there has been no significant improvement at this short interval.

MEDICATIONS:
1. Aspirin 81 mg daily.
2. Proscar 5 mg daily.
3. Plavix 75 mg daily.
4. Zocor 20 mg at h.s.
5. Omeprazole 20 mg daily.
6. Oxybutynin 5 mg at h.s.
7. Toprol XL 25 mg daily.
8. Donepezil 5 mg daily to start today.

PHYSICAL EXAMINATION finds a pleasant, 89-year-old Caucasian gentleman with blood pressure of 146/70, pulse 70, respirations 16, temperature 95.9, height 5 feet 3 inches, and weight 68 kg. Pain is zero. He is not a smoker. Specifically, his neurologic exam shows a slow but intact finger-nose-finger examination. His muscular strength is 5/5 throughout. He has no tremor, and when he walks with his Rolator he has a good step height, cadence, and shows no shuffling gait. Mini Mental status test is less than 10. He is unable to tell me any component of the date. Knows this is Florida but cannot tell me what city or county, and he does not know the name of the building. Further cognitive testing was not continued.

(Continued)

ID#: M-59   PAGE 2

LABORATORY AND X-RAY DATA: None since our last visit.

ASSESSMENT

1. Alzheimer disease: Moderate to advanced, given his current cognitive status. Lack of objective evidence to show vascular dementia, paucity of vascular risk factors, and no clinical signs of Parkinson disease: Otherwise, he is doing fairly well in his current living situation, and it is certainly appropriate for him to be living at home. He is well taken care of and receives good nutrition and support in his ADLs from his wife.
2. Ischemic cardiomyopathy: Doing well with no signs of angina or congestive heart failure. I agree with no objective evidence for fluid overload and appreciate co-management by Cardiology.
3. Nocturia: Overactive bladder versus benign prostatic hypertrophy.
4. Health care maintenance: Up to date.

PLAN

1. Aricept 5 mg p.o. daily for up to 2 months. Discussed potential side effects and expectations.
2. Have started Ditropan. Will continue the current plan.
3. Recommended he get into a regular exercise program with at least ambulating from the house to the corner and back twice daily. Should the family desire, would support a brief course of outpatient physical therapy.
4. Followup plan: Follow up with me in one month. I contacted our schedulers to request assistance with the wait list.

_____

Michael Panagides, MD, Internal Medicine

MP:pai
D:8/10/----
T:8/11/----

c: Martha C. Eaton, MD, Family Practice

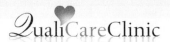

Plastic Surgery Clinic Followup Note

Patient Name: Tashinda Jones   **PCP:** Jean W. Mooney, PA

Date of Exam: 30 Aug ----   **Age/Sex:** 48-year-old female   **ID#:** M-60

HISTORY: The patient is a 48-year-old black female who is now 2 weeks status post bilateral mastectomies for lobular carcinoma in situ. She underwent an immediate tissue expander reconstruction bilaterally, and 100 mL of saline was infiltrated bilaterally at the time of surgery. Patient reports she had very minimal pain. She no longer requires even Tylenol. She is walking 4 miles a day and has found minimal limitation to her range of motion, bilateral upper extremities.

PHYSICAL EXAMINATION

Limited to surgical site: Mastectomy incisions are clean and dry without evidence of infection. There is minimal ecchymosis around the left incision. The incisions are well approximated. She is nontender to palpation.

ASSESSMENT/PLAN

The patient underwent an additional 100 mL expansion to bilateral tissue expanders without difficulty. She had good capillary refill and no pain at the conclusion of the procedure.

She does have slight increased fullness in the left upper outer quadrant adjacent to the axilla, and this will require minor pocket modification on the left at the time of exchange of the implant for the expanders. This is scheduled for 18 Dec ----.

Patient will undergo her next expansion approximately 3 weeks from now with anywhere from 60 mL to 100 mL, depending upon how much she tolerates and the size. She desires a full B cup. Currently the patient appears to be a small B cup. I estimate that she will need a total of 300 mL to 350 mL of volume in her expanders to reach a full B cup, as the patient has a very small-based diameter.

_____

Danila R. Fry, MD
Plastic Surgery

DRF:pai
D:9/1/----
T:9/2/----

c: Jean W. Mooney, MD, Internal Medicine

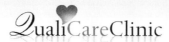

Nephrology Clinic Followup Note

Patient Name: Eduardo Martinez
Date of Exam: 20 Feb ----   **Age/Sex:** 66-year-old male

PCP: Martha C. Eaton, MD
ID#: M-61

CHIEF COMPLAINT: Patient is seen in Nephrology Clinic in followup for multiple renal issues.

HISTORY: Eduardo was last seen by me on 14 Dec last year. He has a history of acute interstitial nephritis, biopsy proven, secondary to antibiotics that were required for osteomyelitis of the great toe in Nov. of last year. He had been treated with vancomycin and ertapenem, then developed the interstitial nephritis with baseline creatinine of 1.2, peaking at 3.5. As the patient had infections, steroids were contraindicated. All we could do was withdraw the 2 antibiotics as the potential offending agents. Antibiotics were changed to Cipro and linezolid, which the patient tolerated very well. He required a few injections of Aranesp for anemia. Since I saw him last Dec, he has completed his course of antibiotics; however, he did have an admission on 15 Feb ---- with infection in another toe. That toe was débrided, the course of antibiotics extended, and he was seen by Infectious Disease this week. They were pleased with his progress. He has stopped antibiotics, and the PICC line has been taken out.

REVIEW OF SYSTEMS: Patient states he generally feels well. He does have some easy fatigability with walking and mild dyspnea on exertion. Denies shortness of breath at rest, denies orthopnea. Has occasional edema but not every day. He does complain of chronic constipation secondary to narcotics. Denies thirstiness, lightheadedness. He has a good appetite.

PAST MEDICAL HISTORY REVIEWED: Type 2 diabetes mellitus with nephropathy and gastropathy. Acute interstitial nephritis. Hypertension. Hyperlipidemia. Obstructive sleep apnea. Seminoma with right orchiectomy. Arthritis. Gastroesophageal reflux disease. Cerebral aneurysm in 2001. Charcot-Marie-Tooth, which is the indication for his chronic pain regimen.

ALLERGIES: IODINE, VANCOMYCIN, ERTAPENEM, and IV CONTRAST DYE.

MEDICATIONS
1. Glynase 3 mg p.o. b.i.d.
2. Reglan 5 mg p.o. q.i.d.
3. Zocor 40 mg p.o. q.h.s.
4. Phenergan 25 mg p.o. q.i.d.
5. Effexor 112.5 mg p.o. daily.
6. Neurontin 600 mg p.o. t.i.d.
7. Fentanyl 75 patch, changed every 2 days.
8. Percocet p.r.n.
9. Prevacid 30 mg p.o. b.i.d.
10. Testosterone gel.

PHYSICAL EXAMINATION

Vitals show blood pressure at 113/76, repeat blood pressure 93/69, pulse 105, repeat pulse 109, respirations 18, temperature 97.1. In general, this is a thin Hispanic male who is nontoxic and in no apparent distress. Alert and oriented x4, cooperative, with a bright affect. He has a slow gait and uses a cane to walk secondary to his recent osteomyelitis in the distal extremity. No respiratory distress. No lower extremity edema, cyanosis, or clubbing. Skin is without rash or other lesion.

LABORATORY DATA: On 16 Feb ---- BUN was 22, creatinine was 1.5, sodium 132, potassium 4.2, phosphorus 3. Hemoglobin was 10.9, which is mildly improved from Hgb 10.3 in Dec. of last year. MCV is 91.6. ESR is 17, CRP 0.5, and Hgb A$_{1C}$ 6.8.

(Continued)

ID#: M-61   PAGE 2

ASSESSMENT/PLAN

1. Acute interstitial nephritis. Surveillance urinalysis was done by another physician on 15 Feb, and that showed no pyuria or hematuria remaining. Also of note, the dipstick was negative for protein. His acute interstitial nephritis has resolved. Recommend that he continue to avoid vancomycin and carbapenems in the future, as we do not know which drug was the culprit.
2. Diabetic nephropathy, biopsy proven. The patient's blood pressures are currently inadequate to start a trial of ACE inhibitors. Will do a spot urine protein-to-creatinine ratio with his next labs. Continue present management with the goal of Hgb A_{1C} of less than 6 to 7 and avoid nephrotoxins.
3. Relative hypotension. Likely exacerbated by his chronic use of narcotics for the Charcot-Marie-Tooth pain. Requested that patient increase his intake of fluids and slightly increase his intake of salt.
4. Anemia. As his kidney function is improving, I would anticipate that his need for erythropoietin would also improve. He is not getting erythropoietin currently, as his hemoglobin came up over goal in December to 13.1 g/dL. I will repeat his H&H with his next labs, follow the trend, and will also order iron studies, B12, and folate to look for other potential etiologies.
5. Type 2 diabetes mellitus, under good control. Continue present management, as that is the only measure we can use at this time to afford him good decrease in his progression of diabetic nephropathy. Patient cannot tolerate ACE inhibitors or ARBs with this level of hypotension.

NOTE: All instructions were given to this patient in writing, and he expressed understanding. We will make him a followup appointment to see me in May.

Patient is to report to the laboratory on 21 Mar ---- at least 1-1/2 hours prior to his appointment with Dr. Eaton. I have ordered a renal function panel, spot urine protein, spot urine creatinine, CBC, iron studies, B12, folate, screening intact PTH, and 25-hydroxy vitamin D. Also, as the patient has a distant history of hyperlipidemia and his past lipid panel was done last August, I have ordered a surveillance lipid panel and LFTs.

The patient will return to the laboratory again one week prior to his appointment with me in May, and I have ordered a renal function panel and an H&H for that time.

_____

Michael Panagides, MD, Nephrology

MP:pai
D:2/20/----
T:2/21/----

c: Martha C. Eaton, MD, Family Practice

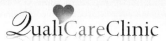

Vascular Clinic Followup Note

Patient Name: Benjamin Dunham **PCP:** Marie Aaron, DO

Date of Exam: 29 Mar --- **Age/Sex:** 58-year-old male **ID#:** M-62

HISTORY: Mr. Dunham is a 58-year-old black man with a history of carotid artery stenosis, status post bilateral CEA in 2001 on the left and in 2003 on the right, both of which were widely patent as of 8 Dec ---- when he had his last duplex. Patient also has a history of peripheral vascular disease. Latest imaging done 8 Dec ---- showed a hemodynamically significant superficial femoral artery and bilateral tibial calcification and claudicant. The patient has been working on an exercise regime. He has no medications for his peripheral vascular disease and states that his tolerance to exercise is increasing. He walks 1 mile a day, 4 to 5 days a week, walking further and faster before the claudication sets in than previously. He now can walk 400 to 500 yards briskly before the claudication sets in, and he then can walk 1+ mile using a normal gait.

PAST MEDICAL HISTORY is significant for increased cholesterol and hypertension.

PAST SURGICAL HISTORY: Has had a hernia repair, Lasik surgery, and a vasectomy.

MEDICATIONS include Zocor.

SOCIAL HISTORY: Does not smoke, has not smoked for 8 years, but he had a 30-year-pack history before he quit. He drinks 2 to 6 beers per day.

PHYSICAL EXAMINATION

VITALS show blood pressure to be 78/43 on the left, 95/48 on the right, pulse 84, respirations 17. He is awake, alert, and oriented. LUNGS are clear to auscultation bilaterally. CARDIOVASCULAR EXAM: S1, S2. Good peripheral pulses. Palpable pulses in the lower extremities. He has good capillary refill. NEUROLOGIC: No focal deficits. Mood is bright.

ASSESSMENT

1. A 58-year-old black male with carotid artery disease, status post bilateral carotid endarterectomies.
2. Peripheral vascular disease, which is improving with exercise.

PLAN

We encouraged Mr. Dunham to continue his exercise and diet regime. We will see him again in approximately 1 month.

_____

Ly An Tabor, MD
Vascular Surgery

LAT:pai
D:3/29/----
T:3/30/----

c: Marie Aaron, DO, Family Practice

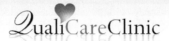

<u>**Neurology/Orthopedics Discharge Summary**</u>

Patient Name: Jennifer Santinos   **PCP:** Ann Basswood, MD

Date of Admission: 29 January ----   **Date of Discharge:** 2 February ---   **Age/Sex:** 30-year-old female   **ID#:** M-63

ADMISSION DIAGNOSIS
Cerebral palsy with progressive neuromuscular scoliosis.

DISCHARGE DIAGNOSIS
Cerebral palsy with progressive neuromuscular scoliosis.

ADMISSION SERVICE: Orthopedics.

PROCEDURES PERFORMED: Posterior spinal instrumented fusion from T2 to pelvis.

HISTORY OF PRESENT ILLNESS: Please see my dictated preoperative history and physical examination.

HOSPITAL COURSE: Patient was admitted to the hospital on 29 January ----. She went to the operating room where she underwent a posterior spinal instrumented fusion without event. She was transferred to the pediatric ICU after surgery for both recovery and continued care. She arrived to the PICU from surgery still intubated. On postop day 1, she was noted to have a mild postoperative anemia, and she received 1 unit of PRBCs, which improved her hematocrit, and she remained with a stable hematocrit after that 1 unit. She also received 6 units of FFP due to a mild postop coagulopathy, and after that another 6-pack, and her coagulopathy improved to the point she had a normal INR on day of discharge. She remained intubated until postop day 3 and was extubated without event in the PICU. The remainder of her hospital course was unremarkable. She transitioned to G-tube feeds without difficulties. Her pain was well managed by day of discharge, per Dr. Fields, with her G-tube pain medicines, and by day of discharge she was doing well and sitting up. Again, her pain was well controlled. She was moving all her extremities very well.

She was discharged to home in good condition on 2 Feb ----, and her operative wound site was checked on the day of discharge. The dressing was changed, and her wound looked very good.

DISCHARGE INSTRUCTIONS: She is to be discharged to home. The mother was instructed on dressing changes. She may do a dry dressing change once a day after she gets a bath. She is allowed to take one bath as long as she is not allowed to soak for long periods of time. There are no restrictions on her activities. Parents will need to contact their wheelchair company to make adjustments to her wheelchair now that her spine is straight. She is instructed to follow up either in the ER or in the ortho clinic if she develops a fever, spreading redness, worsening pain, or any worsening discharge from her surgical wound site. Otherwise, followup will be with either Dr. Fields or his PA on 9 Feb in the ortho clinic.

Discharge meds include Percocet 1 tab p.o. q.4-6 h. p.r.n. via the G tube. Valium 2 mg per G tube q.6 h. p.r.n. painful muscle spasms. Will plan on having the patient seen by Home Health Nursing for assistance on dressing changes.

_____

Gilbert M. Fields, MD
Orthopedic Surgery

GMF:pai
D:2/3/----
T:2/4/----

c: Ann Basswood, MD, Neurology

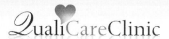

Radiation Oncology Clinic

History and Physical Examination

Patient Name: Rubin Glover **PCP:** Glenn Ruffolo, MD

Date of Exam: 14 June ---- **Age/Sex:** 57-year-old male **ID#:** M-64

DIAGNOSIS: 57-year-old white male with newly diagnosed pathologic stage T1, clinical stage N0, squamous cell carcinoma of the left temple. Patient is referred by Dr. Ruffolo for consideration of radiation therapy.

HISTORY OF PRESENT ILLNESS: Col. Glover is a recently retired psychiatrist who developed a scaling lesion in his left temple approximately 2 to 3 years ago. In February ---- he noted that it began to grow rapidly, and he sought medical attention. He was evaluated by a dermatologist and underwent a biopsy on 26 March ----, which revealed squamous cell carcinoma, moderate to well differentiated. Architecturally it had some features of keratoacanthoma. Subsequently the patient underwent a wide local excision without Mohs support on 17 April ----. This revealed a squamous cell carcinoma that was completely excised. Excised skin measured 6.2 x 1.6 x 0.6 cm. Within this was a 0.9 cm ulcerated nodule. The cancer extended to just less than 1 cm from the deep inked margin. The pathology report does not indicate the presence of or absence of perineural invasion; however, upon my conversation with Dr. Ruffolo, he indicated that the tumor was abutting several nerves. There was no clear evidence of true perineural invasion.

Prior to his surgery, the patient denied any sensation of paresthesias or formication. He also denied any local symptoms in the head and neck area.

PAST MEDICAL HISTORY: Depressive disorder, prehypertension, benign prostatic hypertrophy.

PAST SURGICAL HISTORY: Septoplasty at age 23, inguinal hernia repair x2 ten years ago.

PAST RADIATION HISTORY: None.

FAMILY HISTORY: Patient's father was a smoker and died of lung cancer at the age of 62. His sister has a history of skin cancer.

SOCIAL HISTORY: The patient was the flight commander at the local Air Force Base and retired from the Air Force last week. In July he plans to relocate to New Hampshire. He has 3 adult children. He neither smokes nor drinks.

MEDICATIONS: Prozac, Wellbutrin, Desyrel, Zestril, Uroxatral, baby aspirin.

REVIEW OF SYSTEMS: A 10-point review of systems is documented in the patient's radiation oncology chart with my signature and stamp. There are no pertinent positives.

PHYSICAL EXAMINATION

In general, this is a pleasant, well-appearing Caucasian male in no acute distress.

HEENT: Tympanic membrane clear on the right, obscured by cerumen on the left. Anicteric sclerae. Pupils are equal, round, and reactive to light and accommodation. Extraocular movements are intact. Oral cavity clear. Lymph nodes: No preauricular, postauricular, submandibular, cervical, or supraclavicular adenopathy. Chest: Clear to auscultation bilaterally. Heart: Regular rate and rhythm with no murmurs. Abdomen: Soft, nontender, no hepatosplenomegaly or masses. Extremities: No pedal edema. Skin: There is a very well healed, faintly visible scar in the left temple extending to the hairline. In the center of this scar is a very tiny area of induration, which I presume is postoperative in nature. There is no evidence for local recurrence at this time. There is a small amount of telangiectasias, and hypopigmentation is noted along the scar. No other skin lesions are noted in the head and neck area. Total body scan exam was not performed.

(Continued)

ID#: M-64   PAGE 2

LABORATORY DATA: Normal electrolytes on 29 March ----. Creatinine 1.1, PSA 1.74, and glucose 93.

IMPRESSION/PLAN

Col. Glover is a healthy 57-year-old male with a recently diagnosed pathologic stage T1, clinical stage N0, squamous cell carcinoma of the left temple, well to moderately differentiated. There was no clear-cut evidence of perineural invasion, skeletal muscle invasion, cartilage invasion, or bone invasion. His deep margin was negative but close at less than 1 mm. Given these findings, I estimate that the patient's risk of local recurrence is on the order of 10% to 20%. This risk, in my mind, is sufficiently low to justify omission of postoperative radiotherapy.

Traditional indications for postoperative radiotherapy include skeletal muscle invasion, cartilage invasion, bone invasion, perineural invasion, and/or positive margins. In these instances, radiotherapy is thought to lower the relative risk of local recurrence by approximately 75%. In Col. Glover's case, however, although radiotherapy may confer some additional marginal benefit, I am not certain that the benefit of radiotherapy would justify the risks. Acute risks include fatigue and dermatitis. There are the late risks of skin atrophy, telangiectasias, and a very low risk of damage to the ocular apparatus or the underlying meninges, which could result in a second malignancy. The patient seems very comfortable to be observed at this juncture. He will locate a dermatologist in his new home, and he will obtain regular followup. I will, however, review the patient's pathology slides and contact him via telephone with my final recommendation.

_____

L. (Lonnie) Willem Erwin, MD
Radiation Oncology

LWE:pai
D:6/15/----
T:6/16/----

c: Glenn Ruffolo, MD, Hematology/Oncology

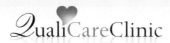

Radiation Oncology Clinic Note

Patient Name: Hilda Schmidt   **PCP:** Eric J. Lopez, MD

Date of Exam: 16 Nov ----   **Age/Sex:** 52-year-old female   **ID#:** M-65

DIAGNOSIS: Squamous cell carcinoma of the nasopharynx with sarcomatoid features, stage IVA, (T4N0M0).

RADIATION THERAPY: Ms. Schmidt initially was irradiated to 44 cGy in 2.0 cGy fractions at Hillcrest Medical Center, completing in February ----. After several months she was then irradiated to the nasopharynx with IMRT technique here with concurrent weekly carboplatin. Dose to the tumor delivered at Quali-Care Clinic was 38 cGy delivered in 2 cGy fractions over 43 lapsed treatment days, completing 10 Aug ----. This resulted in a total estimated dose to the tumor bed of 82 cGy.

INTERVAL HISTORY: She has completed her chemotherapy, during which time she developed discomfort and dysphagia. Patient is unable to swallow because of apparent pharyngeal stenosis from her previous radiation therapy. She also has mild trismus and is unable to completely open her mouth. Sense of taste is preserved, but she has almost complete xerostomia. She uses a feeding tube for all her nutrition. Nasal discharge persists. MRI of the neck 28 Sept ---- showed a right nasopharyngeal mass at skull base and intracranial extension. The mass had not changed compared to 18 July ---- and measured 2.9 cm in the longest dimension at the right nasopharynx. There were no new areas of abnormal enhancement or signal intensity. PET CT scan 5 Oct ---- showed decreased intensity and extent of FDG avidity in the right pharyngeal region medial to the right middle cranial fossa. Maximum standard uptake value (SUV) was 1.7. It favored a response to therapy of decreased but persistent disease.

PHYSICAL EXAMINATION

Patient is not acutely ill. Weight 123.5 pounds, blood pressure 118/69, heart rate 90, temperature 98.4.

HEENT: Conjunctivae pink, sclerae anicteric. Oral cavity shows mild trismus. There is moderate xerostomia with thickened mucus present. No visible tumor seen in the oral cavity or in the oropharynx. Endoscopy through the right nasion shows no tumor mass in the nasopharynx, oropharynx, base of tongue, vallecula, epiglottis, supraglottic larynx, glottic larynx. Vocal folds adduct normally with phonation. **NECK:** I feel no adenopathy in the neck. **LUNGS:** Clear to auscultation. **CARDIOVASCULAR:** Regular rate and rhythm with normal S1, S2. No murmurs heard. **ABDOMEN:** Benign. **EXTREMITIES:** No edema. **NEURO:** Cranial nerves intact except a right cranial VI palsy prevented complete abduction of the right eye on extreme lateral gaze. She is to be evaluated in ophthalmology clinic for this.

(Continued)

ID#: M-65 PAGE 2

IMPRESSION/PLAN

Ms. Schmidt is a 52-year-old woman with stage IVA (T4N0M0) squamous cell carcinoma of the nasopharynx. She completed chemotherapy and radiation. Unfortunately, her October PET scan suggested persistent disease. I am unable to visualize this, and she needs to be seen in the ENT Clinic so Dr. Pittfield can perform endoscopy.

She has a CT scan scheduled by medical oncology, and she will also been seen in the ophthalmology clinic for her cranial nerve palsy, which seems to be causing diplopia on extreme lateral gaze.

I will refer her to speech pathology for her dysphagia and pharyngeal stenosis. We will also try pilocarpine for her xerostomia.

She will follow up with me in two months. I will also discuss her case at the next ENT Tumor Board.

_____

L. (Lonnie) Willem Erwin, MD
Radiation Oncology

LWE:pai
D:11/16/----
T:11/17/----

c: Eric J. Lopez, MD, Oncology
   Leah Pittfield, MD, ENT Clinic

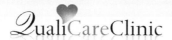

Emergency Department Treatment Record

Patient Name: John Doe

Date of Exam: 11 Nov ----

Age/Sex: Male, age unknown

PCP: Unknown

ID#: M-66

CONSULTING SERVICE: Neurosurgery.

MODE OF ARRIVAL: Code 3 EMS, unresponsive.

HISTORY OF PRESENT ILLNESS: Unknown Hispanic male, 30 to 40 years of age, who was found unresponsive in his bed this morning with urinary incontinence.

REVIEW OF SYSTEMS: Unable to be obtained.

PAST MEDICAL HISTORY: Unknown.

PAST SURGICAL HISTORY: Unknown.

MEDICATIONS: Unknown.

ALLERGIES: Unknown.

IMMUNIZATIONS: Unknown.

SOCIAL HISTORY: Unknown.

FAMILY HISTORY: Unknown.

PHYSICAL EXAMINATION

VITAL SIGNS on presentation: Patient has a Glasgow coma score of 3, is breathing and afebrile, but he is otherwise completely unresponsive. HEENT: Normocephalic, atraumatic. Patient has a dilated, fixed left pupil that is deviated to the left. Funduscopic exam reveals a somewhat blurred disk margin with obvious elevated ectopy. Nares and oropharynx are clear. Neck is supple. Heart is regular without murmur, gallop, or rub. Lungs are clear to auscultation bilaterally. Abdomen is soft and nondistended. Extremities are warm and well perfused. The patient does have multiple areas of ecchymoses noted on his heels and on his toes, concerning for track marks. Patient has no splinter hemorrhages and has no petechiae, but he is rather ecchymotic on his lower extremities. Patient also has some ecchymoses noted near his right nipple. NEUROLOGIC exam: Patient's GCS is 3. He is unresponsive to pain or other stimuli. He is not posturing and has fixed, deviated left eye and pupil.

EMERGENCY DEPARTMENT COURSE/MEDICAL DECISION MAKING: Patient was brought by EMS to the emergency department. Patient had neurologic exam as documented above. Because of a fixed, deviated pupil and a GCS of 3, patient was intubated using rapid sequence intubation. Patient was given 20 mg of etomidate and 100 mg of succinylcholine. Patient had no hypoxic event and no hypotensive event. ET tube placement was confirmed with end-tidal CO_2. The patient was then transferred to CT for head CT scan.

After patient was intubated, Neurosurgery was called. Dr. Youngblood was consulted, given the concerning process for an intraparenchymal hemorrhage and herniation in this patient. Patient was also given 50 g of mannitol. CBC and other blood work were sent, including coags. Patient was afebrile. The head CT revealed a large intraparenchymal bleed with extension into his lateral ventricle, 3rd and 4th ventricles, with midline shift and evidence of uncal herniation. Patient had effacement of his quadrigeminal cisterns. Neurosurgery was then re-paged and Dr. Youngblood notified of the situation. He was asked to come emergently to evaluate the patient for possible ventriculostomy or craniotomy.

(Continued)

CBC returned showing platelet count of 48,000 with an elevated white blood cell count. Toxicology screen revealed positive cocaine and amphetamines.

It is likely that this patient has suffered an intracranial hemorrhage, likely secondary to cocaine and amphetamine use. Patient did have evidence of track marks. I do not know what the significance of this thrombocytopenia was; however, because the patient had 1+ protein, creatinine of 1.5, and a platelet count today of 48,000, with ecchymoses, it is concerning that the patient has TTP. I do not believe he has ITP. Platelets were ordered; however, they were not drawn, given that he had a platelet count of 48,000. Possibly, if he does have TTP, a consumptive process would certainly worsen his dim prognosis.

Arnold R. Youngblood from Neurosurgery evaluated the patient. He felt the patient was not eligible for ventriculostomy as he had no brain stem reflexes except for breathing. The patient was transferred to the ICU under the care of the MICU team with Neurosurgery consultation. The patient certainly could have endocarditis, and his diagnosis certainly can be a reflection of that.

EMERGENCY DEPARTMENT DIAGNOSES

1. Intraparenchymal bleed.
2. Respiratory failure.
3. Thrombotic thrombocytopenic purpura.

DISPOSITION

Admit to ICU under the care of the MICU team. Prognosis is grim.

_____

Samuel Ernest, MD
Emergency Room Physician

SE:pai
D:11/11/----
T:11/11/----

c: Arnold R. Youngblood, MD, Neurosurgery

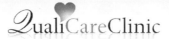

Vascular Surgery Clinic Consult

Patient Name: Fergus Roberts   **PCP:** Trevor Jordan, MD

Date of Exam: 2 Feb ----   **Age/Sex:** 62-year-old male   **ID#:** M-67

REASON FOR REFERRAL: Evaluation for arteriovenous fistula requiring hemodialysis in the near future.

HISTORY OF PRESENT ILLNESS: Mr. Roberts is a delightful 62-year-old black male who has chronic renal insufficiency, stage 5, and who will require hemodialysis in the near future. He is referred from Nephrology for fistula fixation by me. He underwent recent venous duplex to evaluate both upper extremities for fistula placement, and he has a pacemaker on the left side. The patient is followed by the cardiologists, who feel he is fairly stable from a cardiac standpoint.

PAST MEDICAL HISTORY includes coronary artery disease as well as his history of the pacemaker.

PAST SURGICAL HISTORY includes the coronary artery bypass grafting.

PHYSICAL EXAMINATION

PE today reveals a well-developed, well-nourished African American male in no acute distress. VITAL SIGNS show temperature of 93.7, pulse 72, respirations 18, and blood pressure 130/64, equal in both arms. IN GENERAL, he is well developed and well nourished. SKIN: Significant discoloration of his dark skin, most likely long-standing fungal infection changes. LUNGS are clear. HEART is regular. He has a well-healed coronary artery bypass grafting incision as well as a pacemaker in the left subclavian vein area.

X-RAY DATA: Duplex examination today reveals bilateral venous studies with good left cephalic vein at the upper arm, although on physical exam I believe his left cephalic vein distally in the arm would also be usable— although it measured only 2.4 mm by duplex examination. His left arm also has adequate upper extremity basilic vein. His right arm has inadequate cephalic vein both by duplex and by physical examination. His right arm, however, has excellent lower extremity basilic vein and good upper extremity basilic vein.

ASSESSMENT AND PLAN

Mr. Roberts is a delightful gentleman with renal failure and impending dialysis in the near future. We sat and discussed options of dialysis to include peritoneal as well as hemodialysis. It sounds like his nephrology physicians have decided on hemodialysis, and I think that is reasonable. I would like to do a fistula on his right lower extremity basilic vein, a transposition type, which I think we can do under local sedation or a block. He fully understands the risks, benefits, and alternatives of the procedure, the failure of fistula rates, the failure to mature, as well as the requirements for repeat interventions. He understands all this and desires to proceed.

We will do this in the middle of February, and patient will come back on 16 Feb for a preop appointment.

_____

Ly An Tabor, MD
Vascular Surgery

LAT:pai
D:2/3/----
T:2/4/----

c: Trevor Jordan, MD, Nephrology

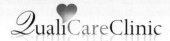

General Surgery Clinic Consult

Patient Name: Brian Arnst   **PCP:** Ken Miller, MD

Date of Exam: 5 Jan ----   **Age/Sex:** 33-year-old male   **ID#:** M-68

REFERRING PROVIDER: Ken Miller, MD, Gastroenterology.

REASON FOR REFERRAL: This 33-year-old white male has recurrent acid reflux after Nissen fundoplication 5 years ago. EGD done by me today confirmed absence of fundoplication with a large, fixed hiatal hernia from about 33 cm to 38 cm. He also had a single erosion at the GE junction despite b.i.d. Prevacid therapy. He requested redo fundoplication and hiatal hernia repair.

HISTORY OF PRESENT ILLNESS: This is a 33-year-old white male with long history of severe acid reflux, for which he underwent a laparoscopic Nissen fundoplication 5 years ago. The patient states he had symptoms recur approximately 1 year later that have been progressively worsening over the last 2 years. He was restarted on AcipHex originally and recently was changed to Prevacid for medical control of his symptoms; however, the patient is still having daily symptoms, worse with spicy or acidic foods and caffeine. The patient states he does not want to be on medications for the rest of his life to control this and desires surgical intervention.

PAST MEDICAL HISTORY: Significant only for gastroesophageal reflux disease.

PAST SURGICAL HISTORY: Significant only for the laparoscopic Nissen fundoplication 5 years ago.

CURRENT MEDICATIONS: Prevacid.

ALLERGIES: NKDA.

SOCIAL HISTORY: He denies tobacco use; admits to only occasional ethanol use. Is single with no children. No unprotected sex.

REVIEW OF SYSTEMS: Negative.

PHYSICAL EXAMINATION

VITAL SIGNS: Temperature 97.1, blood pressure 127/88, pulse 63, respiratory rate 18. GENERAL: He is alert and oriented x3, in no acute distress. LUNGS: Clear to auscultation bilaterally. HEART: He has a regular rate and rhythm with no murmurs, rubs, or gallops. ABDOMEN: His abdomen is soft, nontender, and nondistended. NEURO: No neurologic deficits.

ASSESSMENT

This is a 33-year-old male with severe gastroesophageal reflux disease, symptomatic on Prevacid therapy, status post a failed laparoscopic Nissen fundoplication.

(Continued)

ID#: M-68   PAGE 2

PLAN
Patient is scheduled for an open Nissen fundoplication on 3 Feb ----. His preop was done today in the clinic. He will be scheduled for a preop appointment with Dr. Carl Avalon of anesthesia. Risks, benefits, and alternatives of the procedure were discussed with the patient. All his questions were answered. He expressed understanding and consented to proceed with the operation as planned.

_____
James A. McClure Jr, MD
General Surgery

JAM:pai
D:1/5/----
T:1/7/----

c: Ken Miller, MD, Gastroenterology
    Carl Erickson Avalon, MD, Anesthesiology

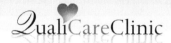

QualiCareClinic

Emergency Department Treatment Record

Patient Name: James E. Stevenson   **PCP:** Unknown

Date of Exam: 3 May ----   **Age/Sex:** Male, age unknown   **ID#:** M-69

MODE OF ARRIVAL: EMS, Code 3 Trauma.

CHIEF COMPLAINT: Status post MVA versus pedestrian.

CONSULTATION: Trauma Surgery Team.

PREHOSPITAL COURSE: Patient was in asystole as per EMS en route. He was placed in a collar and on a back board. He was bleeding from the mouth. On arrival patient was placed in trauma bay 3 in pulseless electrical activity (PEA). No pulses, breathing assisted by bag-valve-mask, in full spinal precautions. Massive amount of blood was coming from oropharynx. Airway was initially assessed by Dr. Ernest, who stated that it was not in the trachea. Until an airway was placed, endotracheal tube 70 at 24 at the teeth was placed. He visualized it going through the trachea. There was no end-tidal CO_2 color change, most likely due to the patient's being in asystole and PEA.

PRIMARY ASSESSMENT

A. Airway: as above.
B. Breathing: lungs clear. Auscultation equal bilaterally following intubation. Midepigastric area with no ventilatory sounds.
C. Circulation: pulses were faint and palpable only with CPR.
D. Disability: patient with Glasgow coma score of 3. Intubated, unconscious.
E. Exposure: patient was fully exposed.

PRIMARY INTERVENTIONS: Patient received epinephrine 1 mg initially. He remained in PEA at multiple stops of chest compressions to reevaluate. With each chest compression there was obvious gross blood from the oropharynx and bilateral nares. Source of bleeding in the oropharynx was not determined; however, suction had to be utilized both during intubation and afterward. Patient received a peripheral IV, and initially 1 liter normal saline was given as a bolus. While several attempts at another IV access were made, finally we were successful in the right femoral vein or artery. By that time, however, Code Blue had been called.

EMERGENCY DEPARTMENT COURSE: Prior to calling the code, an ACLS protocol was performed. A 36-French chest tube was placed in the left chest. No air, no blood. A right subclavian central line was obtained by Surgery. An orogastric tube was placed and connected to suction. At 1251 hours ACLS protocol continued. At 1253 hours infuser switched to right subclavian line. At 1256 hours ACLS protocol continued. At 1257 hours time of death called by Dr. Stolga per the Trauma Surgery Team, and postmortem care was begun at 1259 hours.

At 1331 hours the Chaplain asked the family members to view the patient. At 1341 hours the mother was in to see the patient.

Patient received a total of 3 liters RBCs while in our trauma bay. At 1243 hours patient received a total of 1 mg epinephrine. He received bicarb at 1248 hours, 1 amp. He received epinephrine at 1248 hours, 1 mg, and then epinephrine at 1256 hours, 1 mg. Those were the total medications given.

(Continued)

ID#: M-69   PAGE 2

TIME OF DEATH
Patient was pronounced dead at 1257 hours on May 3, ---- , by Mack Stolga, MD, of the Trauma Surgery Team.

_____
Samuel Ernest, MD
Emergency Room Physician

SE:pai
D:5/3/----
T:5/3/----

c: Mack Stolga, MD, Trauma Surgery Team

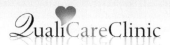

Orthopedic Discharge Summary

Patient Name: Hal Patterson   **PCP:** Ronald Reardon, DO

Date of Admission: 2 March ----   **Date of Discharge:** 6 March ---   **Age/Sex:** 60-year-old male   **ID#:** M-70

ADMITTING SERVICE: Carol Dodds, MD, Orthopedics

ADMITTING DIAGNOSES
1. Left distal radius malunion.
2. Left distal radial ulnar joint incongruity.

DISCHARGE DIAGNOSES
1. Left distal radius malunion.
2. Left distal radial ulnar joint incongruity.

HISTORY OF PRESENT ILLNESS: Patient is a 60-year-old, left-hand dominant white male who sustained a left distal radius fracture on 8 Nov last year that was treated with a closed reduction and a long arm cast, which went on to subsequent malunion. He presents predominantly with ulnar-sided wrist pain and difficulty with his activities of daily living. He desires distal radius osteotomy to improve his wrist range of motion and diminish his pain.

HOSPITAL COURSE: Mr. Patterson underwent left distal radius osteotomy with Acumed volar radius plate through a standard SCR approach with adjuvant iliac crest bone grafting, which was harvested from the left iliac crest. He also underwent a left ulnar Kapandji-Sauvé procedure without complication on 2 March ----. Patient was subsequently admitted for overnight observation and adequate pain control. He proceeded in the usual fashion, exhibiting a neurovascularly intact left upper extremity with some minor difficulties with his postoperative pain regimen. This was appropriately managed with the addition of adjunctive analgesia. On hospital day 2 the patient was noted to be in stable condition, neurovascularly intact, and ambulating about the ward with his pain well controlled. Thus, he was deemed stable for discharge with imminent followup in the outpatient orthopedic clinic on 15 March.

DISCHARGE MEDICATIONS: Patient is instructed to resume his home medications, to include his 25 mg fentanyl TTS patch. Patient will also be given a prescription for Percocet, which he is instructed to take 1 to 2 q.4 h. p.r.n., as well as OxyContin 20 mg p.o. b.i.d. p.r.n.

CONSULTATIONS: None.

OPERATIONS/PROCEDURES: Left distal radius osteotomy. Left distal ulnar Kapandji-Sauvé procedure with iliac crest bone grafting on 2 Mar ---- without complication.

DISCHARGE INSTRUCTIONS: Discharge diet is regular. Discharge activities: He is to keep his left upper extremity elevated. He was given a cheese block to help facilitate this. Again, he is to keep his left upper extremity elevated at all times. Keep his splint clean, dry, and intact. He will refrain from heavy physical activity. He is asked to call the orthopedic clinic during daytime hours with problems, to include increasing pain, elevated temperature, or discharge from his wound. Otherwise, he is to return to Quali-Care Clinic.

(Continued)

ID#: M-70   PAGE 2

Follow up on 15 March ---- in the orthopedic clinic with Dr. Dodds or her PA, and the patient is instructed to call for an appointment date and time.

_____

Gilbert M. Fields, MD
Orthopedic Surgery

GMF:pai
D:3/7/----
T:3/8/----

c: Ronald Reardon, DO, Family Practice
    Carol Dodds, MD, Orthopedics

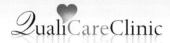

Orthopaedic Clinic Followup Note

Patient Name: Jena Sage DeLeon   **PCP:** Reed Phillips, MD

Date of Exam: 9 Mar ----   **Age/Sex:** 16-year-old female   **ID#:** M-71

HISTORY: Patient is a 16-year-old female, status post right foot lateral column lengthening through calcaneus and opening wedge allograft bone plus percutaneous tendo Achillis lengthening (TAL). Date of surgery 12 Jan ---- for indication of bilateral symptomatic pes planovalgus. Patient has been in a short leg cast. She is supposed to be nonweightbearing; however, she admits that she has been weightbearing as tolerated in her cast as well as even running in her cast without pain. She also has returned to clinic for a wet cast. She has no complaints currently.

PHYSICAL EXAMINATION

On exam the incision is well healed. Supple foot. No erythema or drainage. Neurovascularly intact distally. Nontender to palpation.

X-RAY DATA: There is lateral column lengthening and allograft/plug is intact—not healed yet, but there is no change in alignment.

ASSESSMENT

Status post right foot lateral column lengthening through calcaneus, opening wedge graft and percutaneous tendo Achillis lengthening. Patient is noncompliant.

PLAN

At this time, she will be placed back in a short leg walking cast and is to be nonweightbearing for another 4 weeks. Followup in 4 weeks with x-rays out of plaster.

We discussed with the patient and her parents that if she persists on being noncompliant, we will not perform the surgery on her left side, which is planned to be done in May, two months from now. Hopefully on followup we will be able to see healing and no change in alignment of the allograft site.

_____

Gilbert M. Fields, MD
Orthopedic Surgery

GMF:pai
D:3/09/----
T:3/10/----

c: Reed Phillips, MD, Pediatric Dept.

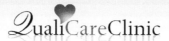

Radiation Oncology Clinic Followup Note

Patient Name: James L. Matthews   **PCP:** A. Leigh Wells, MD

Date of Exam: 14 June ----   **Age/Sex:** 67-year-old male   **ID#:** M-72

DIAGNOSES
1. Pathologic T1 versus T2N2b squamous cell carcinoma of the right lateral oral tongue treated with surgery and postoperative radiotherapy 20 years ago.
2. Squamous cell carcinoma of the posterior pharyngeal wall, pathologic stage T2N0, treated with total laryngopharyngectomy and left neck dissection with free flap reconstruction.

The patient received postoperative radiotherapy to the retropharyngeal lymph nodes to a total dose of 57.6 Gy delivered in 1.8 Gy/fraction, completed on 14 March this year due to the finding of suspicious retropharyngeal lymph nodes on the patient's preoperative MRI scan.

HISTORY: The patient returns today in routine followup. A PET CT obtained on 7 June revealed no suspicious FDG uptake. There was a sclerotic lesion in the right pubic ramus, which was thought to be atypical for metastatic disease. Patient's blood work on 9 May indicated a TSH of 7.59 and a free thyroxine of 0.8.

Currently the patient notes persistent ear drainage, which has been quite troublesome. He is using boric acid drops at this time, and he has bilateral myringotomy tubes in place. Otherwise, he notes mild difficulty swallowing either large pieces of food or very dry food. Nevertheless, he has gained 4 pounds over the past 2 months. He notes moderate xerostomia, which does respond to pilocarpine 5 mg in the morning. His taste is 79% recovered. He denies significant pain in the head and neck region.

PHYSICAL EXAMINATION

In general, this is a pleasant, well-appearing Caucasian male in no acute distress. HEENT: Bilateral ear tubes present with drainage noted. Anicteric sclerae. Pupils are equal, round, and reactive to light and accommodation. Extraocular movements intact. Visual inspection of the oral cavity and oropharynx reveals no suspicious mucosal lesions. The mucosa is somewhat dry. NECK: There is a fullness in the left neck compatible with a free flap placement. No palpable adenopathy. The tracheal stoma is intact with no suspicious changes.

IMPRESSION/PLAN
Mr. Matthews is radiographically and clinically without evidence of recurrent head and neck cancer 3 months after having completed a course of re-irradiation to the retropharyngeal lymph nodes for a second head and neck primary. He does have evidence of biochemical hypothyroidism, and he does report heat intolerance; therefore, I have started him on Synthroid 25 mcg daily.

He is to follow up with his primary care provider tomorrow, and I have asked patient to notify his PCP of this new diagnosis. Either his PCP or I can follow the patient with serial TSH checks to ensure that the patient is on the appropriate dose of Synthroid.

(Continued)

ID#: M-72   PAGE 2

Otherwise, the patient continues to do well. He is followed closely by the ENT clinic with regular fiberoptic endoscopy, then clinical exams. I will see the patient again in 2 months. In the interval, he will be seen by Dr. David Cohen of Hematology to follow his iron deficiency anemia.

_____

L. (Lonnie) Willem Erwin, MD
Radiation Oncology

LWE:pai
D:6/14/----
T:6/15/----

c: A. Leigh Wells, MD, Internal Medicine
    David H. Cohen, MD, Hematology
    Leah Pittfield, MD, ENT Clinic

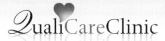

QualiCareClinic

<u>**Vascular Surgery Clinic Consultation**</u>

Patient Name: Mary Margaret Kalter   **PCP:** Jack Zullig, MD

Date of Exam: 24 March ----   **Age/Sex:** 69-year-old female   **ID#:** M-73

REASON FOR CONSULT: It was a pleasure to see Ms. Kalter today in the vascular surgery clinic. Ms. Kalter was referred to us for evaluation of her right lower extremity ulcer.

REFERRING PHYSICIAN: Jack Zullig, MD

HISTORY OF PRESENT ILLNESS: The patient is a 69-year-old woman with a past medical history significant for right lower extremity deep vein thromboses in both 2008 and 2009. The patient has remained on permanent anticoagulation since. The patient comes in now with postphlebitic syndrome complaining of chronic, nonhealing, right lower extremity venous insufficiency ulcer in the medial aspect of her right leg. The ulcer has been there for several months, and the patient has tried multiple forms of wound care with no significant relief. The patient employs leg elevation occasionally, and she uses suboptimal compression stockings. The patient has received no Unna boot therapy for this ulcer.

PAST HISTORY: As in HPI.

PHYSICAL EXAMINATION

This is a healthy-appearing woman in no acute distress. VITAL SIGNS reveal temperature 97.7, blood pressure 147/82, pulse 106, respirations 18. GENERAL: Alert and oriented. HEART: Regular rate and rhythm. LUNGS: Clear to auscultation. ABDOMEN: Soft, nontender, nondistended. PULSE EXAM reveals 2+ carotid and radial pulses, 1+ femoral pulses bilaterally. Patient has no pulses in her right foot but has monophasic signals in her dorsalis pedis artery and biphasic signals in her posterior tibialis artery. In her left foot, she has 1+ pulses in the posterior tibialis and dorsalis pedis arteries. Ankle-brachial index performed in clinic today was 1.4 in the patient's right posterior tibialis artery. Lower extremity exam shows patient has 1+ edema in the right lower extremity with brawny discoloration of the lower leg. She has an approximately 5 cm superficial ulceration just superior to the medial malleolus without significant erythema but with some fibrinous exudate.

X-RAY DATA: Today patient underwent lower extremity venous duplex scan, which revealed evidence of chronic thrombosis throughout her right lower extremity venous system from the superficial femoral down to the peroneal veins. The flow is decreased in the superficial femoral and profunda veins, and there is no evidence of reflux in the greater saphenous vein system. One Cockett perforator is superior to the medial malleolus that connects to the ulcer and to the greater saphenous vein close to it.

ASSESSMENT

A 69-year-old woman with postphlebitic syndrome, status post deep venous thrombosis x2 in the past. Patient comes in with right lower extremity nonhealing ulcer characteristic of venous insufficiency.

PLAN

1. Continued wound care, right lower extremity.
2. Application of an Unna boot in clinic today to allow for ulcer healing.

(Continued)

ID#: M-73   PAGE 2

3. Patient is to follow up in the vascular surgery clinic 4 days after application of the Unna boot for reevaluation.
4. The expectation is that the ulcer will heal with conservative management. If this ulcer remains nonhealing, however, some consideration should be given to addressing this Cockett perforator and/or performing a venogram.

_____

Ly An Tabor, MD
Vascular Surgeon

LAT:pai
D:3/24/---
T:3/25/----

c: Jack Zullig, MD, Orthopedic Surgery

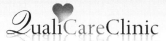

General Surgery Consultation

Patient Name: Rudy Briones

PCP: Ken Miller, MD

Date of Exam: 10 August ----   **Age/Sex:** 38-year-old male   **ID#:** M-74

REASON FOR CONSULT: Left inguinal hernia.

HISTORY OF PRESENT ILLNESS: Capt. Briones is a 38-year-old, single, active-duty Hispanic male who complains of an approximately 6-month history of left groin discomfort. He recalls nothing specific that brought it on, but he says that it is worse with sports activities, such as basketball, running, and lifting. He says he has noted no bulge, but on CT there was a finding that prompted his referral.

PAST MEDICAL HISTORY significant for some right upper quadrant discomfort that may be related to gastritis or GERD, followed by Gastroenterology.

PAST SURGICAL HISTORY: Lasik eye surgery last year.

MEDICATIONS: None.

ALLERGIES: NKDA.

SOCIAL HISTORY: Patient drinks 2 to 3 beers a month. Denies tobacco and illicit drugs. Denies unprotected sexual encounters.

PHYSICAL EXAMINATION

Temp 97.3, blood pressure 112/74, pulse 65, respirations 14. GENERAL: Patient is an alert and oriented Hispanic male who is in no apparent distress. He appears well developed and well nourished. ABDOMEN: Soft, nontender, nondistended. No surgical scars. GU/RECTAL: Patient has a normal, circumcised male phallus. He has bilaterally descended testes, which are without tenderness. No palpable cord tenderness. On the right side he has a small, palpable inguinal hernia that is asymptomatic. On the left side he has an inguinal hernia that elicits discomfort when palpated and during Valsalva. No blood in the vault, prostate WNL.

X-RAY DATA: CT abdomen and pelvis with contrast on 24 July ---- demonstrated a fat-containing left inguinal hernia that descends into the scrotum without signs of incarceration or strangulation.

ASSESSMENT/PLAN

This is a 38-year-old male with a symptomatic left inguinal hernia and a small asymptomatic right inguinal hernia. I discussed with him the options, including laparoscopic inguinal hernia repair of both as well as an open left inguinal hernia repair for the symptomatic side. He opts for observing the small asymptomatic right-sided hernia and open repair of the left inguinal hernia. Plan is to accomplish this on Tuesday, 18 Sept ----. The patient will return for a preoperative visit prior to that time, given that it is more than a month away.

(Continued)

I discussed with the patient the risks, benefits, and alternatives to surgery, including the risk of bleeding, infection, and recurrence—which is slightly higher with laparoscopic than with open surgery—and the reasonable postop activity restrictions. He understands and agrees to proceed with surgery. I consider him informed.

_____
James A. McClure Jr, MD
General Surgery

JAM:pai
D:8/10/----
T:8/11/----

c: Ken Miller, MD, Gastroenterology

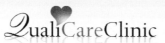

QualiCareClinic

Orthopedic Clinic Followup Note

Patient Name: Albert Erwin Bernard   **PCP:** Nancy Lawrence, MD

Date of Exam: 7 July ----   **Age/Sex:** 25-year-old male   **ID#:** M-75

HISTORY OF PRESENT ILLNESS: Master Sgt Bernard presents for evaluation with a longstanding history of an L2 compression fracture sustained while deployed in Iraq when he fell approximately 15 to 20 feet from a guard tower. The patient reports that an L2 compression fracture was seen and treated at that time with conservative measures. He continues to complain of significant pain on a regular basis that rates 4-10/10. He has difficulty performing his normal active duty requirements. As a training instructor, he has had difficulty with activities and with running. He has been pondering whether or not to pursue treatment from a surgical standpoint.

PHYSICAL EXAMINATION

Exam today is unchanged. He continues to have prominence on the right side with tenderness to palpation and deviation of the right spinous process of L2; however, he has a normal neurologic exam with 5/5 strength throughout and normal sensibility in the bilateral lower extremities.

RADIOGRAPHIC DATA: X-ray and CT scan and MRI done in March do reveal significant compression deformity of the L2 vertebral body with more prominent right-sided compression and advanced degenerative changes of L1-2 and L2-3. The patient is also noted to have degenerative changes of L3-4 and L4-5 and L5-S1 with grade 1 L3 retrolisthesis. At this point the patient has decided to pursue surgical intervention as a result of his persistent pain.

IMPRESSION

L2 compression fracture, multilevel lumbar spondylosis with continuing back pain.

PLAN

Plan at this time is to schedule the patient for consideration of surgical procedure, including L2 corpectomy with posterior instrumented fusion versus anterior plate fixation. The patient was counseled that it is possible that over time he will have persistent degeneration of the L3-L4 level with potential for increased instability, as he is already noted to have hypermobility at this time.

Patient is aware that we will decide the final surgical plan on my return from Iraq in the next four months, and he is to schedule an appointment for evaluation at that time.

_____

Gilbert M. Fields, MD
Orthopedic Surgery

GMF:pai
D:7/7/----
T:7/8/----

c: Nancy Lawrence, MD, Internal Medicine

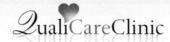

Initial Colorectal Surgery Consultation

Patient Name: Janet Ruth Evans   **PCP:** Don Richards, MD

Date of Exam: 5 Jan ----   **Age/Sex:** 50-year-old female   **ID#:** M-76

REASON FOR CONSULTATION: Rectal prolapse.

HISTORY OF PRESENT ILLNESS: Patient is a 50-year-old female who recently underwent colonoscopy for bright red blood per rectum. She describes a practically 2-week history of prolapsing anal mass prior to her colonoscopy. This had been diagnosed by another physician as prolapsing hemorrhoids; however, patient now describes a prolapse of greater length than would be expected with hemorrhoids. In total she has had an approximately 2-month prolapse. She denies diarrhea and constipation, but she does have to strain at stools. She has not used digital splinting in order to achieve bowel movements, but she does have a sensation of incomplete emptying after bowel movements.

PAST SURGICAL HISTORY: Total abdominal hysterectomy and bilateral salpingo-oophorectomy 10 years ago. Left-sided breast biopsy for a benign tumor last year.

PAST MEDICAL HISTORY: Hypertension.

MEDICATIONS: Atenolol, aspirin, vitamins.

ALLERGIES: PENICILLIN and IODINE, which cause a rash.

SOCIAL HISTORY: One pack per day of tobacco for 20 years. No alcohol use.

REVIEW OF SYSTEMS: During the winter months, patient occasionally develops a cough, which resolves spontaneously. She has no chest pain, arrhythmias, or shortness of breath. She does have wheezing at rest, according to her husband, but this has not been properly evaluated. Patient denies renal and/or hepatic disease. Denies diabetes. No symptoms of connective tissue disease.

PHYSICAL EXAMINATION

VITALS show temperature 97.9, blood pressure 120/77, pulse 89, respirations 16.

ABDOMEN is soft, flat, and nontender with a well-healed lower midline abdominal incision. no hernia is present, no palpable mass.

RECTAL EXAM shows an approximately 3 to 4 cm low rectocele. She has a small amount of anal gaping at rest but good squeeze pressure and good voluntary control of the anal sphincters. On severe straining she does have an approximately 3 to 4 cm full-thickness rectal prolapse.

ASSESSMENT

Rectocele and rectal prolapse. Patient most likely developed loss of vaginal support following her hysterectomy, then physically developed a large rectocele. I believe that over time the rectocele has caused a degree of straining, which has led to rectal prolapse. I encouraged the patient to begin a high-fiber diet, trying to achieve 30 g per day with supplements in addition. Also adequate hydration to try to achieve 1 to 2 soft bowel movements daily. I counseled patient to avoid straining at all times in order to decrease the severity of the rectal prolapse.

(Continued)

ID#: M-76   PAGE 2

PLAN
Patient will return to see me in 1 to 2 months for followup appointment regarding further evaluation of this rectal prolapse.

_____
James A. McClure Jr, MD
General Surgery

JAM:pai
D:1/6/----
T:1/7/----

c: Don Richards, MD
     Gastroenterology/Endoscopy

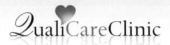

Internal Medicine Clinic Followup Note

Patient Name: Blanche Winters   **PCP:** Martha C. Eaton, MD

Date of Exam: 16 March ----   **Age/Sex:** 80-year-old female   **ID#:** M-77

REASON FOR VISIT: Evaluation of right shoulder, right hip, and right knee pain.

HISTORY OF PRESENT ILLNESS: Ms. Winters is a pleasant, 80-year-old, widowed black lady with a past medical history significant for hypertension, depression with anxiety, and osteoarthritis. Patient reports that she has been having significant pain in her right shoulder, right knee, and right hip. She states that she has had no recent trauma or falls to start this. She states that it is just her underlying osteoarthritis acting up. She has been taking occasional Aleve with relief of the pain. She has had no stomach discomfort with taking the Aleve. Has had no redness, warmth, or swelling over the joints. Has had no symptoms on the other joints on the left side.

Patient reports that she continues to have significant anxiety. We had started her on Celexa last year with some improvement. Somehow, this medication has been discontinued. She continues to have difficulty sleeping with awakening at 2 a.m. or 3 a.m. and having difficulty falling back to sleep. Her interest level has decreased. Her energy level has decreased. She is cheerful at times.

REVIEW OF SYSTEMS: Denies fevers, chills, night sweats. Weight has been stable. Has had no chest pain, no orthopnea, no paroxysmal nocturnal dyspnea. She has decreased her smoking. She smokes only about 2 cigarettes per day currently. Has had no nausea or vomiting. No abdominal pain. Her mood is as discussed above.

MEDICATIONS

1. Lisinopril 40 mg daily.
2. Atenolol 50 mg daily.
3. Adalat 30 mg daily.
4. Aspirin 81 mg daily.

PHYSICAL EXAMINATION

Blood pressure is 129/82, pulse 98, respirations 20, temperature 98.9, height 51 inches, weight 136 pounds. She reports 8/10 pain in her right hip. In general, she walks with a right-sided limp. HEENT: Unremarkable. NECK: Supple without bruits. CV: Regular rate and rhythm. Normal S1, S2. No S3 or S4. No murmurs. CHEST: Clear to auscultation bilaterally. EXTREMITIES: No clubbing, cyanosis, or edema. Right shoulder— patient has tenderness over the acromion. She has pain with abduction greater than 100 degrees. She has good external and internal rotation. She does have a slightly positive Apley scratch test. Right hip—patient is significantly tender over the greater trochanter. She does not let me fully internally or externally rotate her hip. Normal flexion and extension. Right knee—she has full flexion and extension. There is no ligamentous instability. No significant joint line tenderness.

X-RAY DATA: Right hip film showed osteoarthritic changes with superior joint space narrowing, subchondral sclerosis, and prominent marginal osteophytes. There is a bone spur at the greater trochanter. There is no notable fracture. Bilateral knee films show osteoarthritic changes, most significantly involving the medial compartment. The left knee is more significantly involved than the right.

(Continued)

ID#: M-77   PAGE 2

CLINICAL COURSE: Patient was significantly tender over the greater trochanter consistent with left trochanter bursitis. Patient was offered a therapeutic corticosteroid injection. After discussing the risks and benefits to include infection and bleeding, patient agreed to therapeutic corticosteroid injection.

PROCEDURE: Patient was examined and appropriate landmarks were obtained. Her skin was prepped and draped in the usual sterile fashion with ChloraPrep. An injection of 1 mL of 1% lidocaine, 1 mL of 0.5% Marcaine, and 1 mL of 80 mg/mL Depo-Medrol was injected into the right trochanteric bursa. Patient had good initial improvement in her pain. She had no complications.

ASSESSMENT

An 80-year-old black female with right hip pain secondary to trochanteric bursitis from underlying osteoarthritis. Patient also with pain in her right knee secondary to osteoarthritis that has been improved since a corticosteroid injection given earlier this year. Patient also with mild evidence of right shoulder impingement, likely secondary to underlying osteoarthritis.

PLAN

1. Significant osteoarthritis, limiting mobility: Will have the patient begin Naproxen 250 mg b.i.d. Patient was counseled to take the medication with food and to discontinue it with any indication of stomach upset, to include nausea or vomiting. She verbalized understanding. Will see patient back in a couple of weeks to see if her pain is improved and discuss further treatment options as appropriate at that time. Patient was offered a cane but deferred at this time.
2. Right trochanteric bursitis: Patient with good initial improvement in her pain. She was counseled to use ice on the area twice daily for the next 4 to 5 days. She is to avoid a lot of bending and twisting. She is to avoid sleeping on that side. Call or return to Clinic if she has any indication of infection, to include redness, warmth, or increased pain over the site of injection. She verbalized understanding.
3. Hypertension: Well controlled on current agents. Continue lisinopril and Adalat at current doses.
4. Depression with anxiety: Patient is to restart her Celexa. Start with 10 mg daily for 5 days and increase to 20 mg daily as tolerated.
5. Health care maintenance: Patient is due for a screening bone mineral density, which was ordered. She is up to date otherwise, other than screening labs that she is to have prior to her followup appointment in approximately 2 weeks. She verbalized understanding with the above plan.

_____

Michael Panagides, MD
Internal Medicine

MP:pai
D:3/16/----
T:3/17/----

c: Martha C. Eaton, MD, Geriatrics

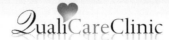

Orthopaedic Clinic Followup Note

Patient Name: Wayne M. Emerson   **PCP:** Sherman Loyd, MD

Date of Exam: 18 Jan ----   **Age/Sex:** 44-year-old male   **ID#:** M-78

HISTORY: Col. Emerson, a 44-year-old black male, is status post right ACL graft with Achilles tendon reconstruction on 25 Oct ---- by Dr. Fields and team. Patient is 12 weeks postop at this time and states that he is doing very well. He has decreasing pain and good range of motion. He feels like he is getting good strength back in his quadriceps. He states he still has some paresthesias on the anterior lateral aspect of his shin, but he had been told preoperatively that this was a possible occurrence. Patient is undergoing PT with resistance training, is full weightbearing, and feels like he has good range of motion.

PHYSICAL EXAMINATION

He is alert and oriented x3, in no acute distress. He is in no respiratory distress. Vision, speech, and hearing are all grossly intact. Exam is limited to the lower extremities. Right knee shows a well-healing incision site with no signs of infection, effusion, erythema, or skin abnormalities. No tenderness to palpation above his knee, with negative patellar grind. He has a stable knee on exam, with negative Lachman and good end point. Negative anterior and posterior drawer testing. Negative instability at 0 and 30 degrees of varus and valgus testing. Range of motion, right knee, is 0 to 145 degrees. The left knee range of motion is 0 to 160 degrees. Distal sensation is intact in saphenous, sural, tibial, deep peroneal, and superficial peroneal nerve distributions. He does have some decreased sensation over the anterior lateral aspect of his tibia. No significant quadriceps atrophy is noted, and he has 5/5 strength in all muscle groups of the right lower extremity.

IMPRESSION
Twelve weeks status post right anterior cruciate ligament allograft reconstruction. Doing well at this time.

PLAN
1. The patient will continue with his physical therapy and his other strengthening exercises as directed. He was given a profile as directed by Dr. Fields.
2. Patient will follow up at the 6-month point —sooner should there be any complications or concerns.
3. Dr. Loyd has been contacted and is in agreement with the assessment and plan for this patient.

_____

Gilbert M. Fields, MD
Orthopedic Surgery

GMF:pai
D:1/18/----
T:1/19/----

c: Sherman Loyd, MD, Internal Medicine

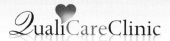

Hematology/Oncology Clinic Followup Note

Patient Name: Margaret Barger   **PCP:** Martha C. Eaton, MD

Date of Exam: 28 Feb ----   **Age/Sex:** 75-year-old female   **ID#:** M-79

REASON FOR VISIT: Anemia.

HISTORY OF PRESENT ILLNESS: Patient is a delightful 75-year-old white female, well known to our clinic, who is followed for anemia. She has been followed in the past for recurrent anemia and hemolytic anemia. She was last seen 6 months ago. She was recently admitted to the hospital on 18 Jan for cellulitis after a cat bite. It was quite extensive. Her hemoglobin during that hospitalization decreased to 8.4 g/dL on 27 Jan from her baseline, which is in the mid-10 g/dL range.

Of note, patient underwent a spinal fusion and laminectomy in December of last year, requiring 2 units of packed red blood cells postop.

Patient has recovered from her cat bite and cellulitis, and she has no complaints today.

PHYSICAL EXAMINATION

VITALS show blood pressure 148/50, pulse 68, temperature 98.6, height 68 inches, and weight 241 pounds. GENERAL: Elderly female in no acute distress. HEENT: Sclerae nonicteric. Conjunctivae pink. Oral mucosa clear. LUNGS: Clear to auscultation bilaterally. HEART: Regular rate and rhythm. ABDOMEN: Obese, soft, nontender, nondistended without splenomegaly. EXTREMITIES are without edema.

LABORATORY DATA: WBCs 4.7, Hgb 10 g/dL, platelets 227,000. Hemoglobin is increased from 8.4 grams on 27 Jan without transfusions. Peripheral smear shows 1+ macrocytes and polychromasia.

IMPRESSION/PLAN

A 75-year-old white female with a history of recurrent hemolytic anemia. Patient has had a decrease in her hemoglobin with acute cellulitis. This likely represented anemia of chronic disease. Her hemoglobin currently is back at baseline with polychromasia on the peripheral blood smear. This may represent regenerating marrow or ongoing mild hemolytic anemia. No intervention necessary at this time; however, I will start patient on folate 1 mg daily. Patient can follow up in the hematology/oncology clinic p.r.n.

_____

Solomon T. Fisher, MD
Hematology/Oncology

STF:pai
D:2/28/----
T:3/01/----

c: Martha C. Eaton, MD, Geriatrics

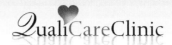

Internal Medicine Clinic Followup

Patient Name: James Sebastian Wright   **PCP:** Sherman Loyd, MD

Date of Exam: 16 March ----   **Age/Sex:** 77-year-old male   **ID#:** M-80

REASON FOR VISIT: Followup of sleep study and echocardiogram.

HISTORY OF PRESENT ILLNESS: Mr. Wright is a pleasant, 77-year-old white gentleman with a past medical history significant for chronic obstructive pulmonary disease and asthma, restrictive lung disease secondary to significant scoliosis, Barrett esophagus, hypertension, and a history of prostate cancer. Patient reports an approximately 6-month history of increased dyspnea on exertion. He also has been noticeably tachycardic in the high 90s to low 100s at each visit for 2 years. EKG done at our last visit showed only sinus tachycardia at 101 bpm. Given his underlying pulmonary disease, I have had concern for right heart strain from pulmonary hypertension. I referred patient to a cardiologist. He was deferred to the network. He had an echocardiogram done that showed a normal left ventricle with mild left ventricular systolic dysfunction with an ejection fraction of 40%. He had a followup nuclear perfusion study that showed an ejection fraction of 48% with no significant ischemia. There was no comment on an estimated pulmonary artery pressure. Patient was also started on lisinopril 10 mg daily for his blood pressure. He has done well with the addition of this medication.

Patient has had a sleep study done since our last visit by Dr. Gatlin of Pulmonology. The sleep study revealed sleep apnea with abnormal oxygen desaturation, snoring, hypertension, and cardiac arrhythmia with fragmented sleep. It was recommended that he start nasal CPAP at 15 cm of water. Patient states that he received the equipment last week but has not yet begun using it.

CURRENT MEDICATIONS
1. Aspirin 81 mg daily.
2. Maxzide 25 mg daily.
3. Lisinopril 10 mg daily.
4. Zocor 10 mg daily.
5. Singulair 10 mg daily.
6. Tylenol p.r.n.
7. Os-Cal Plus D b.i.d.
8. Prevacid 30 mg daily.
9. Patanol eye drops p.r.n.
10. Flonase daily.
11. Detrol LA 4 mg h.s.
12. Combivent 2 puffs t.i.d.
13. Flovent 220 mcg b.i.d.

PHYSICAL EXAMINATION

Blood pressure is 127/77, pulse 108, respirations 16, temperature 98.9, height 72 inches, and weight 139 kg. In general he is an obese gentleman with significant kyphoscoliosis. HEENT: Unremarkable. NECK: Supple without bruits. CARDIOVASCULAR: Regular rate and rhythm. Normal S1, S2. No S3 or S4. No murmurs. CHEST: Clear to auscultation bilaterally. EXTREMITIES: No cyanosis, clubbing, or edema. BACK: Patient has an area on his right lower back consistent with folliculitis.

(Continued)

ID#: M-80   PAGE 2

LABORATORY DATA: On 13 March white blood cells were 6.2, hemoglobin 14, hematocrit 40.7, and platelets 212,000. TSH 1.48, glucose 102, BUN 31, creatinine 1, sodium 139, potassium 4.4, magnesium 2.1.

ASSESSMENT

77-year-old white gentleman with past medical history as listed above with the new findings of obstructive sleep apnea and mildly depressed ejection fraction of unclear etiology as well as persistent sinus tachycardia.

PLAN

1. Sinus tachycardia: Patient has had a 6-minute walk in the Pulmonary Clinic and shows no evidence of hypoxemia with ambulation. He does have significant nighttime oxygen desaturation, and we are beginning CPAP to treat this. Again, given patient's body habitus and underlying lung disease, I am concerned that he is having right heart strain from pulmonary hypertension. I will try to contact the clinic where he had his echocardiogram done and see if they are able to estimate his pulmonary artery pressures before trying to refer him for another study. In the meantime, he also may be somewhat volume depleted, given his use of Maxzide and his increased BUN. Will have patient discontinue Maxzide and begin hydrochlorothiazide 12.5 mg daily. He is to have a followup chem panel in approximately 1 week.
2. Hypertension: Well controlled with use of lisinopril and Maxzide. Will continue lisinopril and change Maxzide to hydrochlorothiazide 12.5 mg as discussed above.
3. Mildly depressed ejection fraction: Patient with no evidence of ischemia on nuclear perfusion testing. He has also been asymptomatic other than the dyspnea on exertion, which may be related to tachycardia. His ejection fraction actually may be depressed secondary to his sinus tachycardia. Will continue to investigate the sinus tachycardia and pursue further ischemic evaluation as appropriate at a later date.
4. Obstructive sleep apnea: Patient is to begin using nasal CPAP on a regular basis. He is to call or notify me if he has difficulty tolerating this.
5. Barrett esophagus: Patient is to continue his Prevacid as listed above. He is up to date on his screening.
6. Health care maintenance is up to date.

DISPOSITION: Patient is to follow up with me in 4 to 6 weeks, sooner as needed.

Michael Panagides, MD, Internal Medicine

MP:pai
D:3/16/----
T:3/17/----

c: Joshua Stephen Gatlin, MD, Pulmonology
   Saul Thompson, MD, Cardiology
   Sherman Loyd, MD, Internal Medicine

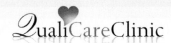

QualiCareClinic

Orthopedic Surgery Hand Team Preoperative History and Physical Examination

Patient Name: Jose Tijerina   **PCP:** Marie Aaron, DO

Date of Exam: 7 Feb ----   **Age/Sex:** 19-year-old male   **ID#:** M-81

DIAGNOSIS
Left index finger metacarpal nonunion.

HISTORY OF PRESENT ILLNESS: The patient is a pleasant 19-year-old right-hand dominant male who was in a motor vehicle accident in December last year. He was noted to have a left index finger metacarpal open fracture. He underwent I&D and open reduction, internal fixation on 1 December. The patient's index finger metacarpal was severely comminuted. He has shown no evidence of healing to date.

ALLERGIES: He is allergic to AMOXICILLIN, which causes hives.

PAST MEDICAL HISTORY: The patient has asthma.

PAST SURGICAL HISTORY: He has had wisdom teeth extracted.

PHYSICAL EXAMINATION

HEENT: The pupils are equal and reactive to light. NECK: There is no lymphadenopathy. LUNGS are clear to auscultation bilaterally. HEART: There is a regular rate and rhythm. ABDOMEN is soft, nontender, and nondistended. EXTREMITIES: The patient's left hand shows a left index finger with well-healed surgical incisions. There is decreased range of motion of the metacarpophalangeal joint of the index finger. There is brisk capillary refill. There is positive extrinsic tightness. His radial, ulnar, median, AIN, and PIN nerves are intact.

DIAGNOSTIC DATA: Films show minimal healing of a comminuted left index finger metacarpal fracture.

IMPRESSION AND PLAN
Left index finger metacarpal revision, open reduction, internal fixation with iliac cross-bone grafting to be done on 9 February ----. The patient is to have his preop labs drawn and consult with Anesthesiology tomorrow.

_____
Raquel Rodriguez, MD
Orthopedic Surgery

RR:pai
D:2/7/----
T:2/7/----

c: Marie Aaron, DO, Family Practice

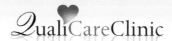

Hematology/Oncology Clinic Followup Note

Patient Name: Linda Klemeyer   **PCP:** Martha C. Eaton, MD

Date of Exam: 7 March ----   **Age/Sex:** 62-year-old female   **ID#:** M-82

DIAGNOSIS
Stage I (T1N0M0) right breast cancer, ER/PR-positive, HER2/neu-negative.

TREATMENT
1. Right modified radical mastectomy and axillary lymph node dissection in October two years ago.
2. MA.27 protocol. Patient was randomized to exemestane, initiated in December two years ago.

PAST MEDICAL HISTORY
1. Type 2 diabetes.
2. Hypertension.
3. Osteoarthritis.
4. Neurogenic bladder requiring routine self-catheterization associated with recurrent urinary tract infections.
5. Obesity.

CURRENT MEDICATIONS
1. Aspirin 81 mg daily.
2. Hydrochlorothiazide 25 mg daily.
3. Lisinopril 40 mg daily.
4. Metformin 500 mg t.i.d.
5. Zocor 5 mg daily.
6. Claritin 10 mg daily.
7. Motrin 600 mg, 1 to 2 times daily.
8. Ciprofloxacin 250 mg daily.
9. Actonel 135 mg weekly.
10. Exemestane 25 mg daily.
11. Calcium + vitamin D.
12. Centrum Silver.
13. Flexeril 5 mg q.h.s.

HISTORY OF PRESENT ILLNESS: Since our last visit, patient has done well. Denies new breast masses or adenopathy. Denies bone pain, abdominal pain, nausea, and vomiting. She does note occasional hot flashes.

PHYSICAL EXAMINATION

Blood pressure 154/77, pulse 94, temperature 96.8, height 59.75 inches, weight 230 pounds. General: Awake, alert, oriented, in no acute distress. HEENT: Sclerae nonicteric. Conjunctivae pink. Oral mucosa clear. LYMPH NODES: No cervical, supraclavicular, infraclavicular, or axillary adenopathy. LUNGS are clear to auscultation bilaterally. HEART: Regular rate and rhythm. ABDOMEN: Soft, obese, nontender. EXTREMITIES: Without clubbing, clots, or edema. BREAST EXAM: Right mastectomy scar without nodules or ulcerations. No right chest wall masses. Left breast has normal contour. No skin changes or palpable masses. No nipple discharge. NEUROLOGIC: No neurologic deficits.

(Continued)

X-RAY DATA: Left mammogram from Sept ---- reveals scattered fibroglandular elements without mass or suspicious calcification. No areas of architectural distortion. Negative **BI-RADS I.**

IMPRESSION

A 63-year-old white female with a history of stage I breast cancer, currently receiving adjuvant exemestane on MA.27 protocol, currently without evidence of disease.

PLAN

1. Continue monthly self-examination of breast.
2. Continue osteoporosis prophylaxis with Actonel, calcium, and vitamin D.
3. Surveillance DEXA scan due in 2 years. I have ordered this for patient.
4. Followup visit with me in 3 months.

_____

Solomon T. Fisher, MD
Oncology

STF:pai
D:3/8/----
T:3/9/----

c: Martha C. Eaton, MD, Family Practice

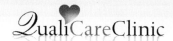

Orthopedic Clinic Preop History & Physical

Patient Name: Maria Irene Flores   **PCP:** Susan McGinnis, MD

Date of Exam: 26 Oct ----   **Age/Sex:** 68-year-old female   **ID#:** M-83

HISTORY OF PRESENT ILLNESS: Maria is a 68-year-old right-hand dominant Hispanic female who sustained a fall on 21 October ----. The patient has a left distal radius and ulnar fracture. Patient with minimal pain and discomfort to her left wrist. The patient was placed in a sugar-tong splint when seen in the emergency room at the time of injury. The patient is compliant with her posterior splint/sling.

ALLERGIES: None.

MEDICATIONS: Aspirin, atenolol, hydrochlorothiazide, potassium, Zyrtec, and Fosamax.

Past medical history includes hypertension, osteopenia, seasonal allergic rhinitis.

PAST SURGICAL HISTORY: Tonsils and adenoids and wisdom teeth in childhood.

SOCIAL HISTORY: Positive tobacco, half a pack per day for 40 years. The patient denies EtOH and illicit drug use. A widow, she is not sexually active.

PHYSICAL EXAMINATION

GENERAL: The patient is alert and in no apparent distress. She is a well-developed, well-nourished female. **HEAD AND NECK EXAM:** Unremarkable. **HEART:** Regular rate and rhythm without murmurs, rubs, or gallops. **PULMONARY:** Clear to auscultation bilaterally without wheezes, rales, or rhonchi noted. **ABDOMEN:** Soft, nondistended, nontender, with positive bowel sounds and no hepatosplenomegaly noted. **EXTREMITIES:** Left arm/wrist reveals minimal edema to the radial aspect of the wrist. No ecchymoses or open lesions noted. Minimal tenderness to palpation at distal radius, radial side. Capillary refill is less than 2 seconds. Sensation and motor intact to radial, ulnar, median, AIN, PIN distributions. Left elbow reveals no tenderness to palpation, with full range of motion.

IMPRESSION
Left distal radius and ulnar fractures.

PLAN
We plan open reduction, external fixation versus open reduction, internal fixation of the left distal radius and ulnar fracture. Patient to go to the OR on 27 October ----. Will set up a consult with the anesthesiologist right away. Preop labs to be drawn today.

_____

Gilbert M. Fields, MD
Orthopedic Surgery

GMF:pai
D:10/26/----
T:10/26/----

c: Susan McGinnis, MD, Family Practice

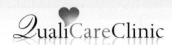

Emergency Department Treatment Record

Patient Name: Steve Fowler   **PCP:** James A. McClure Jr, MD

Date of Exam: 19 March ----   **Age/Sex:** 24-year-old male   **ID#:** M-84

MODE OF ARRIVAL: Privately owned vehicle.

CONSULTING SERVICE: General Surgery.

CHIEF COMPLAINT: Rectal prolapse.

HISTORY OF PRESENT ILLNESS: This 24-year-old male presents to the ED today for the third time in 3 days for complaints of recurrent rectal prolapse. Patient states that he had his initial rectal prolapse 3 days ago. He came to the ED at that time where he was taught to reduce it on his own. Since that time patient has been able to reduce the prolapse on his own with the exception of one time, causing presentation yesterday, as well as a prolapse at 0700 hours this morning, resulting in his current presentation. Patient reports that he was eating breakfast when he began to feel the sharp, sudden umbilical pain associated with his prolapses in the past. Patient states that the prolapse is often exacerbated by running and by bowel movements. His last bowel movement was "normal" today. He admits to chronic constipation with bowel movement approximately every 10 days. He also states that he has been taking Colace as prescribed since his last ED visit. He has had no hematochezia or melena, no abdominal pain, fever, chills, or other complaints currently.

REVIEW OF SYSTEMS: As per HPI. Patient denies visual changes, cough, cold, congestion, sore throat, headaches, chest pain, shortness of breath, abdominal pain, back pain, dysuria, weakness, or numbness of extremities.

PAST MEDICAL HISTORY: Chronic constipation.

PAST SURGICAL HISTORY: None.

MEDICATIONS: Motrin p.r.n. pain.

ALLERGIES: No known drug allergies.

SOCIAL HISTORY: Does not drink, denies tobacco use. Is single, lives alone. Denies unprotected sexual encounters.

FAMILY HISTORY: Colon cancer in his grandmother. No history of kidney disease or diabetes.

PHYSICAL EXAMINATION

VITAL SIGNS on presentation: Heart rate 77, BP 131/76, R 20, T 98.4, saturating 99% on room air. In general, patient is a well-developed, well-nourished 24-year-old white male lying supine on the bed in no apparent distress. HEAD: Normocephalic, atraumatic. EYES: Pupils are equal, round, and reactive to light and accommodation. ENT: Oropharynx clear. Nares patent. NECK: Supple. HEART: Regular rate and rhythm with no murmurs, rubs, or gallops. LUNGS: Clear to auscultation bilaterally. ABDOMEN: Soft, nontender, nondistended. Bowel sounds present. No back pain, no flank pain. EXTREMITIES: Two-plus distal pulses bilaterally. No clubbing, cyanosis, or edema. RECTAL exam: Patient has a full-thickness rectal prolapse. Edematous and with moderate bleeding.

(Continued)

EMERGENCY DEPARTMENT COURSE: Patient's rectal prolapse was partially reduced by the ED staff before consulting General Surgery at roughly 1100 hours. Dr. McClure came down to see the patient. He easily reduced the prolapse and recommended that the patient be put on Lactulose, titrated to 1 bowel movement per day. They also recommended no physical activity, and they arranged for followup with Dr. McClure on Monday at 1300 hours in the general surgery clinic. Official consult has been placed on the chart.

MEDICAL DECISION MAKING: This 24-year-old male patient presents for the third time in 3 days with recurrent rectal prolapse. Given his third presentation in 3 days, General Surgery was consulted, as above, and it has been agreed that the patient needs to be placed on med hold until further disposition can be arranged with General Surgery. Given his otherwise normal physical exam, with his history of chronic constipation, the recurrent prolapse is likely due to chronic constipation.

EMERGENCY DEPARTMENT DIAGNOSIS
Rectal prolapse, now reduced.

DISPOSITION
To general surgery clinic on Monday afternoon.

PLAN
1. Patient is to follow up at the general surgery clinic with Dr. McClure on Monday at 1300 hours. Report to the front desk, give his name, and give his ED discharge papers. We have recommended that the patient be on med hold until that time.
2. Patient is to partake in no physical activity. Physical activity will only increase the incidence of prolapse.
3. Continue taking Colace as directed and start Lactulose as directed, approximately 15 mL to 30 mL daily. Change as needed for goal of 1 bowel movement daily.
4. Return to ED immediately with recurrent symptoms, pain, rectal bleeding, prolapse, fever, or any concerns.
5. Patient was informed of his followup appointment, and he voiced complete understanding of the instructions given and agreement with the plan. He was released from the ED in good condition.

_____
Samuel Ernest, MD
Emergency Room Physician

SE:pai
D:3/19/----
T:3/19/----

c: James A. McClure Jr, MD, General Surgery

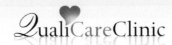

Hematology/Oncology Clinic Followup Note

Patient Name: Barbara Ann Tinka   **PCP:** Chris Salem, DO

Date of Exam: 2 March ----   **Age/Sex:** 50-year-old female   **ID#:** M-85

DIAGNOSIS
Stage IIA left breast cancer, ER/PR-positive, HER2/neu-negative, diagnosed in January one year ago.

TREATMENT
1. Lumpectomy and sentinel lymph node dissection.
2. Adjuvant dose density AC for 4 cycles followed by every-2-week Taxol for 4 cycles.
3. Post lumpectomy radiation completed 28 Feb this year.
4. Letrozole.

CURRENT MEDICATIONS
1. Fosamax 70 mg weekly.
2. Letrozole.
3. Calcium + vitamin D.
4. Hydrochlorothiazide.
5. Vitamin E.
6. Vitamin B.
7. Vitamin C.
8. Multivitamin.
9. Potassium chloride 10 mEq daily.

HISTORY OF PRESENT ILLNESS: At our last visit, patient complained of insomnia and depression related to financial issues and work. She states that her financial concerns and work concerns continue. She continues to have insomnia but would not like medication for this at this time. She complains of leg cramps. She complains of vaginal dryness and decreased sexual drive.

Patient has concerns about possible osteonecrosis of the jaw related to her Fosamax use. This was started for osteopenia of her spine, which she had at the initiation of letrozole.

Patient denies new masses in her breasts, has no lymphadenopathy. Denies bone and abdominal pain. Patient continues to complain of arthralgias from her letrozole.

PHYSICAL EXAMINATION

Blood pressure 120/79, pulse 106, temperature 98.1, height 63-1/2 inches, weight 155 pounds. **GENERAL:** Middle-aged female in no acute distress. **HEENT:** Sclerae clear. Conjunctivae pink. Oral mucosa clear. **LYMPH NODES:** No cervical, supraclavicular, infraclavicular, or axillary adenopathy. **LUNGS** are clear to auscultation bilaterally. **HEART** has regular rate and rhythm without murmurs, rubs, or gallops. **ABDOMEN:** Soft, nontender without hepatosplenomegaly. **EXTREMITIES** are without edema. **BREAST EXAM:** There are lumpectomy changes in the left breast. Otherwise, there is normal contour to the right breast. No other skin changes. No palpable masses on breast exam. No nipple discharge.

(Continued)

ID#: M-85   PAGE 2

LABORATORY DATA: Creatinine 0.7, potassium 3.3, magnesium 1.8.

IMPRESSION

A 50-year-old female with stage IIA breast cancer, currently with no evidence of disease.

PLAN

1. Barbara appears to be quite distressed about the arthralgias regarding her letrozole as well as the use of Fosamax. We reviewed her original tumor pathology. She had a 1.2 cm, well-differentiated tumor with no lymphovascular invasion. She was ER-70%- positive, PR-90%-positive, and HER2/neu-negative. She had 1 lymph node involved. I discussed that perhaps her arthralgias could get better with tamoxifen. In addition, she would not need a bisphosphonate with tamoxifen. However, she would have a slightly increased risk of disease relapse on tamoxifen compared to letrozole. At this time, patient wishes to continue with letrozole.
2. We decreased Fosamax from 70 mg weekly to 35 mg weekly. Again, she is concerned with osteonecrosis of the jaw. I am not sure that decreasing the dose will affect her overall risk; however, she is in only the osteopenic range. I think 35 mg as a prophylactic dose is reasonable.
3. Of note, she will be due for repeat DEXA scan in December. Mammogram is due in November.
4. Leg cramps, possibly secondary to low potassium. We increased potassium to 30 mEq daily. Repeat chemistries in 1 week.
5. Vaginal dryness. I recommended a trial of Replens.
6. Insomnia, depression, lack of sexual drive. I again discussed an antidepressant with the patient. She is not interested at this time. Her decreased sexual drive is due at least in part to her letrozole; however, it may also be related to her depression. Again, patient declines antidepressant at this time.
7. Patient will follow up in 3 months.

_____

Solomon T. Fisher, MD
Oncology

STF:pai
D:3/3/----
T:3/4/----

c: Chris Salem, DO, Family Practice

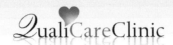

QualiCareClinic

Orthopaedic Surgery Spine Consultation

Patient Name: Tomas Garza   **PCP:** Mack Stolga, MD

Date of Exam: 7 Jan ----   **Age/Sex:** 27-year-old male   **ID#:** M-86

TRAUMA TEAM ADMITTING PHYSICIAN: Mack Stolga, MD

CONSULTANT: Gilbert M. Fields, MD, Orthopaedic Spine Surgeon.

REASON FOR CONSULT: A 27-year-old Hispanic male involved in an MVA with multiple C-spine fractures. Patient was the restrained driver involved in a rollover MVA and was transferred to our ED for our orthopedic and trauma team management.

HISTORY OF PRESENT ILLNESS: At the time of my evaluation, the patient complains only of neck pain. He denies other orthopedic problems or complaints, such as numbness, tingling, or other radicular problems. He has been stable from the Trauma Team standpoint thus far. Please see the handwritten orthopedic notes from the residents, which I have co-signed, regarding the remainder of this patient's history.

PHYSICAL EXAMINATION

Initial

At the time of my initial exam, the patient has appropriate midline tenderness for his injuries involving the cervical spine. No other midline tenderness of the thoracic or lumbar spine. He does have some tenderness off to the left paraspinal region of the lumbar spine correlating with his transverse process fractures. No abrasions, other contusions, or other problems about the posterior aspect of the cervical spine, thoracic spine, or lumbar spine.

Head and Neck

Some abrasions and a small hematoma around the left temporal and parietal regions. He does have a small amount of dried blood in the right ear, which, again, would be appropriate given the fact that he has basilar skull fractures as well.

Musculoskeletal/Neurologic

Exam demonstrates 5/5 strength in the deltoids, biceps, triceps, grip strength, hand intrinsics, wrist flexors and extensors. He has sensation symmetrically in C3, C4, C5, C6, C7, and T1 dermatomal distributions. Negative Hoffman. Symmetric deep tendon reflexes in both upper extremities. Lower extremities demonstrate 5/5 in flexors, quadriceps, hamstrings, dorsiflexors, plantar flexors, and extensor hallucis longus. He has symmetric light touch in L2, L3, L4, L5, and S1 dermatomal distributions. Symmetric deep tendon reflexes in the patellar and Achilles tendons. Again, no other gross upper or lower extremity abnormalities, deformities, swelling, etc.

X-RAY DATA: Multiple radiographs were reviewed today. The C-spine, T-spine, L-spine films, and plain films were completed; however, some are inadequate and need to be repeated at this time.

The transverse process fractures of L2, L3, L4 on the left are identified. No other fractures about the lumbar spine are noted. The AP thoracic x-ray is unremarkable for significant findings.

The lateral C-spine x-ray demonstrates the teardrop fracture, which is barely noticed on the lateral at C5 due to the patient's body habitus; otherwise, overall good alignment. No evidence for distraction injury, jumped facets, or significant angular deformities.

(Continued)

ID#: M-86   PAGE 2

CT scan of cervical spine reveals multiple fractures.

- There is a right occipital condyle impaction fracture noted without significant displacement or instability.
- Nondisplaced posterior arch fractures of C1 are noted bilaterally.
- C2 right lateral mass body fracture with mild displacement and left pedicle vertebral foramen fracture, which is essentially nondisplaced.
- Nondisplaced right C3 superior facet fracture.
- Nondisplaced bilateral C5 lamina fractures at the level of the base of the spinous process. There is also a teardrop fracture involving the body of C5, again with significant angular deformity.

IMPRESSION/PLAN

1. Motor vehicle accident with rollover in a restrained passenger with multiple cervical spine fractures. None of these appear to be significantly displaced, but due to multiple levels of involvement as well as the C2 lateral mass body fracture, as well as the teardrop fracture of C5, I feel that halo immobilization for approximately 3 months would be indicated.
2. Long discussion with the patient and his wife and brother-in-law today regarding the findings. We also discussed treatment options involving the continued Minerva immobilization versus halo versus surgical intervention. Again, I think halo is the best option at this time. This will hopefully allow us to avoid surgical intervention. The patient and his family do understand that at the 3-month mark, if he still has evidence of instability, we may still be required to perform surgery at either one or all levels. Risks, benefits, and alternatives to all procedures were discussed. We obtained consent today for halo immobilization.
3. In light of the hematoma overlying the left temporal and parietal bones, which is in the area of our halo pin placement trauma, we will continue immobilization right now in the Minerva and will follow this hematoma. As his hematoma resolves and his abrasions improve, we will convert him to a halo at that time. We will also continue to follow his neurologic status closely.
4. At this time, we plan repeat lateral thoracic and lumbar films for improved visualization of these levels. We will review his outside head CT to assess for any other issues that may contraindicate our using a halo. At this time, however, I see no problem with halo immobilization other than the above-mentioned hematoma.

_____
Gilbert M. Fields, MD
Orthopedic Surgery

GMF:pai
D:1/7/----
T:1/8/----

c: Mack Stolga, MD, Trauma Team

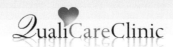

QualiCareClinic

Emergency Department Treatment Record

Patient Name: Paul Travis Overton   **PCP:** Reed Phillips, MD

Date of Exam: 26 Dec ----   **Age/Sex:** 11-month-old male   **ID#:** M-87

CHIEF COMPLAINT: Diarrhea and fever.

MODE OF ARRIVAL: Privately owned vehicle.

HISTORY OF PRESENT ILLNESS: This 11-month-old male child with no significant comorbidities presents to the ED complaining of approximately 4 to 5 days of diarrhea, then fever for the past day or two. Mom reports that he has had approximately 2 days of decreased p.o. intake for solids but is tolerating p.o. liquids with a mild decrease in the number of wet diapers. He is still producing anywhere from 3 to 5 per day. They report only mild upper respiratory-type symptoms, including some minor sinus congestion and rhinorrhea; otherwise, they deny tugging at the ears, persistent nausea, or history of vomiting. They report maybe some mild cough. The child is otherwise well appearing. Mother denies any history of sick contacts, although the child is a daycare dweller. HPI is otherwise unremarkable.

REVIEW OF SYSTEMS: Negative except as dictated in the HPI.

PAST MEDICAL HISTORY: None.

PAST SURGICAL HISTORY: None. Circumcised at 10 days of age.

MEDICATIONS: Motrin and Tylenol.

ALLERGIES: No known drug allergies.

IMMUNIZATIONS: Up to date.

SOCIAL HISTORY: No smokers in the home. He does go to daycare 5 days a week.

PHYSICAL EXAMINATION

VITAL SIGNS on presentation: P 158, R 28, T 102.6, O2 saturation of 97% on room air. **CONSTITUTIONAL:** This is a well-developed, well-nourished 11-month-old playful, interactive child who is nontoxic appearing at the time of my evaluation in bed #23. **HEENT:** Normocephalic, atraumatic. Pupils are equal, round, and reactive to light. TMs clear. No erythema or effusion appreciable on exam. Oropharynx is clear and moist without exudates or lymphadenopathy. **NECK:** Supple. Trachea midline. No lymphadenopathy. **CHEST:** Clear to auscultation. No wheezes, rales, or rhonchi are audible on exam. **ABDOMEN:** Soft, nondistended, nontender without rebound or guarding. There is no evidence of mass or pulsatile mass at the time of my exam. **EXTREMITIES:** No rash is visible.

EMERGENCY DEPARTMENT COURSE/MEDICAL DECISION MAKING: This is an 11-month-old male child, well appearing and nontoxic, who presented to the ED with 4 to 5 days of diarrhea, a couple days of vomiting, and 1 or 2 days of fever subjectively—102 F at home and 102.6 F in the ED. This child is otherwise nontoxic, well appearing, hydrating well in the ED. Given his presentation and the duration of his symptoms, PA and lateral chest x-ray was obtained to rule out an infiltrative pneumonia. This revealed no evidence of an infiltrative process, no effusion, no other focal consolidation. However, the lateral view revealed a suspicious

(Continued)

ID#: M-87   PAGE 2

opacified coin-shaped lesion somewhere in the abdomen. Repeat abdominal films, PA and cross-table lateral, revealed a coin within the gastric space. It appears to be proximal to the pylorus. Mom reports no known history of foreign body ingestion, no history of choking, no repeated drooling. We have no clear date for exact onset of this foreign body ingestion; however, given that the patient is otherwise well appearing, tolerating p.o. liquids and solids without difficulty, having no bloody bowel movements, we feel that the child is safe to be discharged to home with his mother.

Follow up here in the ED in 24 hours for repeat films to assess the coin's passage through the pylorus. If the coin does not pass through the pylorus within 24 hours, pediatric gastroenterology consult will be warranted for endoscopic removal.

EMERGENCY DEPARTMENT DIAGNOSES
1. Diarrhea.
2. Acute febrile illness.
3. Gastric foreign body.

DISPOSITION
Medications: None. Discharge instructions are as follows.

1. Continue to use Motrin and Tylenol p.r.n. symptom control of any fever.
2. Return to the ED in 24 hours for repeat abdominal and flat plate images of the abdomen to ensure passage of the foreign body.
3. Discharge to home.
4. Parents given aftercare handout on acute febrile illness in children and gastric foreign body. They are instructed to return to the ED for the indications listed above or for any additional concerns.

_____
Samuel Ernest, MD
Emergency Room Physician

SE:pai
D:12/26/----
T:12/26/----

c: Reed Phillips, MD, Pediatrics

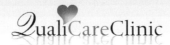

Internal Medicine Initial Visit

Patient Name: Roseanne Erickson	**PCP:** Linda Galbraith, FNP
Date of Exam: 27 Oct ---- **Age/Sex:** 50-year-old female	**ID#:** M-88

Outpatient Record: Unavailable.

Time Allotted for Visit: 30 minutes.

REASON FOR VISIT: 50-year-old white female establishing care. Notes an inability to sleep. She has used amitriptyline for this.

HISTORY OF PRESENT ILLNESS: The patient states that she has been plagued by sweating at night. She states that she will go to bed and will be able to get off to sleep; however, she will awaken with sweating that is intense. She will sweat through her night clothes and need to get up and change the night clothes. She then will remain awake. She has found the use of amitriptyline up to 50 mg ineffective. She is from England and admits that she will never be able to regard America as her home. She was last back to England a year ago when her 27-year-old daughter was killed in a nightclub. Apparently a date rape drug had been added to her daughter's drink, and she had an allergic reaction.

The patient does not wake up with headaches, but she does suffer from these. She describes this as beginning early in her life. She states that she had parental abuse very early on that eventuated in a head trauma. These headaches can awaken her, though not usually, and they are associated with bitemporal pressure to pounding. She prefers inactivity. The headache will last days without her medications. Years and years ago she saw neurology for this. She describes the pain as pulsating—almost like 2 electric wires on either side of her head that are connecting. There is tense nausea that goes along with this, and she can vomit.

The patient has not attempted any of the newer abortive migraine headache medicines. She states that she had brought her night sweats to previous providers' attention, and she was given estrogen replacement therapy; however, there was no decrease in her night sweats despite an increase to 0.9 mg of Premarin taken each day. This dose was maintained for 4 months.

PAST MEDICAL HISTORY
1. "Emphysema."
2. Migraines.
3. Nicotine dependence.
4. Blood clot, left calf, while on birth control pills.

PAST SURGICAL HISTORY: Hysterectomy 20 years ago without bilateral salpingo-oophorectomy.

ALLERGIES: SULFA.

MEDICATIONS: Fiorinal p.r.n., Proventil p.r.n., baby aspirin each day.

SOCIAL HISTORY: She lives here in the Miami area. Her husband is a retired Master Sergeant from the Air Force. He has had recurrence of his Hodgkin disease after a 17-year remission. They have had 3 children in toto. She is not a drinker, is a smoker.

FAMILY HISTORY: No migraines, but there is heart disease and diabetes as well as alcoholism. She did not know her dad well.

(Continued)

REVIEW OF SYSTEMS: Generally, her weight has gone up over the years. Neurologic: She gets headaches as described above. She denies the description of warning signs with her headaches. She does have a follow-on washed-out day after resolution of the headache. No seizures or faints. HEENT: Vision and hearing are stable. Endocrine: No diabetes or thyroid disease. Heart: No prior heart attack or fast heart rate. Pulmonary: She is not exercise-limited by her apparent lung disease. She does have wheezing and shortness of breath that is alleviated with Proventil. Gastrointestinal: No ulcer disease. Gynecologic: Normal vaginal deliveries. Approximately 9 years ago she was told that she was entering "the change," as her blood tests had indicated such.

PHYSICAL EXAMINATION

Vitals show blood pressure 136/75, pulse 92, respirations 12, temperature 96.5, height 67 inches, weight 170 pounds. She is comfortable in the exam chair. Her speech is effortless. NECK is without cervical lymphadenopathy, thyromegaly, or nodules. HAIR: She wears her hair long. It has been dyed blond. She does have gray roots. EYES are without injection. HEART: Regular. S1, S2 are within normal limits. I could appreciate no diastolic or systolic sounds today. EXTREMITIES are without cyanosis, clubbing, or edema.

ANCILLARY DATABASE: 26 Oct ---- laboratory results show creatinine 1.1 and calcium (without albumin) 9.4. White blood cells showed a steady decrease, going outside the normal range with WBC count of 4.2. MCV was 101.7, MCH 34.1, and platelets were 189,000. H&H were 13.9 g and 41.5%.

Labs from 9 years ago: Gonadotropins—follicle stimulating hormone of 147 (0-12 mIU/mL) with luteinizing hormone 43 (0-14 mIU/mL).

ASSESSMENT WITH MEDICAL DECISION-MAKING

1. Night sweats, an established problem. Additional diagnostics and therapeutics required. The patient states this condition has worsened over the last year.
2. Menopause, an established problem. Additional therapeutics required.
3. Leukopenia, new problem. Additional diagnostics and therapeutics required.

PLAN

1. We have discussed the role of triptans in abortive vascular headache therapy. Since she gets less than 1 a week, we will not start preventive medicine at this point.
2. We renewed her Fiorinal but advised her to begin using Zomig 2.5 mg tablets.
3. We have prescribed Zomig 2.5, one now and then one 2 hours later at the first sign of headache.
4. We recommend that she stop the amitriptyline.
5. Today we obtained a chest x-ray. (For her piece of mind, I went ahead and looked at the 2-view.) The x-ray was without active pulmonary disease. I could appreciate no bony disease. Her heart size was within normal limits, pulmonary vessels within normal limits. I appreciate no masses and no adenopathy.
6. We prescribed Ambien 5 mg, 1 p.o. to get to sleep but not to return to sleep.
7. We have entered a consult to Hematology, noting the sweating at night, which seems to meet "night sweats" criteria for myself. It is atypical in that it has not responded to estrogen replacement therapy and now is associated with a low white count in a smoker. Smokers can actually have an increase in their white blood cell count.
8. At this juncture I would not recommend estrogen replacement therapy for this patient, only because there is a relative contraindication of ERT in those who have migraines plus her past history of blood clot on estrogen.
9. We advised patient to follow up with either myself or Linda Galbraith, FNP, in approximately 1 month to review her laboratory results and the response to the initial therapies.

(Continued)

ID#: M-88   PAGE 3

I entered the room at 1405, and I exited at 1440. We spent over half of this time in counseling and education and the coordination of the patient's care.

_____
Michael Panagides, MD
Internal Medicine

MP:pai
D:10/27/----
T:10/28/----

c: Linda Galbraith, FNP, Family Nurse Practitioner
    Stephen C. Gordon, MD, Hematology Clinic

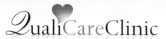

Orthopedics Shoulder Clinic Consult

Patient Name: Patrick Joseph Flynn   **PCP:** Nancy Lawrence, MD

Date of Exam: 21 May ----   **Age/Sex:** 20-year-old male   **ID#:** M-89

NOTE: This patient is a dog handler.

HISTORY OF PRESENT ILLNESS: This 28-year-old right-hand dominant male has bilateral shoulder dislocations. The left shoulder was first dislocated after a fall on a confidence course in basic training. The right shoulder first dislocated with military press after that time. The left shoulder dislocates on a regular basis. The last time was 3 days ago with no exertion or force applied, and the patient states that he has dislocated it so many times that he can place it back himself or a friend of his can help by pulling for 10 minutes to put the shoulder back in place. The right shoulder has dislocated x3, the last time after a fall 4 years ago. He states that he put the shoulder back into its place on his own. He states that the left shoulder subluxes with overhead activity, throwing, and military press. There is no history of trauma for the right shoulder, and he has done no rehabilitation up to this time. Both of the patient's shoulders dislocated before he became a dog handler.

REVIEW OF SYSTEMS: There is no night pain. It is positive for subluxation on the left at night. Otherwise, the review of systems is negative.

PAST MEDICAL HISTORY: There is no past medical history other than that listed in the Present Illness.

PAST SURGICAL HISTORY: None other than tonsils and adenoids in childhood.

ALLERGIES: There are no known drug allergies.

SOCIAL HISTORY: He has smoked a pack per day for the past year. He does not drink. He is a member of the United States Marine Corps. He is single. No prostitute contact, no unprotected sex.

PHYSICAL EXAMINATION

Exam of the right shoulder shows forward elevation from 0 to 160 degrees without pain. Abduction from 0 to 180 degrees without pain. External rotation to 45 degrees and internal rotation to T6. Supraspinatus and external rotators are 5/5. Subscapularis was measured at 4+/5. He had negative Neer, Hawkins, cross-arm, sulcus, apprehension, and relocation tests. Negative load shift test and no tenderness.

Exam of the left shoulder shows forward elevation from 0 to 160 degrees without pain. Abduction from 0 to 180 degrees without pain. External rotation to 20 degrees and internal rotation to T6. Supraspinatus and external rotators and subscapularis were 5/5. He had a negative Neer test. He had positive pain with the Hawkins test along the anterolateral border of the acromion. He had a negative cross-arm test, positive sulcus test, positive apprehension test with relocation. Patient could not tolerate a load shift test, and he was nontender to palpation.

Both upper extremities were intact to sensory and motor along the musculocutaneous, axillary, radial, ulnar, and median nerve distributions. Ligamentous laxity test showed the elbow to be minimally hyperextended. The index finger was able to be extended to 90 degrees without pain bilaterally. He could not place his palms on the floor with the legs extended and the hips flexed. There was no genu rockerbottom bilaterally.

X-RAY DATA: X-ray examination of the left shoulder shows a bony Bankart lesion along the anterior inferior glenoid. MRI of the left shoulder confirms the bony Bankart lesion with what appears to be global erosion of the glenoid in that region. There is an inferior humeral osteophyte, a small Hill-Sachs lesion. The rotator cuff was noted to be intact. There was no SLAP lesion.

IMPRESSION
Bilateral shoulder multidirectional instability with a left shoulder Bankart lesion (TUBS).

(Continued)

ID#: M-89   PAGE 2

PLAN
The plan at this time is to rehab bilateral shoulders with Thera-Band for the next 10 weeks, progressing from yellow to gray. These exercises were explained to the patient by me, and he is to do them 4 to 5 times a day. He is to obtain a Stryker notch view of the left shoulder today as well as right shoulder films. Patient is to follow up in Dr. Rodriguez's clinic in 6 to 8 weeks for repeat evaluation.

_____

Raquel Rodriguez, MD
Orthopedic Surgery

RR:pai
D:5/21/----
T:5/22/----

c: Nancy Lawrence, MD
    Internal Medicine

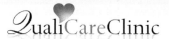

Emergency Department Treatment Record

Patient Name: Michael John Babjak   **PCP:** Nancy Lawrence, MD

Date of Exam: 16 June ----   **Age/Sex:** 63-year-old male   **ID#:** M-90

CONSULTATION: Internal Medicine, admission pending.

CHIEF COMPLAINT: A 63-year-old male with chief complaint of bilateral lower extremity edema and shortness of breath.

HISTORY OF PRESENT ILLNESS: Over the past 2 weeks patient has noticed increased shortness of breath with more difficulty lying flat. Patient with increased orthopnea, using up to 3 pillows at night to remain comfortable. Patient has noted increased swelling acutely in his legs over the past 2 weeks. He has a history of congestive heart failure. Patient is without fever, chills, nausea, vomiting, cough, chest pain. No numbness or tingling.

REVIEW OF SYSTEMS: All systems negative except as mentioned in HPI.

PAST MEDICAL HISTORY: Significant for sarcoidosis, congestive heart failure, chronic renal failure, back pain, glaucoma, diabetes.

PAST SURGICAL HISTORY: Significant for cyst and appendix removal.

PHYSICAL EXAMINATION

VITAL SIGNS on presentation: Pulse 58, blood pressure 128/68, respirations 20, saturating 96% on room air, temperature 97.2. HEENT: Pupils are equal, round, and reactive to light and accommodation. Extraocular movements intact. Moist mucous membranes. Oropharynx clear. NECK: Supple. CARDIOVASCULAR: Regular rate and rhythm without murmurs. No gallops or rubs. LUNGS: Some crackles in the bases bilaterally. ABDOMEN: Soft, nontender, nondistended. Positive bowel sounds. EXTREMITIES: Patient with 2+ to 3+ pitting edema bilaterally. NEURO: Cranial nerves II through XII intact. Strength 5/5 bilaterally.

EMERGENCY DEPARTMENT COURSE: Labs were ordered, including white count of 9.1, hemoglobin 12.6, and hematocrit 37.3, platelets 165,000. Chemistry panel: Sodium 136, potassium 4.3, chloride 100, bicarb 25, BUN 40, creatinine 2.8, glucose 164. ProBNP was 249.1. Cardiac enzymes were ordered with CK 135, MB 3.4, troponin 0.01. Patient with LFTs that have been within normal limits. Chest x-ray with slight cephalization but no acute findings, no pneumonia. No mediastinal widening. EKG with sinus bradycardia; otherwise, within normal limits. No ST-segment changes. Patient given Lasix in the ED. Patient refused aspirin. Patient was given nitro and Plavix and morphine in the ED with improvement in his symptoms.

MEDICAL DECISION MAKING: With a history of congestive heart failure, patient is likely having some sort of exacerbation. ProBNP is only 249.1 at this time. Still, I think the patient needs inpatient evaluation and treatment.

(Continued)

ID#: M-90

EMERGENCY DEPARTMENT DIAGNOSIS
Acute dyspnea and anginal variant.

DISPOSITION
Plan is to be admitted to Internal Medicine Service. Set up consult with Pulmonary Services.

_____
Samuel Ernest, MD
Emergency Room Physician

SE:pai
D:12/3/----
T:12/3/----

c: Nancy Lawrence, MD, Internal Medicine
    Lloyd Verlin, MD, Pulmonary Clinic

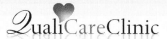

QualiCareClinic

Internal Medicine Clinic Followup Note

Patient Name: Rosemary George   **PCP:** Patrick Keathley, MD

Date of Exam: 3 Feb ----   **Age/Sex:** 54-year-old female   **ID#:** M-91

OUTPATIENT RECORD: Unavailable; we did take advantage of the electronic database.

CHIEF COMPLAINT: A 54-year-old white female called in by me for elevated blood sugars.

HISTORY OF PRESENT ILLNESS: A 54-year-old retired master sergeant brought in when elevated fasting blood sugar was noted. She has had no polyuria, polydipsia. Admits to intentional weight loss.

PAST MEDICAL HISTORY: Seasonal allergic rhinitis. Congestion, etiology unclear. She describes it as a sinusitis, though recent CT scans are reportedly without sinus disease.

PAST SURGICAL HISTORY: Bilateral carpal tunnel releases.

ALLERGIES: PENICILLIN and CODEINE.

MEDICATIONS
1. Flonase, recently stopped.
2. Claritin as needed.

FAMILY HISTORY: Family history of leukemias, mainly in her father and a daughter.

SOCIAL HISTORY: She is not a smoker, rarely drinks. Has children and lives in town with her husband. Until recently she was employed in medical credentialing.

REVIEW OF SYSTEMS

GENERAL: Weight loss, as described. There has been no weakness. HEENT: Congestion, as described. NEUROLOGIC: There has been no headache. ENDOCRINE: There has been no thyroid disease or hypertension. No treatment for cholesterol. HEART/LUNG/GASTROINTESTINAL DISEASE: Denied.

PHYSICAL EXAMINATION

VITAL SIGNS show blood pressure 123/81, pulse 73, respirations 18, temperature 99, height 5 feet 6 inches, weight 87 kg.

GENERAL: Patient is comfortable in the exam chair. She is somewhat tearful as she recalls processes leading to losing her recent job.

HEENT: She has no dominant facial or skin lesions. Eyes are without injection. Speech is effortless.

NECK: Without cervical lymphadenopathy, thyromegaly, or nodules. There are no carotid bruits or murmurs. Her thyroid I would estimate to be less than 20 g.

LUNGS: Clear to auscultation.

HEART: Regular. S1, S2 are normal.

ABDOMEN: Minimally obese, flat, soft, nontender. Bowel sounds present without organomegaly, masses, bruits, or unusual abdominal pulsations.

(Continued)

ID#: M-91   PAGE 2

SKIN: No evidence of acanthosis nigricans.

EXTREMITIES: Without cyanosis, clubbing, or edema.

LABORATORY DATA: Fasting blood sugar 113. Normal thyroid function tests, both TSH and free T4.

ASSESSMENT

1. Impaired fasting glucose.
2. Obesity, mild.
3. Seasonal allergic rhinitis.

PLAN

1. Diagnostically, we will ask for oral glucose tolerance test.
2. Counseling/Education.
   • We reviewed the statistics regarding impaired fasting glucose.
   • We reviewed the relationship between obesity and diabetes.
   • We tried to encourage her in this recent loss of job.
   • There is no additional therapy at this point.
   • We did not specifically outline a weight loss program, given the described success she has had.

TIME SPENT WITH THIS PATIENT

Some 28 minutes 20 seconds. None of this dictation was done in her presence. It was done immediately after her leaving the exam room.

_____
Jean W. Mooney, PA
Internal Medicine

JWM:pai
D:2/3/----
T:2/3/----

c: Patrick Keathley, MD, Endocrinology

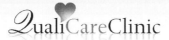

<u>**Orthopedic Spine Clinic Followup Note**</u>

Patient Name: Tracy M. Dooley   **PCP:** Carol Dodds, MD

Date of Exam: 10 Nov ----   **Age/Sex:** 49-year-old male   **ID#:** M-92

HISTORY: Tracy is a 49-year-old male who has been seen over the years by Dr. Lee and me in the spine clinic. He presents now with progressive low back pain and gait difficulty over the past 4 to 5 months. Patient underwent diskectomy and decompression of the lower lumbar region approximately 6 or 7 years ago. We do not have an operative report for all the detailed information. Patient suffered a closed head injury in an MVA in the early 1980s and has a leg-length discrepancy that is of concern to the patient and his father.

Today his primary issues include worsening low back pain and clumsiness of gait. Since his last visit 2 years ago, patient has not been on a regimented physical therapy program. He has had no injections. He denies radicular or bowel/bladder dysfunction.

ALLERGIES: None.

MEDICATIONS: None.

PAST MEDICAL HISTORY: As in HPI. Closed head injury with subsequent spasticity and issues related to that.

PAST SURGICAL HISTORY: Multiple right femur procedures. Left foot procedures. Lumbar spine decompression.

PHYSICAL EXAMINATION

Patient is awake, alert, oriented, in no acute distress. Examination of the back reveals a well-healed surgical midline scar in the lumbar region. He has mild tenderness to palpation in the paraspinal musculature. Patient has slightly more lordosis at the lumbar region. He has 5/5 strength in extensor hallucis longus, tibialis anterior, gastrocnemius soleus, hamstrings bilaterally. Sensation is intact to light touch in all distributions. He has bilateral flexion contractures of the knees. He has left forefoot deformities from previous surgeries, with some overlap of the digits. Patient has 2+ Achilles and hamstring deep tendon reflexes. There is no clonus. Patient has a pelvic obliquity with left leg discrepancy, with the right leg being short.

ASSESSMENT
Increasing low back pain in a patient with previous closed head injury and a previous lumbar decompressive surgery.

PLAN
1. Today we will obtain x-rays of the lumbar spine. He has had no x-rays for the past 2 years.
2. Previous films showed some degenerative changes as well as bilateral L5 spondylolysis.
3. Magnetic resonance scan of the L-spine (with gadolinium) will be performed as well to ensure no nerve root compression or disk disease.
4. Neurology consult was placed for evaluation and possible nonsurgical management of his gait disturbance.
5. Physical Therapy consult was placed so patient could have instruction on core stabilization and paraspinal strengthening exercises.

(Continued)

ID#: M-92   PAGE 2

6. Patient will follow up after these studies have been performed, at which time (depending on what our evaluation shows) he is interested in having an evaluation for his left forefoot deformities. These have been treated in the past.

_____
Gilbert M. Fields, MD
Orthopedic Spine Clinic

GMF:pai
D:11/10/----
T:11/11/----

c: T. Washington King, MD, Neurology
    Michael Baker, MD, Physical Medicine & Rehabilitation
    Carol Dodds, MD, Orthopedics

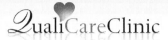

<u>**Emergency Department Treatment Record**</u>

Patient Name: Salvatore Menchaca   **PCP:** Unknown

Date of Exam: 29 Oct ----   **Age/Sex:** 30ish Hispanic male   **ID#:** M-93

MODE OF ARRIVAL: Level III EMS transfer.

CONSULTING SERVICE: Trauma Surgery.

HISTORY OF PRESENT ILLNESS: This is a Hispanic male, 30 years old or so, who was allegedly assaulted at approximately 0300 hours and found south of the city, from where he was taken to the nearest hospital and stabilized. Apparently some CT scans and x-rays were done. Patient was diagnosed with multiple facial fractures and intoxication, and he was transferred here for further evaluation and care.

On arrival the patient is agitated, combative. He was not boarded or collared by EMS. They stated that they had to give him several rounds of Ativan to keep this patient asleep. Also, they had to restrain him with a 5-point restraint.

MEDICATIONS: Unknown and unable to obtain.

ALLERGIES: Unknown.

REVIEW OF SYSTEMS: Unable to obtain.

PAST MEDICAL/SURGICAL HISTORY: Unknown.

SOCIAL HISTORY: Unknown, although apparently by report this patient is either a crack or a cocaine user.

FAMILY HISTORY: Also unable to obtain. Historian is EMS.

PHYSICAL EXAMINATION

VITAL SIGNS on presentation: Blood pressure 136/68, heart rate 89, respirations 12, temperature 100.1, saturations 100% on nonrebreather. Vital signs prior to transfer to CT scan by Surgery were blood pressure of 170/88, heart rate 92, respirations 12, saturations 100% via endotracheal tube. In general, this is a combative, restrained, somnolent man with obvious massive trauma to his face who is neither collared nor boarded. HEENT: The conjunctivae are completely edematous and periorbital area is edematous, and so we cannot actually see his eyes. Nose is full of blood with a lot of edema. Tympanic membranes are clear. His oropharynx reveals teeth to be normally aligned. There are no broken teeth. He does have a lot of blood pooled in the back of his throat and on his tongue. Buccal mucosa is intact. Head shows notable edema and ecchymoses throughout his anterior face, particularly on his left maxilla and zygomatic arch. NECK: Supple, nontender, trachea midline. No cervical spine tenderness. LUNGS are clear to auscultation bilaterally. ABDOMEN is soft, nontender, nondistended. HEART: Normal heart tones. BACK: No obvious injury. His thoracic, lumbar, and sacral spines are without step-off. We do not know if there is tenderness because patient is intubated during back exam. GENITALIA are without injury. EXTREMITIES: His hips are stable and nontender. His 4 extremities also are without injuries except for slight abrasion to his proximal left forearm. Patient is moving all 4 extremities spontaneously. He is combative. His Glasgow coma score initially was approximately a 6 or 7. Upon awakening, patient did relate his name and was moving all 4 extremities spontaneously, probably likely more of a 10, one for eyes, four for verbal, and five for musculoskeletal.

(Continued)

ID#: M-93   PAGE 2

DIAGNOSTIC STUDIES: Chest x-ray was without a fracture, pneumothorax, or infiltrate. Endotracheal tube was in good place. FAST exam was negative.

EMERGENCY DEPARTMENT DIAGNOSES
1. Status post alleged assault with multiple facial injuries.
2. Endotracheal intubation.
3. Altered mental status.

MEDICAL DECISION MAKING: Differential diagnosis on his altered mental status is alcohol withdrawal, some other drug intoxication or withdrawal, as well as possible Ativan sequelae. It is also possible that this patient has intracranial bleed from his assault. Patient was intubated for airway protection as he was very agitated and combative in the trauma bay and needed to have his cervical spine protected, airway protected, as well as have some decisive imaging.

PROCEDURE NOTE: Patient was intubated on the second attempt by Dr. McClure with a 7.5 endotracheal tube at 22 at the teeth. Cords were visualized. We had end-tidal CO_2 change in bilateral breath sounds, and no sounds over his gastric. Chest x-ray verified the endotracheal tube in place.

DISPOSITION: Patient was escorted by Dr. Stolga of Trauma Surgery to the CT scan and will be admitted to the surgical intensive care unit (SICU).

TRAUMA BAY COURSE: Patient was initially given 20 mg of etomidate, then 100 mg of succinylcholine. Post intubation he was given another 2 mg of Ativan as well as 40 mcg/kg/min of propofol and 10 mg of vecuronium. Tetanus status had been updated at the previous hospital.

Patient was seen and discussed with Dr. Stolga, who was in attendance during the entire trauma resuscitation.

_____
Samuel Ernest, MD
Emergency Room Physician

SE:pai
D:10/29/----
T:10/29/----

c: Mack Stolga, MD, Trauma Surgery

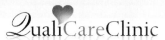

Internal Medicine Geriatrics Clinic Followup Note

Patient Name: Paul DuBose **PCP:** Martha C. Eaton, MD

Date of Exam: 3 Feb ----   **Age/Sex:** 84-year-old male   **ID#:** M-94

CHIEF COMPLAINT: Mr. DuBose presents in routine followup to discuss diabetes mellitus, type 2.

HISTORY OF PRESENT ILLNESS
1. Diabetes mellitus, type 2: All of his blood sugars have been in an excellent range, from 113 to 126. He feels well and most days he does not take glyburide. If his blood sugar rises above 130, he will generally take 1 tablet.
2. Sinus bradycardia: He had a pacemaker placed on 30 Aug last year. He continues to do well. Has excellent energy. No signs of congestive heart failure, has regained all of his weight lost during his overriding illness. He is active, healthy, and will follow up with Cardiology in 3 weeks' time.
3. Atrial fibrillation: Continues with a controlled ventricular rate and feels well. No angina or congestive heart failure.
4. Iron deficiency anemia, for which he had a full workup last year: He had an esophagogastroduodenoscopy and colonoscopy. He was seen by Hematology/Oncology and started on Procrit. He was given intravenous iron twice. His last several blood counts showed good replacement of lost blood volume. Coumadin was stopped briefly but has been reinstituted, and he continues to take iron.
5. Hypertension: Excellent control on the current medications. He did not bring in blood pressures today but says most of them are in the 120 to 140 range.
6. Benign prostatic hypertrophy: He takes Flomax for this and is doing well.

MEDICATIONS
1. Isordil 20 mg t.i.d.
2. Flomax 0.4 mg daily.
3. Lasix 60 mg in a.m. and 40 mg in p.m.
4. Zocor 80 mg at bedtime.
5. Candesartan 32 mg at bedtime.
6. Lopressor 100 mg b.i.d.
7. Iron 325 mg b.i.d.
8. Coumadin as directed by the Coumadin Clinic.
9. Lisinopril 40 mg daily.
10. Calcitriol 0.25 mcg daily.

REVIEW OF SYSTEMS

CONSTITUTIONAL: No fevers, chills, or weight change.

RESPIRATORY: No shortness of breath, cough, or hemoptysis.

CARDIOVASCULAR: No chest pain, palpitations, or edema.

GASTROENTEROLOGY: No abdominal pain, nausea, vomiting, diarrhea, constipation, melena, or hematochezia. No hematemesis.

GENITOURINARY: No dysuria, incontinence, or hematuria.

(Continued)

ID#: M-94   PAGE 2

PHYSICAL EXAMINATION found a pleasant 84-year-old gentleman with blood pressure 155/70, heart rate 78, respirations 18, temperature 97.1, height 71 inches, weight 88 kg. He is in no pain and is not a smoker.

HEENT exam found extraocular muscles intact. Pupils are equal, round, and reactive. No scleral icterus. Oral exam is benign with moist mucous membranes. No pharyngitis.

NECK: Supple with no adenopathy or thyromegaly.

LUNGS: Clear to auscultation bilaterally with no wheeze, rales, or rhonchi.

HEART is irregularly irregular with a 2/6 systolic murmur best heard in the upper left sternal border.

ABDOMEN: Soft, nontender, with normoactive bowel sounds.

EXTREMITIES are without edema.

NEUROLOGIC exam is nonfocal, with normal gait and stance. No abnormal movements. He is fully intact cognitively. Mood is euthymic.

DIAGNOSTIC DATA on 11 Jan ---- showed iron 61, total iron-binding capacity 225, iron saturation 27%, ferritin normal at 342. PT and INR 27.1 and 2.5, respectively. Hemoglobin 14.6, hematocrit 42.1. Previous H&H on 30 Nov ---- were 15.2 and 43.8.

ASSESSMENT
1. Diabetes mellitus, type 2: Excellent control without medication. He takes a small dose of glyburide as needed if blood sugars become elevated, most likely from dietary indiscretions. Will continue the current plan and follow.
2. Bradycardia with a pacemaker and overall doing well. No signs of congestive failure or angina.
3. Atrial fibrillation with a controlled ventricular rate. Overall doing well.
4. Iron deficiency anemia, for which he has remained with an excellent hemoglobin and hematocrit off Procrit.

PLAN
1. Stop iron.
2. In 2 months will recheck hemoglobin and hematocrit and iron panel to determine whether he still needs to be taking iron. If a significant decrease is noted in either H&H or iron levels, will reconsider starting.
3. Hypertension. Blood pressures appear from his description to be in good control but blood pressure is elevated today. Check blood pressures for 1 week, then contact me.
4. Benign prostatic hypertrophy, for which he takes Flomax. That is being changed to Uroxatral (alfuzosin). Will change over his medication today.
5. Health care maintenance: Up to date. Follow up with me in 2 to 3 months, sooner as needed.

_____

Jean W. Mooney, PA
Endocrinology

JWM:pai
D:2/3/----
T:2/4/----

c: Martha C. Eaton, MD, Family Practice/Geriatrics

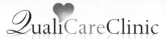

Orthopedic Clinic Followup Note

Patient Name: Jimmy Wu   **CP:** Marie Aaron, DO

Date of Exam: 19 June ----   **Age/Sex:** 50-year-old male   **ID#:** M-95

HISTORY: This is a 50-year-old right-hand dominant Asian male who sustained an injury to his right middle finger while playing softball on 3 June. He was placed in an AlumaFoam splint in the ED and is at the orthopedic clinic today. The patient denies any other injuries.

PAST MEDICAL/SURGICAL HISTORY: The patient has a past history of a hernia.

SOCIAL HISTORY: The patient works in a finance office.

MEDICATIONS: None.

ALLERGIES: He has no known drug allergies.

REVIEW OF SYSTEMS: Negative for any other complaints.

PHYSICAL EXAMINATION

The patient is right-hand dominant. The exam reveals that he has tenderness to palpation and swelling involving the distal phalanx and distal interphalangeal joint of his middle finger. He is able to flex and extend the DIP joint with some pain. He has brisk capillary refill and intact sensation in his finger. Otherwise, his AI, PI, radial, medial, and ulnar nerves are intact. Motor and sensation are intact.

X-ray reveals a nondisplaced fracture at the base of the distal phalanx, right middle finger.

IMPRESSION

Right middle finger nondisplaced P3 (third phalanx) fracture.

PLAN

We will place Mr. Wu in a Stax splint, which he is to wear for an additional 2 weeks. He may then come out of it and start range of motion to his distal interphalangeal joint. Follow up with us if he has any complaints.

_____

Raquel Rodriguez, MD
Orthopedics Hand Clinic

RR:pai
D:6/20/----
T:6/21/----

c: Marie Aaron, DO, Family Practice

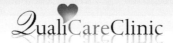

Emergency Department Treatment Record

Patient Name: Leonard Gonzales   **PCP:** Unknown

Date of Exam: 16 Oct ----   **Age/Sex:** 41-year-old male   **ID#:** M-96

Date of Birth: 23 June ----

MODE OF ARRIVAL: Code 3, EMS.

HISTORY OF PRESENT ILLNESS: This is a 41-year-old male who was brought unresponsive to the ED after having been found pinned underneath a large truck. It appears that he may have been working underneath the truck; however, the events surrounding this are unknown. EMS was called, arrived, found the patient under the vehicle. He was extracted, and he was found to have no pulses and no vital signs at that time. Therefore, CPR was initiated. He was intubated in the field, placed on a gurney, placed in the ambulance, and brought Code 3 to our facility with CPR throughout en route. Upon arrival patient had a GCS of 3.

PRIMARY SURVEY

    A: Patient was intubated.
    B: He had clear breath sounds bilaterally. Blood was noted in the ET tube.
    C: He had no pulses without CPR; however, he did have good femoral and carotid pulses with CPR.
    D: Again, his Glasgow coma score was 3.
    E: He has multiple abrasions and lacerations over his chest. No asymmetrical chest motion noted.

SECONDARY SURVEY

VITAL SIGNS on presentation: Blood pressure was not obtainable. He had no pulse and no electrical activity on the monitor. We were unable to get saturation.

EMERGENCY DEPARTMENT COURSE: Patient had approximately 20 minutes of CPR in the field and en route prior to arriving at the ED. After approximately 5 minutes of CPR in our facility, we had no return of spontaneous circulation. Bilateral chest tubes were placed, one by Dr. McClure of Emergency Medicine and one by the general surgery intern, on the left and on the right. For procedure notes, please see the written chart. The chest tube put out approximately 350 mL of gross blood immediately after placement.

FAST exam was performed, which showed no blood in Morrison pouch, no organized cardiac activity, and no evidence of tamponade. Cardiac windows: On the spleen, splenorenal recess was hard to visualize secondary to interference and subcutaneous tissue air. Urinary bladder was normal. Abdomen was not distended. At this time, with no organized cardiac activity on echo and electrically and with the prolonged CPR, we opted to pronounce the patient with a time of death of 1614 hours.

Radiology, none. Labs, none.

EMERGENCY DEPARTMENT DIAGNOSES
    1. Massive blunt chest trauma.
    2. Hemothorax.

(Continued)

ID#: M-96

DISPOSITION
Patient died at 1614 hours, and medical examiners were notified for investigation of the case. The City Police were present on arrival as well.

_____

Samuel Ernest, MD
Emergency Room Physician

SE:pai
D:10/16/----
T:10/16/----

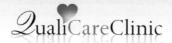

Internal Medicine Clinic Followup Note

Patient Name: Oma Gaye Enderle   **PCP:** Joshua Gatlin, MD

Date of Exam: 28 July ----   **Age/Sex:** 69-year-old female   **ID#:** M-97

REASON FOR VISIT: Annual preventive visit.

HISTORY: Ms. Enderle is a pleasant 69-year-old lady with a past medical history significant for ankylosing spondylitis with restrictive lung disease, gastroesophageal reflux disease, hypertension, and depression. Patient reports that she has been doing okay recently. She has had no acute changes in her health. She states that she will be moving to Ohio in the middle of next month. She will be coming back to Miami intermittently.

Patient reports no significant change in her shortness of breath. She does not wear oxygen during the day. She does wear oxygen at night. She has previously been followed in the pulmonary clinic. She has restrictive lung disease secondary to her kyphosis from her ankylosing spondylitis.

REVIEW OF SYSTEMS: Ms. Enderle denies headaches and visual changes. She has had no difficulty swallowing or speaking. She has had no pain with swallowing. Denies epigastric pain, nausea, vomiting, abdominal pain, bright red blood per rectum, and melena. She has had no cough or hemoptysis. She has had no urinary incontinence or dysuria. No new musculoskeletal complaints. She is sleeping okay, and her mood has been okay.

PAST MEDICAL HISTORY
1. Ankylosing spondylitis.
2. Restrictive lung disease.
3. Gastroesophageal reflux disease.
4. Hypertension.
5. Depression.
6. Likely osteoporosis. (Patient has been unable to perform a bone mineral density test secondary to her limited ability to lie flat secondary to her ankylosing spondylitis.)

PAST SURGICAL HISTORY: Has had cataracts removed from both eyes.

FAMILY HISTORY: She has a daughter with diabetes. Her sister has a history of breast cancer. There is no family history of coronary artery disease.

SOCIAL HISTORY: Patient quit tobacco in 1985. She had an approximate 8-pack-year history. She has never been a drinker. Is not sexually active.

MEDICATIONS
1. Fosamax 70 mg weekly.
2. Tolmetin VS 400 mg t.i.d. p.r.n.
3. Flexeril 10 mg p.r.n.
4. Lopressor 100 mg b.i.d.
5. Hydrochlorothiazide 25 mg daily.
6. Prevacid 30 mg daily.
7. Combivent 2 to 4 puffs p.r.n.
8. Advair Diskus 250/50 mcg, 1 puff b.i.d.
9. Celexa 40 mg daily.

ALLERGIES: No known drug allergies.

(Continued)

ID#: M-97   PAGE 2

PHYSICAL EXAMINATION

Blood pressure 132/58, pulse 83, respirations 20, temperature 99.1, height 5 feet 3 inches, weight 65.5 kg.
She denies pain. In general she is a well-nourished, well-developed Caucasian lady in no acute distress.
HEENT: Pupils are equal, round, and reactive to light and accommodation. Extraocular muscles intact.
Tympanic membranes clear bilaterally. Oropharynx is moist and pink without erythema or exudates.
NECK: Supple without bruits. CARDIOVASCULAR EXAM: Regular rate and rhythm with normal S1,
S2 and no S3 or S4. No murmur. CHEST: Clear to auscultation bilaterally. ABDOMEN: Soft, nontender,
nondistended with no organomegaly. LOWER EXTREMITIES: No clubbing, cyanosis, or edema.
MUSCULOSKELETAL: Patient has notable kyphosis to approximately 30 degrees. BREAST EXAM: Patient
has no skin changes. There is no palpable axillary lymphadenopathy. No palpable masses.

LABORATORY DATA: Recent laboratory studies dated 18 July: Vitamin B12 330, folate 13.6. White blood cells
7.1, hemoglobin 11.2, hematocrit 35, MCV 79.3, platelets 355. Reticulocyte fraction is elevated at 0.380. LFTs are
within normal limits. Glucose 79, BUN 28, creatinine of 0.9, sodium of 139, potassium 4.2, calcium 9.3, albumin
4.3. Iron 24, TIBC is elevated at 419, iron saturation at 6%, and ferritin is low at 21.

ASSESSMENT
A 69-year-old white lady with past medical history as listed above. She is doing okay at this time with new finding
of iron deficiency anemia.

PLAN
1. Iron deficiency anemia: Patient had a colonoscopy in the early 1990s. She has had no recent screening.
   Discussed with her the importance of followup gastroenterology appointment for consideration of upper and
   lower endoscopy. In the meantime, she is to begin iron 325 mg b.i.d. She is currently asymptomatic with no
   chest pain, shortness of breath, or lightheadedness.
2. Ankylosing spondylitis: Patient has been followed in the rheumatology clinic. She takes tolmetin and Flexeril
   p.r.n. pain. She has no acute complaints, and these meds have worked for her in the past.
3. Gastroesophageal reflux disease: Patient's symptoms are well controlled with Prevacid 30 mg daily. She is to
   continue this at the current dose.
4. Hypertension: Good control on Lopressor and hydrochlorothiazide. Will continue these at their current doses.
5. Depression: Patient is euthymic. She is to continue her Celexa 40 mg daily.
6. Osteoporosis: Patient is to continue her Fosamax 70 mg once daily with calcium and vitamin D. She has had
   no recent falls.
7. Restrictive lung disease: No recent change in her symptoms. She is to continue to wear her oxygen at night as
   directed by the pulmonary clinic.
8. Healthcare maintenance: Patient had a pneumococcal vaccine 3 years ago. She receives the influenza vaccine
   annually. She had an eye exam 2 years ago. Her last mammogram was in February last year. Her annual
   screening mammogram has been ordered. Patient's lipid profile was checked this January and was at goal.

(Continued)

ID#: M-97 PAGE 3

DISPOSITION: Patient is to follow up with her new PCP in Ohio as soon as she establishes residency. We will forward her records on request. I told her that she is welcome to follow up with me at any time she returns to Miami.

_____

Jean W. Mooney, PA
Internal Medicine

JWM:pai
D:7/28/----
T:7/29/----

c: Luke Mosbacker, MD, Rheumatology Clinic
   Joshua Gatlin, MD, Pulmonology Clinic

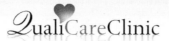

Orthopedic Spine Clinic Followup Note

Patient Name: Bernadette Dolly   **PCP:** Susan McGinnis, MD

Date of Exam: 10 June ----   **Age/Sex:** 22-year-old female   **ID#:** M-99

HISTORY: Bernadette is a 22-year-old female who has been followed in the past by Dr. Fields for a bilateral L5 pars defect and anterolisthesis. There has been a stable listhesis since the age of 12 when she was first evaluated. She performed in gymnastics for several years and has had intermittent pain over the course of her career. States that she was working in a cheerleading camp last week when she developed an exacerbation of her back pain. Patient denies any pain into her lower extremities. Denies any difficulty with bladder or bowel function. She returns today for evaluation.

PHYSICAL EXAMINATION

Patient has no midline tenderness to palpation. She has good range of motion of the lumbar spine. Has pain on extension of the lumbar spine. She is able to ambulate and toe-heel walk without difficulty. She has negative straight-leg raise and cross straight-leg raise tests. Neurologic exam reveals that she has 5/5 strength of her iliopsoas, quad, hamstring, anterior tibialis, extensor hallucis longus, gastric psoas, and peroneals. Sensation is intact to light touch throughout the lower extremities. She has downgoing toes and no clonus.

X-RAY DATA: X-rays of lumbar spine were obtained and compared with previous x-rays since she was 12 years old. These revealed bilateral L5 pars defect with anterolisthesis of L5-S1 measuring approximately 27% in anterolisthesis. This is unchanged from all previous films.

ASSESSMENT/PLAN

A 22-year-old female with L5-S1 anterolisthesis secondary to bilateral pars defect with exacerbation of her back pain. She has no radicular symptoms, no neurologic deficits.

At this time, Bernadette was counseled that she should treat her back pain conservatively with antiinflammatories, rest, ice, heat, and massage. She should be stretching and strengthening her trunk muscles. She was warned that she has a small risk of this progressing and was instructed to follow up with us if she develops severe back pain that causes her to limit her activities of daily living or if she develops neurologic or radicular-type symptoms.

There were no barriers to communication, and patient agreed to the above plan.

_____

Gilbert M. Fields, MD
Orthopedic Surgeon

GMF:pai
D:6/10/----
T:6/11/----

c: Susan McGinnis, MD, Family Practice

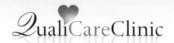

Emergency Department Treatment Record

Patient Name: Barbara Christine Anello   **PCP:** Reed Phillips, MD

Date of Exam: 31 Oct ----   **Age/Sex:** 8-month-old female   **ID#:** M-100

CHIEF COMPLAINT: Possible shaken baby syndrome.

CONSULTATION: Pediatrics and Trauma Surgery Service. Taken to CT scanner at 1230 hours.

MODE OF ARRIVAL: EMS, Code 3.

HISTORY OF PRESENT ILLNESS: An 8-month-old female child was seen at a rural ED today for fever and decreased mental status. Patient underwent a lumbar puncture, which showed gross blood in cerebrospinal fluid. She underwent CT scan of the head, which revealed no blood at that time. Patient was also noted to have retinal hemorrhage in both fundi. Patient with bulging fontanels at the rural ED. Patient was transported Code 3 trauma to our facility for evaluation and admission. Patient with one IV in place during transport. During transport EMS placed patient on spine board with cervical collar in place.

PRIMARY SURVEY

    A: Airway was patent and protected.
    B: Breathing spontaneous bilaterally with equal lung sounds present.
    C: Circulation with good pulses in all 4 extremities.
    D: Disability—patient irritable but awake and responsive to any painful stimuli administered.
    E: Exposure—with log rolling precautions, no additional evidence of trauma was found.

PRIMARY INTERVENTIONS: Oxygen continued, second IV established.

REVIEW OF SYSTEMS: Unobtainable as patient is a minor in the ED.

PAST MEDICAL HISTORY: Unobtainable.

PAST SURGICAL HISTORY: Unobtainable.

MEDICATIONS: Unknown.

ALLERGIES: Unknown.

SOCIAL HISTORY: Patient lives with both parents according to EMS personnel.

SECONDARY SURVEY

VITAL SIGNS on presentation: BP 97/39, HR 185, R 38, T 102 rectally, O_2 sat. 100% with oxygen. In general, the patient appears to be in no acute distress at this time, is nontoxic appearing. She is responsive to all stimulation, though she is very irritable. HEENT: Normocephalic with bulging fontanels noted. Patient with bilateral retinal hemorrhages noted on funduscopic exam. Pupils are equal, round, and reactive to light and accommodation. Extraocular movements intact without strabismus or ptosis. No scleral icterus noted. No external evidence of trauma noted. NECK: No jugular venous distention noted. Trachea is midline without deviation. No C-spine tenderness to palpation noted. CHEST: Equal chest expansion with respirations. Clavicles intact. No deformities to chest wall are noted. CV: Heart tones show regular rate and rhythm without clicks, rubs, or murmurs. RESPIRATORY: Lungs clear to auscultation without adventitious sounds. ABDOMEN is soft, nontender to palpation x4 quadrants. No rebound or guarding noted. Pelvis is intact on inward, downward palpation. EXTREMITIES: No deformities noted to all 4 extremities. She is moving all 4 extremities and has good pulses in all 4 extremities. NEUROLOGIC: Patient is awake, alert, moving all 4 extremities, and is irritable in our ED.

(Continued)

ID#: M-100

EMERGENCY DEPARTMENT COURSE: Patient is taken to trauma bay #3 where she was evaluated. Cervical collar was removed. Patient log rolled with C-spine precautions. A second IV was established. Retinal hemorrhages were confirmed on our exam also. Patient received Claforan with a normal saline bolus of 280 mL while at the rural ED. Laboratory tests were drawn and sent, which will be followed by Pediatrics and Trauma Surgery Service. Patient was then taken to the CT scanner by Trauma Surgery and Pediatrics for further evaluation.

MEDICAL DECISION MAKING: Patient presents with retinal hemorrhages with an expanding fontanel, most likely secondary to shaken baby syndrome. No other evidence of trauma was noted on this patient. She will be admitted to Trauma Surgery Service with Pediatrics to follow all labs and radiographic findings.

PROCEDURES: None.

EMERGENCY DEPARTMENT DIAGNOSES
1. Retinal hemorrhages.
2. Expanding fontanel.
3. Shaken baby syndrome.

DISPOSITION/PLAN
Admission to Pediatrics and Trauma Surgery Service. Dr. Stolga was present for the entire case and agreed with the treatment and plan. Per protocol, the proper officials were notified: Children's Protective Service and the local police.

_____

Samuel Ernest, MD
Emergency Room Physician

SE:pai
D:10/31/----
T:10/31/----

c: Reed Phillips, MD, Pediatrics
   Mack Stolga, MD, Trauma Team

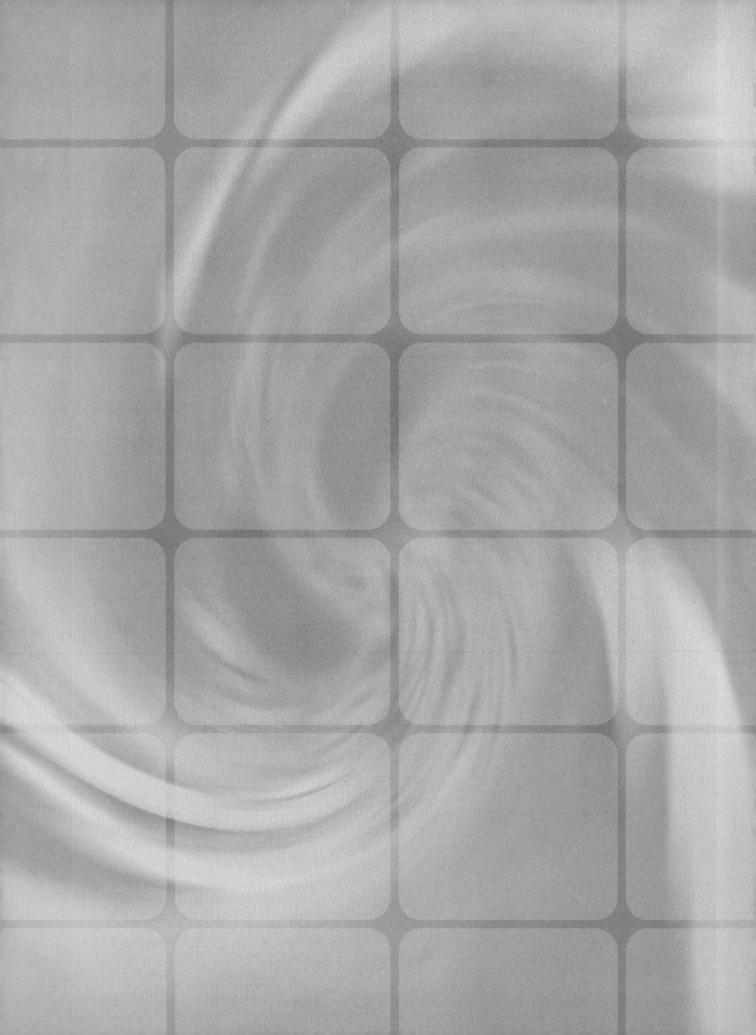

SECTION 2

RADIOLOGY REPORTS

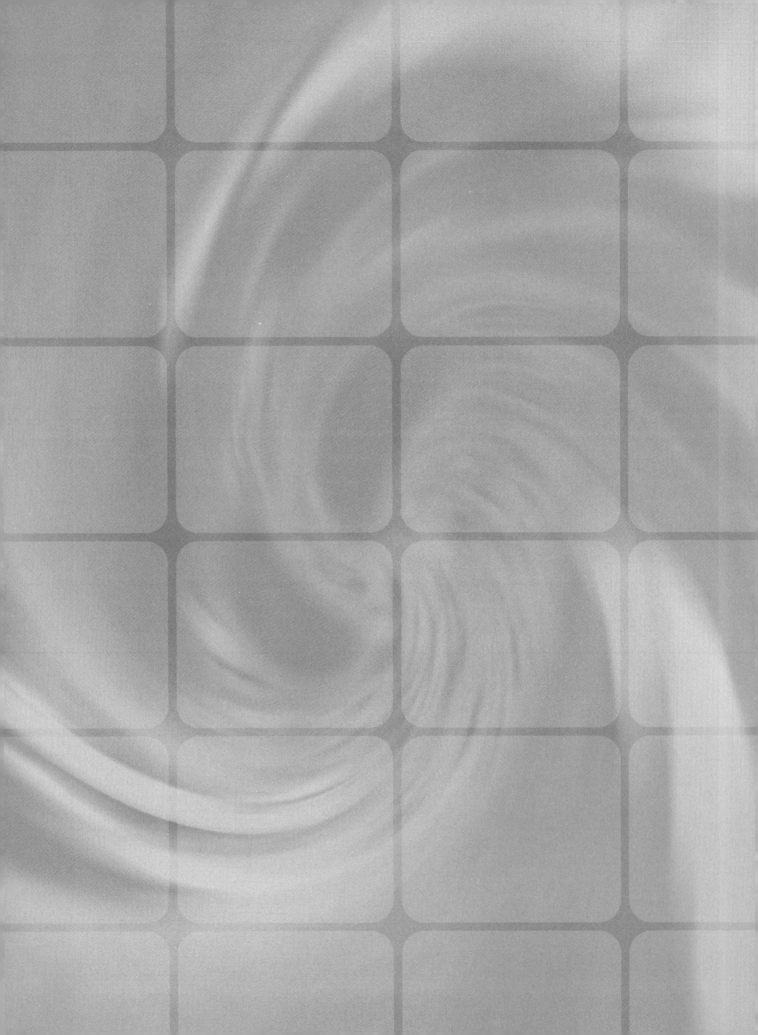

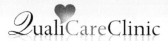

CT Brain Scan

Patient Name: Agnes Wenceslas **PCP:** Marie Aaron, DO

Date of Exam: 22 Mar ---- **Age/Sex:** 52-year-old female **ID#:** R-1

CLINICAL INFORMATION: Migraine headache with aura.

The brain parenchyma demonstrates uniform attenuation. The ventricles, basal cisterns, and cortical sulci appear normal and symmetrical with no evidence of increased intracranial pressure, midline shift, or hydrocephalus. The orbits, sella turcica, and skull base along with the frontal, ethmoid, and sphenoid sinuses appear normal. No extra-axial fluid collection is present.

Postcontrast study demonstrates the major vascular structures within the circle of Willis to be unremarkable. There is no unusual parenchymal enhancement. No aneurysm is seen.

IMPRESSION
Normal study.

_____

George Murray, MD
Radiology

GM:pai
D:3/22/----
T:3/22/----

c: Marie Aaron, DO, Family Practice

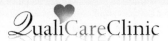

Bilateral Low-Dose Mammograms

Patient Name: Lois Jensen   **PCP:** Rosemary Bumbak, MD

Date of Exam: 29 Apr ----   **Age/Sex:** 51-year-old female   **ID#:** R-2

CLINICAL INFORMATION: Routine yearly mammogram.

There is a small, nonaggressive-appearing mass noted just medial to the level of the nipple deep in the superior aspect of the right breast. This measures 7 mm in diameter. Perhaps a followup study could be obtained in 6 or 7 months to be certain the appearance is stable, assuming that there is no palpable abnormality suggesting the need for biopsy at this time.

No other dominant masses are delineated. There are no clusters of calcification to suggest malignancy.

IMPRESSION
There is a small, nonaggressive-appearing mass deep in the medial superior aspect of the right breast measuring 7 mm in maximum diameter. Perhaps a followup study of only the right breast could be obtained in 6 to 7 months.

NOTE
A negative x-ray report should not delay biopsy if a dominant or clinically suspicious mass is present. Some 4% to 8% of cancers are not identified by x-ray.

Dr. Bumbak has been called and notified of these findings.

_____

George Murray, MD
Radiology

GM:pai
D:4/29/----
T:4/29/----

c: Rosemary Bumbak, MD, OB/GYN Clinic

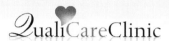

Right Breast Mammogram

Patient Name: Lois Jensen   **PCP:** Rosemary Bumbak, MD

Date of Exam: 9 Aug ----   **Age/Sex:** 51-year-old female   **ID#:** R-3

CLINICAL INFORMATION: Followup study, right breast.

ADDENDUM: The small mass deep in the medial superior aspect of the right breast is very difficult to identify in the outside mammograms from 2 years ago, which have been obtained for comparison. I believe the mass was probably there, although I cannot be completely certain, and I still believe that it would be advisable to obtain followup radiographs of the right breast 6 to 7 months from the study done on 29 April of this year to be certain that the appearance is stable.

There was a question of a small mass in the left breast on the outside study of 30 July two years ago, but I cannot identify this with certainty on our study from this year in April.

_____

George Murray, MD
Radiology

GM:pai
D:9/8/----
T:9/8/----

c: Rosemary Bumbak, MD, OB/GYN Clinic

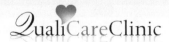

Pain Management

Patient Name: Christopher Lorenes   **PCP:** Mark L. Haskill, MD
Date of Exam: 10 Aug ----   **Age/Sex:** 44-year-old male   **ID#:** R-4

Pain management utilizing steroid injection, intermediate joint. Fluoroscopic-guided anesthetic steroid injection to talonavicular joint, calcaneocuboid joint, and cubonavicular joint.

After obtaining informed consent, the patient was prepped and draped in the usual sterile fashion. Using fluoroscopic guidance, a 25-gauge needle was placed into the 3 individual joints: talonavicular joint, calcaneocuboid joint, and cubonavicular joint.

Each joint was infused with a solution containing Marcaine and Kenalog. The patient tolerated the procedure well, and there were no immediate complications. The patient's preprocedure pain level was 10 on a scale from 0 to 10. The postprocedural pain level was reduced to zero. The patient was given a pain diary and instructed to follow up with Dr. Haskill as per his instructions.

IMPRESSION
Successful anesthetic steroid injection of the talonavicular, calcaneocuboid, and cubonavicular joints.

_____
George Murray, MD
Radiology
Electronically signed: 10 Aug ---- at 3:08 p.m.

GM:pai
D:8/10/----
T:8/10/----

c: Mark L. Haskill, MD, Orthopedic Surgery

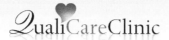

MRI, Left Knee

Patient Name: Benjamin Helland   **PCP:** Jesse D. Smith, MD

Date of Exam: 4 Aug ----   **Age/Sex:** 40-year-old male   **ID#:** R-5

CLINICAL INDICATION: Sprained ankle and knee pain. Status post fracture, age 14, with left ankle surgery.

TECHNIQUE: Sagittal T1-weighted and STIR images. Axial proton-density and STIR images. Coronal proton-density fat-saturated FSE images.

FINDINGS: The Achilles tendon and plantar fascia are intact. There are mild degenerative changes in the dorsal aspect of the calcaneocuboid joint with subchondral bone marrow reaction in the cuboid and anterior process to the calcaneus. The tarsometatarsal joints are intact.

Degenerative changes are seen in the talonavicular joint with joint space narrowing and dorsal osteophyte formation. A focal 5 mm subchondral bone marrow reaction is seen in the center of the distal talar articular surface with corresponding changes in the proximal navicular. A joint effusion is present with an additional fluid collection at the dorsolateral aspect of the talonavicular joint measuring 1 x 2 cm. There is a small 3 mm marrow-containing loose body at the lateral aspect of the joint with an additional 5 mm loose body within the dorsolateral fluid collection adjacent to the extensor retinaculum.

The subtalar joints and sinus tarsi are intact. The ankle joint shows no evidence of significant effusion. There is a small 5 mm osteochondral lesion on the anterior aspect of the distal tibial articular surface. A small bone island is seen in the center of the talar dome without osteochondral lesion of the talar dome. Small metal artifacts are seen near the medial malleolus and near the lateral aspect of the extensor retinaculum—present from previous surgery.

The ligaments about the ankle are intact. There is a large, 1 cm accessory navicular bone in the distal insertion to posterior tibial tendon without bone marrow edema or tendon abnormality. The rest of the medial, lateral, and anterior tendons about the ankle are intact.

IMPRESSION

1. Small osteochondral lesion on the anterior aspect of the distal tibial articular surface as well as postoperative changes at the medial and lateral aspects of the ankle joint.
2. Degenerative changes involving the dorsal aspect of the calcaneocuboid joint and the entire talonavicular joint. Small loose body in the lateral aspect of the talonavicular joint with additional loose body within a dorsolateral fluid collection adjacent to the extensor retinaculum. This finding may represent a synovial cyst or bursal fluid collection.

_____

George Murray, MD
Radiology

GM:pai
D:8/4/----
T:8/4/----

c: Jesse D. Smith, Orthopedic Surgery

QualiCareClinic

Carotid Ultrasound

Patient Name: J. Bruce Randolph   **PCP:** Nancy Lawrence, MD

Date of Exam: 18 April ----   **Age/Sex:** 82-year-old male   **ID#:** R-6

B-Mode Ultrasound/Color Flow-Directed Pulsed Doppler evaluation was performed. Real-time spectral waveform analysis performed at 7.5 and/or 5.0 MHz with Doppler angle optimized to 60 degrees when possible.*

Duplex assessment of the carotid bifurcations performed. Calcific plaquing noted at the take-off of the right ICA. There is some plaquing along the take-off of the left ECA. Spectral analysis shows peak-systolic velocity in the right CC of 154 cm/sec, end-diastolic velocity of 16 cm/sec.

Peak-systolic velocity in the left CCA is 106 cm/sec, end-diastolic velocity of 10 cm/sec. Peak left bulb/ICA velocity of 112 cm/sec, end-diastolic velocity of 19 cm/sec.

Cephalad flow noted in both vertebral arteries.

No hemodynamically significant flow-reducing stenosis detected.

CONCLUSION
Duplex assessment of the carotid bifurcations negative for hemodynamically significant flow-reduction stenosis.

*TECHNICAL NOTE
Doppler percent stenosis estimates are based upon Strandness duplex criteria. Correlation with angiographic percent stenosis should be based upon the ratio of the residual bulb diameter to the distal normal ICA diameter as in NASCET.

_____

George Murray, MD
Radiology

GM:pai
D:4/18/----
T:4/18/----

c: Nancy Lawrence, MD, Internal Medicine

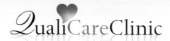

Bilateral Mammograms

Patient Name: Bonnie Gentry Parker   **PCP:** Rosemary Bumbak, MD

Date of Exam: 15 Feb ----   **Age/Sex:** 58-year-old female   **ID#:** R-7

PERTINENT HISTORY: No current symptoms. Correlation is made with previous examination of one year ago.

DISCUSSION: No interval change. The faint outline of a small, bean-shaped, 10 x 8 mm nodule projects medially in the posterior third of the right breast. It was present before. A few subtle, ill-defined, nodular densities can be seen in the left breast, but they, too, were present before. There is no lobulated or spiculated mass suggestive of malignancy. No suspicious calcification or architectural distortion identified.

RECOMMENDATION: Monthly patient self-breast exam (SBE), annual screening mammogram, and annual clinical evaluation.

IMPRESSION
No evidence for malignancy.
BI-RADS Category 2.
Benign findings.

_____

George Murray, MD
Radiology

GM:pai
D:2/15/----
T:2/15/----

c: Rosemary Bumbak, MD, OB/GYN Clinic

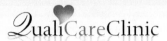

Right Upper Quadrant Sonogram

Patient Name: Yolanda Benavides   **PCP:** Don Richards, MD

Date of Exam: 2 Sept ----   **Age/Sex:** 45-year-old female   **ID#:** R-8

CLINICAL INDICATION: Abdominal pain.

Multiple sonographic images of the right upper quadrant of the abdomen were obtained in the usual fashion. The gallbladder has multiple stones present within it, which cast acoustical shadows. There is no evidence of thickening of the gallbladder wall. The common bile duct is dilated, measuring 8.5 mm in diameter, but no stones can be seen in the common bile duct. The pancreas is within normal limits. There is no free fluid in the upper abdomen. The right kidney is normal.

IMPRESSION

1. Gallstones present within the gallbladder.
2. Dilated common bile duct of 8.5 mm, but no stone can be identified in the common bile duct.
3. The remainder of the study is within normal limits.

_____

George Murray, MD
Radiology

GM:pai
D:9/2/----
T:9/2/----

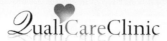

Acute Abdominal Series

Patient Name: Yolanda Benavides   **PCP:** Don Richards, MD

Date of Exam: 2 Sept ----   **Age/Sex:** 45-year-old female   **ID#:** R-9

CLINICAL INDICATION: Abdominal pain.

CHEST: Mediastinal structures within normal limits. The lungs are clear.

ABDOMEN: Supine and Upright Views: Bowel gas pattern is nonspecific. Large amount of fecal material is seen throughout the colon. No obstruction or ileus. The bony structures and soft tissues are otherwise unremarkable.

IMPRESSION
Retained fecal material in the colon but negative exam otherwise.

_____

George Murray, MD
Radiology

GM:pai
D:9/2/----
T:9/2/----

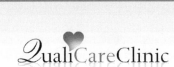

Ultrasound-Guided Left Hip Aspiration

Patient Name: Lula Belle Shaefer   **PCP:** Martha C. Eaton, MD

Date of Exam: 11/30/----   **Age/Sex:** 85/Female   **ID#:** R-10

HISTORY: Joint effusion.

COMPARISON: CT of the left hip from 11/28/----.

CONSENT: Procedure was explained to the patient and written informed consent was obtained.

TECHNIQUE—DESCRIPTION OF PROCEDURE: Patient's left hip was prepped and draped in the usual sterile fashion. One percent lidocaine used as a local anesthetic. Under direct fluoroscopic visualization, a 14-gauge catheter was advanced into the left hip joint effusion. Approximately 75 mL of thick, chocolate-colored fluid was removed. Needle was removed and bandage applied. Patient tolerated the procedure with no complications.

IMPRESSION
Technically successful ultrasound-guided aspiration of left hip with removal of approximately 75 mL of chocolate-colored fluid. Patient reported 100% relief of her typical symptoms immediately post procedure.

_____

George Murray, MD
Radiology

GM:cks
D:11/30/----
T:11/30/----

cc: Jesse D. Smith, MD, Orthopedic Surgery
    Martha C. Eaton, MD, Family Practice

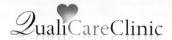

Whole Body Bone Scan

Patient Name: Martha Whitsall   **PCP:** Chris Salem, DO

Date of Exam: 11/13/----   **Age/Sex:** 67/Female   **ID#:** R-11

CLINICAL STATEMENT: DJD.

COMPARISON: Lateral lumbar spine radiograph from one year prior.

TECHNIQUE: Anterior and posterior whole body osseous phase imaging was acquired following intravenous administration of 29.0 mCi Tc 99m labeled MDP.

FINDINGS: Patient gives a history of left hip arthroplasty in 1992 and right hip arthroplasty for revision in 2005.

There is mildly increased activity about the right hip arthroplasty, including some laterally about the expected greater trochanter, possibly within heterotopic bone. The photopenic portion of the femoral head and acetabular cup are somewhat laterally positioned, perhaps by intention. At the left hip, there is moderate to intense abnormal uptake at the DeLee-Charnley zone 1 and moderate increased uptake at zone 3. Centrally the uptake about the acetabular component is thin and very minimal. Radiographic correlation for protrusion is suggested. There is only mild increased uptake about the proximal left hip total arthroplasty femoral component.

Patchy foci of mildly increased uptake at the right mid to distal femoral diaphysis could be postsurgical or related to central medullary infarcts.

There is intense abnormal uptake at the right mid to upper cervical spine in the region of one of the facet joints consistent with metabolically active facet arthritis. Moderate heterogeneous uptake is seen throughout the thoracic spine. There are intense abnormal linear areas of uptake at T12-L3 corresponding to extensive diskogenic change seen on the previous lumbar radiograph. A superimposed compression fracture cannot be excluded—again, radiographic correlation is suggested.

There is moderate arthritic uptake at the acromioclavicular joints, right greater than left. Mild left sternoclavicular arthritic uptake is present. There is mild arthritic uptake at the visualized right elbow joint. Minimal arthritic uptake at both knees and moderate arthritic uptake at both mid feet, right greater than left. Mildly arthritic uptake is seen at the forefeet.

Normal renal uptake is present and no abnormal soft tissue uptake is identified.

IMPRESSION
1. Status post bilateral total hip arthroplasties, as above, most significant for moderate to intense abnormal uptake about the acetabular components of the left hip arthroplasty. Correlation for loosening/acetabular protrusion is suggested on conventional radiographs.
2. Multifocal arthritic changes, as detailed above.
3. Moderate to intense abnormal areas of spondylosis/diskogenic uptake. Specifically, at the T12-L3 levels, there are intense, band-like areas of uptake probably related to metabolically active degenerative disk disease, but correlation with lumbar radiographs is suggested to exclude underlying compression fracture at these levels.

George Murray, MD
Radiology

GM:cks
D:11/13/----
T:11/14/----

cc: Chris Salem, DO, Family Practice
    Carol Dodd, MD, Orthopedic Surgery

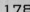

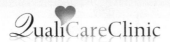

CT of Left Hip

Patient Name: Harold Hines   **PCP:** Susan McGinnis, MD

Date of Exam: 07/24/----   **Age/Sex:** 54/Male   **ID#:** R-12

CLINICAL HISTORY: Patient with history of arthrogryposis. Left hip pain. Evaluate.

High-resolution scans were performed from the left hip joint through the tip of the custom long-stem femoral prosthesis.

FINDINGS: The patient has a custom long-stem left total hip prosthesis. The femoral stem extends to the level of the distal femoral metaphysis. There are 3 cerclage wires in the proximal subtrochanteric left femur. The calcar is eroded but this appears chronic. There is also a prominent 3.5 x 2.0 cm erosion of the undersurface of the tip of the greater trochanter. This appears to be direct erosion secondary to a massive hip joint effusion. There are no definite CT changes of loosening of the femoral component. Very mild asymmetric polyethylene wear is present with 1 mm to 2 mm of differential between superior weight-bearing portion and medial cup. Patient has moderate acetabulum protrusion. No definite CT findings for loosening of the acetabular cup. There is an oval 1.5 x 1.0 cm cyst in the superolateral acetabulum that corresponds to the area of marked increased uptake on bone scan. This could be related to either small-particle disease or to a marginal erosion.

There is a massive presumed left hip joint effusion. Marked soft tissue density circumferentially surrounds the left hip prosthesis. There is extension of fluid into the deep pelvis along the iliopectineal line. There also is a bilobed 6.0 x 3.5 cm mass in the interval between the left gluteus medius and maximus. This measures just above fluid density and probably is a massive joint effusion. Recommend arthrocentesis and evaluation of the fluid.

Associated with the fluid densities are some marginal areas of ossification, both deep in the pelvis and in the gluteal region. The cystic mass in the buttocks lies anterolateral to the sciatic nerve. No visible pubic insufficiency fractures.

There is complete fatty infiltration of the entire extensor musculature. Moderate fatty infiltration of the medial hamstrings and adductor muscles is present. Patient's biceps femoris is relatively unaffected.

IMPRESSION
1. Massive left hip joint effusion with dissection of fluid into the deep pelvis and gluteal region. Consider arthrocentesis.
2. A 1.5 x 1.0 cm area of either small-particle disease or marginal erosion in the superolateral acetabulum.
3. Custom hip prosthesis, which shows no CT evidence for loosening.
4. Moderate acetabulum protrusion of the acetabular cup.
5. Eroded and deficient calcar.
6. A 3.5 x 2.0 cm erosion in the greater trochanter appears to be related to the large joint effusion.
7. Severe muscle atrophy of the left thigh. See above.

_____

George Murray, MD
Radiology

GM:cks
D:07/25/----
T:07/26/----

c: Susan McGinnis, MD, Family Practice
   Jesse D. Smith, MD, Orthopedic Surgery

SECTION 3

SURGICAL REPORTS

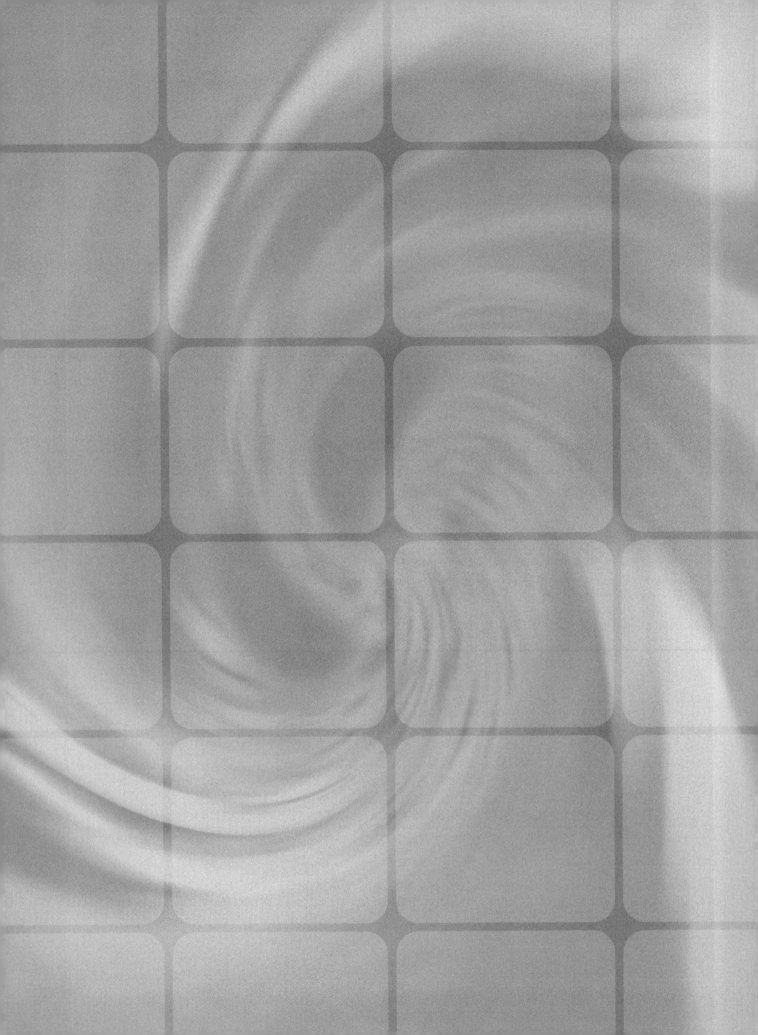

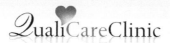

Oromaxillofacial Surgery

Patient Name: Lilly Grace   **ID#:** S-1

Date of Operation: 13 March ----   **Age:** 55   **Sex:** Female

PREOPERATIVE DIAGNOSIS
Obstructive sleep apnea.

POSTOPERATIVE DIAGNOSIS
Obstructive sleep apnea.

SURGEON: Jon Kyle Daily, MD

ASSISTANT: Leela Pivari, MD

ANESTHESIA: General anesthesia given by Dr. Thorner.

OPERATION PERFORMED: Anterior horizontal mandibular osteotomy with genioglossus advancement and suction-assisted submental liposuction.

SPECIMEN REMOVED: None.

MEDICATIONS: Some 3.6 mL of 2% lidocaine with 1:100,000 epinephrine was injected into the surgical sites to establish hemostasis and local anesthesia for the anterior horizontal mandibular osteotomy; 20 mL of a tumescent solution was injected into the submental region to establish hemostasis and local anesthesia for the submental liposuction.

INDICATIONS: This patient was referred to us after having a sleep study done at an outside facility. Her apnea/hypopnea index was 15.1, giving her the diagnosis of moderate sleep apnea. She was first referred to an outside oromaxillofacial surgeon for this procedure; however, the patient discovered that we accept her insurance coverage and asked to be referred to our facility for treatment. She does have mild or moderate obstructive sleep apnea, and this surgery is part of a combined treatment approach to help cure her of her obstructive sleep apnea symptoms.

PROCEDURE IN DETAIL: The patient was identified in the preoperative holding area and was brought to oral surgery operating room #7. Intravenous access had been previously obtained, and after induction of an adequate level of general anesthesia, nasotracheal intubation was accomplished via the right naris atraumatically. The patient was then prepped and draped in the usual sterile manner for a sterile intraoral surgical procedure.

An omega-style incision was made in the anterior mandibular vestibule dissecting down through the muscle to bone. The mental foramen was identified bilaterally, and the nerve was protected. An osteotomy was created 5 mm inferior to the mental foramen as it came up and anterior to the canine. The osteotomy was ramped higher anteriorly in order to preserve as much of the genioglossus attachments as possible. This was accomplished bilaterally. After the osteotomy was completed, the chin was inspected to verify that, in fact, there were attachments of the genioglossus muscles to the genial tubercles after the osteotomy.

The chin was then advanced with a Stryker-Leibinger 8 mm step plate. This was secured in with 6 screws, and the lateral aspects were verified for symmetry. The site was then irrigated thoroughly with sterile saline solution, suctioned free of saliva and debris, and closed with 4-0 Vicryl deep and 3-0 chromic in the mucosa.

A dilute tumescent solution was then injected into the chin. Some 20 mL was used in this tumescent hydrodissection technique. A small puncture site was made directly in the center of the submental area just posterior to the chin in a skin crease. The plane of dissection was just beneath the skin. The suction cannulae were then utilized. A suction-assisted submental liposuction was created in an equal plane bilaterally. Once this was completed, the area was cleaned off, and the site was closed with one 5-0 Prolene suture.

(Continued)

A head wrap and Jobst jaw bra were placed at the end of the procedure, and the patient was then awakened in the operating room. Patient followed commands appropriately and was taken to PAR.

The patient tolerated the procedure well, and there were no apparent complications.

_____
Leela Pivari, MD, for Jon Kyle Daily, MD
Oromaxillofacial Surgery

LP:pai
D:3/13/----
T:3/14/----

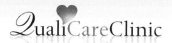

Orthopedic Surgery

Patient Name: Christopher Lee   **ID#:** S-2

Date of Operation: 22 Feb ----   **Age:** 17   **Sex:** Male

PREOPERATIVE DIAGNOSIS
Right ankle chronic instability.

POSTOPERATIVE DIAGNOSIS
Right ankle chronic instability.

SURGEON: Gilbert M. Fields, MD

ASSISTANT: Jack Zullig, MD

ANESTHESIA: General endotracheal with 5 mL Marcaine injected.

OPERATION PERFORMED: Right ankle lateral ligament reconstruction with augmentation with the inferior extensor retinaculum.

SPECIMEN REMOVED: None.

INDICATIONS: Christopher is a 17-year-old male who is a semiprofessional skateboarder and who has sustained multiple right ankle sprains. He now has complained for several months of ankle instability with his skateboarding activities. He has undergone immobilization as well as physical therapy in the past, and he continues to have the instability. The decision was made preoperatively to proceed with anatomic right ankle ligament reconstruction. The risks were discussed with the patient and his mother, including the risk of recurrence, failure to repair, loss of function, decreased range of motion of the ankle, infection, bleeding, damage to adjacent structures, need for further surgery. After we discussed these options and answered all questions, they agreed to proceed with the surgery.

PROCEDURE IN DETAIL: Patient was identified in the holding area by the operating team. The correct limb was marked. Consent was reviewed with the patient and his mother, and they had no further questions and agreed to proceed. The patient was intubated by Anesthesia and taken back to the operating room. He was placed upon the operating room table where induction of general anesthesia with intubation was accomplished without difficulty. Patient was given 1 gram of Ancef prior to the procedure starting. Proximal thigh tourniquet was placed on his right thigh. Sandbag was placed underneath the right hip. The right lower extremity was prepped and draped in the usual sterile fashion.

A curvilinear incision was made just anterior to the fibula. This incision was carried down through skin and subcutaneous tissue to the level of the ankle capsule. Superficial nerves and veins were identified and retracted out of the way. Incision was made midway between the talus and the fibula, curving around to the tip of the fibula. The anterior talofibular ligament (ATFL) was identified within the fibers of the capsule. The calcaneofibular ligament (CFL) was identified. The incision was stopped just prior to entering the peroneal tendon sheath. The ATFL and CFL were then overlapped with the foot held in a dorsiflexed, slightly everted position and a bump under the heel to prevent an anterior drawer. The capsular ligament was then overlapped in a pants-over-vest fashion and sutured using 2-0 Ethibond, which resulted in a very nice repair. The extensor retinaculum was identified and sutured to the tip of the fibula, again using 2-0 Ethibond sutures.

The wound was thoroughly irrigated with normal saline, and the skin was closed with 3-0 Vicryl and 3-0 Monocryl sutures. Steri-Strips were placed as well as Xeroform. Patient was placed into a well-padded AO splint with the foot in dorsiflexion and slight eversion. Patient was awakened from anesthesia without difficulty and taken to PACU for recovery.

(Continued)

ID#: S-2

SPONGE COUNT: All counts verified x2.

TOURNIQUET TIME: 67 minutes at 250 mmHg.

ESTIMATED BLOOD LOSS: Minimal.

URINE OUTPUT: Not recorded.

INTRAVENOUS FLUIDS: 1100 mL.

POSTOPERATIVE PLAN will be for patient to be nonweightbearing and in a splint for 2 weeks. We will then place him into a short leg walking cast for an additional 4 weeks. At the 6-week point, we will allow him to start working on ankle range of motion. He is to have no formal physical therapy until the 3-month point.

_____

Gilbert M. Fields, MD
Orthopedic Surgery

GMF:pai
D:2/22/----
T:2/23/----

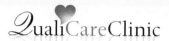

Genitourinary Surgery

Patient Name: Raul Armando Rodriguez
Date of Operation: 3 Feb ----

Age: 16 months old

ID#: S-3
Sex: Male

PREOPERATIVE DIAGNOSIS
Distal shaft hypospadias.

POSTOPERATIVE DIAGNOSIS
Distal shaft hypospadias.

SURGEON: Charles Mendesz, MD

ASSISTANT: Anna Marie Iaccarino, RN, Scrub Nurse

ANESTHESIA: General endotracheal by Chuck Delaney, MD

OPERATIONS PERFORMED
1. Transverse island prepucial flap hypospadias repair.
2. Circumcision.

SPECIMEN REMOVED: Foreskin.

INDICATIONS: Raul is an otherwise healthy 16-month-old, 40-week term infant who now meets appropriate anesthesia criteria for distal shaft hypospadias repair. He has no urinary tract history. Parents note a bit of ventral curve to the penis upon erection, and the patient has no circumcision.

PROCEDURE IN DETAIL: Patient is fully examined, identified, consented, and taken to the operating room where appropriate intravenous antibiotics were administered preoperatively. Patient was sterilely prepped and draped in the usual sterile fashion after general anesthesia had been induced, with all pressure points adequately padded. A Prolene suture was then placed through the glans in a horizontal manner as a grasping suture for manipulation of the penis. An 8-French feeding tube was placed into the proximal meatus of the hypospadias, demonstrating ease of entry into the urinary bladder. The urinary bladder was then drained to completion.

A circumscribed incision just proximal to the meatus was then performed with degloving of the penis, of the tunica dartos off underlying Buck fascia with sharp dissection. This was performed to the base of the penis without event. The length of the glans to the meatus was approximately 1.4 cm; therefore, a transverse island prepucial flap was fashioned out of the dorsal hooded inner prepucial skin for an approximately 1.8 cm length, so as to adequately tailor this to fit upon repair. A transverse island flap was then taken off the inner prepucial skin of 1.8 x 0.8 cm. Once the skin was incised, the shaft skin was deepithelialized so as to maintain the tunica dartos with the transverse island prepucial flap to the point of the base of the penis. This vascular attachment to the dartos fascia was then swung around the left lateral aspect of the penis so as to place the transverse island flap in a longitudinal fashion from the meatus to the tip of the glans.

Two lateral incising incisions just to each side of the urethral plate were performed on the glans to the point of the proximal urethral meatus so as to gain adequate, fresh new edges of skin to which to attach the transverse island flap. This was performed after a partially constricting tourniquet was placed at the base of the penis with a sterile rubber band. The incision was then developed laterally so as to raise glans flaps bilaterally in order to reapproximate these in the midline after the fascia was repaired. The transverse island flap was then swung into appropriate position, being pexed proximally with 7-0 Vicryl suture being run on the lateral aspect of the urethral plate to the meatal tip on each side after appropriate tailoring. The neomeatus was then fashioned and matured to the glans flaps that had been developed previously. The flaps were then swung medially after a dartos interposition of material was pexed over the suture line so as to ensure adequate layering of the hypospadias repair.

(Continued)

ID#: S-3   PAGE 2

The glans wings were then approximated in the midline using 6-0 Vicryl suture material along the ventrum. Once this was performed to the point of the circumcising collar, Byars flaps were then fashioned with a midline incision on the dorsal aspect of the prepucial and penile shaft skin so as to tailor this in a manner that would remove the redundant foreskin. This was then pexed to the dorsum of the skin where the Byars flaps were rotated medially and then pexed in the midline. The Byars flaps were then incised and fashioned so as to reapproximate the rotational flap along the midline of the penis in a circumcising collar. All incisions were reapproximated with 5-0 chromic suture material. It is important to note that prior to doing so, a Zaontz urethral catheter was placed into the urethra without evidence of constriction. This was draining clear urine at the conclusion of the case.

Once all suture lines and flaps had been reapproximated in an adequate manner, Telfa and Tegaderm dressings were placed. Catheter was allowed to drain into a diaper. Patient was awakened and extubated and transported to the postanesthesia care unit in otherwise appropriate condition.

ESTIMATED BLOOD LOSS: Minimal.

INTRAVENOUS FLUIDS: 400 mL.

COMPLICATIONS: None.

DISPOSITION: We will see the patient back in 1 week for catheter removal, sooner if any problems, questions, or concerns arise.

_____
Charles Mendesz, MD
Urology Surgery

CM:pai
D:2/3/----
T:2/4/----

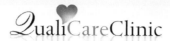

QualiCareClinic

Plastic Surgery

Patient Name: Zoe Maude Gideon   **ID#:** S-4

Date of Operation: 15 Feb ----   **Age:** 43   **Sex:** Female

PREOPERATIVE DIAGNOSIS
Brow ptosis.

POSTOPERATIVE DIAGNOSIS
Brow ptosis.

SURGEON: Danila R. Fry, MD

ASSISTANT: Jimmy Dale Jett, RN, Circulating Nurse

ANESTHESIA: General endotracheal by Carl Erickson Avalon, MD

OPERATION PERFORMED: Endoscopic brow lift.

SPECIMEN REMOVED: None.

INDICATIONS: Patient is unhappy with her brows, feels they have drooped too low, requests they be lifted.

ESTIMATED BLOOD LOSS: 10 mL.

INTRAVENOUS FLUIDS: 1100 mL of lactated Ringer's.

COMPLICATIONS: None.

FINDINGS: Brow ptosis. No significant blepharochalasis.

PROCEDURE IN DETAIL: Patient is brought back by Anesthesia. General endotracheal was induced. The head of the bed was rotated 180 degrees. The patient was prepped and draped in the usual sterile fashion for brow surgery. Endoscopic guidance was used during the entire case. The tumescent solution was injected along the subperiosteal aspect of the entire brow prior to beginning the procedure.

The planned incision sites were injected with approximately 10 mL of 1% lidocaine with 1:100,000 epinephrine total. Five ports were created, 2 laterally along the temporalis muscle and 3 medially—one in the midline and two 4 cm lateral to the midline. The incisions in the midline went down to the bone. Subperiosteal dissection was carried out bluntly using subperiosteal elevators. The lateral incisions were carried down to the superficial layer of the deep temporalis fascia. The fascial elevator was then used to elevate the fascia to the level of the conjoined tendon and to the orbital rim.

Endoscopic guidance was then used to complete the elevation of the subperiosteal flaps over the orbital rim, identifying the supraorbital complex. The supraorbital complex was left intact. The arcus marginalis was incised using the periosteal elevator and was then released on both orbits and in the midline. The corrugators and procerus were incised. The forehead flap was then pulled superiorly and laterally. Then 2-0 nylon sutures were used laterally to tack the temporoparietal fascia down to the superficial layer of the deep temporalis fascia. The Endotine forehead lift prostheses were implanted at the 2 midline incision sites, after burring the appropriate-sized hole using the Endotine instrument. The Endotines were snapped into place, and the periosteal flap was elevated and secured onto the Endotines.

The incisions were closed with deep 4-0 PDS sutures and cutaneous 5-0 chromic interrupted sutures. Thirty units of botulinum toxin had been injected along the lateral canthus region and the corrugator and procerus regions

(Continued)

immediately prior to the procedure. The patient's hair was washed and combed to remove any blood clots and debris. The head was toweled off, and a Kerlix and Coban head drape was fashioned. The wound incisions were covered with bacitracin. The patient was then returned to the anesthesia team, extubated and stable.

DISPOSITION: Patient went awake, alert, stable, and without any event to the recovery room in good condition.

_____
Danila R. Fry, MD
Plastic Surgery

DRF:pai
D:2/15/----
T:2/16/----

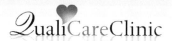

Obstetrics/Gynecology Surgery

Patient Name: Julie Tustolana   **ID#:** S-5
Date of Operation: 9 Feb ----   **Age:** 35   **Sex:** Female

PREOPERATIVE DIAGNOSES
1. Primary infertility.
2. Bilateral hydrosalpinges.

POSTOPERATIVE DIAGNOSES
1. Primary infertility.
2. Bilateral hydrosalpinges.
3. Bilateral severe tubal disease.

SURGEON: Tillman Risha, MD

ASSISTANT: Rosemary Bumbak, MD

ANESTHESIA: General endotracheal by Dr. Avalon.

OPERATION PERFORMED: Operative laparoscopy with bilateral salpingectomies.

MATERIAL FORWARDED TO LABORATORY FOR EXAMINATION: Left and right tubes.

FINDINGS: Severe tubal disease—left tube with distal hydrosalpinx and afimbria, right tube filled to the midampulla only, no fimbria or distal fill. Paratubal cyst and perihepatic adhesions were noted.

PROCEDURE IN DETAIL: Patient was taken to the operating room where general endotracheal anesthesia was found to be adequate. She was prepped and draped in the usual sterile fashion in dorsal lithotomy position. Foley catheter was placed. Speculum was placed into the vagina, which allowed the cervix to be visualized. It was grasped with a tenaculum, and a uterine manipulator was then inserted. Speculum was removed.

Attention was turned to the abdominal portion of the case where an 11-blade scalpel was used to make an incision in the umbilicus, through which an 11 mm Xcel trocar was passed under direct visualization. This was confirmed to be in the abdomen, and the abdomen was insufflated. Thorough inspection of the abdomen revealed what appeared to be hydrosalpinges bilaterally. Two lateral operative ports were placed approximately 2 cm superior and medial to the anterior superior iliac crest bilaterally. These were 5 mm ports, and they were placed under visualization from inside the abdomen. Once these ports were placed, the Maryland graspers and a blunt probe were used to more thoroughly inspect the tubes bilaterally. The tube on the right was noted to have no spill, and there appeared to be no fimbria. EndoShears scissors were then used to make a cruciate incision at the most distal portion of fill in the tube. Inspection of this incision revealed no fimbria.

Attention was turned to the left tube, which was grasped with the Marylands. Again the tubes were filled with dye. The point where the most distal fill of dye was seen was incised with cruciate incision. Once again, no fimbriae were seen. Decision was made at this point to remove the tubes to make the patient a better candidate for IVF.

The ACE Harmonic scalpel was then introduced, and the tubes were taken bilaterally from the cornua down the mesosalpinx as close to the tube as possible. Excellent hemostasis was noted. The tubes were then removed through the 10 mm port. Further inspection of the abdomen revealed a normal appendix and multiple filmy adhesions between the liver and the anterior abdominal wall. The 5 mm ports were removed. Excellent hemostasis was noted. The 10 mm port was then removed after the abdomen had been relieved of all gas.

(Continued)

ID#: S-5   PAGE 2

Attention was then turned to the vagina where the tenaculum and the uterine manipulator were removed. The Foley was removed. The umbilical incision was closed with 3-0 Monocryl and Dermabond. The two 5 mm ports were closed with Dermabond. The patient tolerated the procedure well. Sponge, lap, and needle counts were correct x2. Patient was then transferred to the PACU in stable condition.

SPONGE COUNT VERIFIED: Correct x2.

ESTIMATED BLOOD LOSS: 10 mL.

REPLACEMENT: None.

COMPLICATIONS: None.

_____
Tillman Risha, MD
Obstetrics/Gynecology

TR:pai
D:2/9/----
T:2/9/----

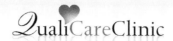

General/Plastic Surgery

Patient Name: Martha Ellen Smith   **ID#:** S-6

Date of Operation: 11 Jan ----   **Age:** 69   **Sex:** Female

PREOPERATIVE DIAGNOSIS
Right breast cancer, scheduled for bilateral mastectomies with immediate reconstruction.

POSTOPERATIVE DIAGNOSIS
Right breast cancer.

SURGEON: Danila R. Fry, MD

ASSISTANT: James A. McClure Jr, MD

ANESTHESIA: General endotracheal by Dr. Delaney.

OPERATIONS PERFORMED
1. Right modified radical mastectomy.
2. Left simple mastectomy.
3. Immediate bilateral breast reconstructions with tissue expanders.

MATERIAL FORWARDED TO LABORATORY FOR EXAMINATION: Mastectomy specimens.

INDICATIONS: Patient is a 69-year-old female with a previously diagnosed right breast cancer that was incompletely excised at the previous biopsy with sentinel node sampling. She was scheduled for return to the OR for completion mastectomy on the right and prophylactic mastectomy on the left. Patient desired immediate breast reconstruction. She was expected to receive no postoperative irradiation. The use of tissue expanders with subsequent implants was discussed with her as well as other options. She agreed to proceed with immediate tissue expander reconstruction. Risks and benefits were discussed. Questions were answered to the satisfaction of the patient and her husband. Informed consent was obtained to proceed.

PROCEDURE IN DETAIL: Patient was marked in the preoperative holding area. She was taken to the operating room where she was placed on the operating table in supine position. Cardiac monitors were attached and general endotracheal anesthesia was induced. Patient's selected mastectomy incisions were demarcated on each breast to include the previous biopsy sites. Mastectomies were performed by Dr. McClure, and that portion of the case will be dictated by the general surgery service.

Once the mastectomies were completed, the plastic surgery team assumed care of the patient. The pectoralis muscle was incised along the direction of the fibers at the lateral aspect, and dissection was carried laterally beneath the serratus fascia and medially beneath the pectoralis major. Inferiorly, the pectoralis muscle was left attached to the overlying dermis. The pocket was dissected down to the level of the inframammary fold. Once an adequate pocket had been created, the tissue expander was brought up onto the field and placed in an antibiotic irrigation solution. It was tested for manufacturing defects. None were found. It was degassed in standard fashion and filled with 50 mL of normal saline through a closed system.

The expanders were prepared and placed in identical fashion on both sides in the pockets previously created. The split pectoralis muscle was reapproximated over the implant, and total muscle coverage was achieved over both implants. A 7 mm flat Blake drain was placed along the inframammary fold and in the axillae bilaterally, then brought up through separate stab incisions in the lateral inframammary fold. They were secured in place with 3-0 nylon sutures. The wounds were copiously irrigated with normal saline, and meticulous hemostasis was assured.

(Continued)

ID#: S-6   PAGE 2

Wounds were closed with interrupted 3-0 Monocryl dermal sutures followed by a running 4-0 Monocryl subcuticular suture. The ports were accessed percutaneously using the magnetic port finders included with the expanders using the supplied 23-gauge needles. Saline was immediately aspirated from both expanders. An additional 50 mL of saline was placed into each expander, and absolutely no tension was identified on the skin flaps. At the completion of the operation, the skin flaps appeared healthy to the flap margins. Drains were placed to bulb suction. Patient was extubated and transferred to the recovery room in good condition. No known complications evident at the time of this dictation.

SPONGE COUNT VERIFIED: Final correct.

DRAINS: 7 mm flat Blake x4 (two in each breast).

INTRAVENOUS FLUIDS: 3300 mL crystalloid.

ESTIMATED BLOOD LOSS: 150 mL.

URINE OUTPUT: 350 mL.

PROSTHETIC DEVICES
- Right breast: Mentor REF No. 354-6224, lot #5625290, serial #5625267-034
- Left breast: Mentor REF No. 354-6224, lot #5596178, serial #5596117-078

_____

Danila R. Fry, MD
Plastic Surgery

DRF:pai
D:1/11/----
T:1/12/----

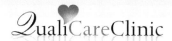

General Surgery

Patient Name: Emma Guzman

Date of Operation: 20 June ----   **Age:** 75

ID#: S-7

Sex: Female

PREOPERATIVE DIAGNOSIS
Peritonitis, possible gastric versus duodenal perforation.

POSTOPERATIVE DIAGNOSES
1. Duodenal perforation.
2. Bowel adhesion.

SURGEON: James A. McClure Jr, MD

ASSISTANT: Rosemary Bumbak, MD

ANESTHESIA: General endotracheal by Chuck Delaney, MD

OPERATIONS PERFORMED
1. Exploratory laparotomy.
2. Lysis of adhesions.
3. Grand patch placement over the duodenal ulcer.

INDICATIONS: This 75-year-old female presents with a 2-day history of midepigastric then diffuse abdominal pain without fever, nausea, vomiting, or diarrhea. She underwent radiographic studies in order to find free air and diffuse intraabdominal fluid. Based on her history of recent chemotherapy for her breast cancer and other indications for possible stress ulcer, the decision was made to take her to the operating room for exploration for a likely perforated gastric or duodenal ulcer.

PROCEDURE IN DETAIL: After all risks, benefits, complications, and alternatives had been explained to the patient and her family and all of their questions had been answered, she freely consented to the above operation. She was placed under general anesthesia without complication. A midline incision was made over her prior midline incision. The peritoneum was entered without difficulty. Adhesions of the omentum and small bowel were encountered, and these adhesions were sequentially ligated with Bovie electrocautery and suture ligation.

Upon entering the abdomen, approximately 2 L of free gastric bilious effluent was found. Culture and Gram stain were sent. We were unable to run the length of the small intestine due to the serial aspects of her gross adhesion to the abdominal cavity. However, we did find an approximately 2 cm ulceration in her proximal duodenum.

The ulcer was without evidence of bleeding on the edges. Interrupted 3-0 Vicryl sutures were placed along the length of the duodenal ulcer, and silk Lembert sutures were placed overlying the area of ulceration. A piece of omentum was freed up from the adhesions, and we patched over this area of duodenal ulceration. The abdominal cavity was irrigated copiously with 3 L of warm saline irrigation until clear fluid returned. Her fascia was closed with running PDS. The subcutaneous tissues were once again irrigated with saline irrigation, and hemostasis was achieved. Her skin was stapled closed. She was taken back to the SICU in stable condition but intubated.

SPONGE COUNT verified x2 at end of case.

MATERIAL FORWARDED TO THE LABORATORY FOR EXAMINATION: Gram stain and culture.

ESTIMATED BLOOD LOSS: Less than 100 mL.

(Continued)

ID#: S-7   PAGE 2

INTRAVENOUS FLUIDS IN: Approximately 2 L.

ANTIBIOTICS USED: Zosyn.

COMPLICATIONS: None.

_____

James A. McClure Jr, MD
General Surgery

JAM:pai
D:6/20/----
T:6/21/----

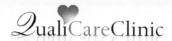

Orthopedic/Plastic Surgery

Patient Name: John Doyle Rice   **ID#:** S-8

Date of Operation: 29 July ----   **Age:** 21   **Sex:** Male

PREOPERATIVE DIAGNOSIS
Left lower extremity fasciotomy wound status post a blast injury while in Iraq on deployment, which led to an open wound with requirements for formal fasciotomies that have been done previously.

POSTOPERATIVE DIAGNOSIS
Left lower extremity fasciotomy wound status post a blast injury while in Iraq on deployment, which led to an open wound with requirements for formal fasciotomies that have been done previously.

SURGEON: Raquel Rodriguez, MD

ASSISTANT: Danila R. Fry, MD

ANESTHESIA: General endotracheal by Dr. Avalon.

OPERATIONS PERFORMED
1. Exploration of wounds.
2. Irrigation and debridement with Wound-Evac change to left lower extremity.

SPECIMEN REMOVED: None.

INDICATIONS: This 21-year-old active duty Air Force male is status post an IED injury sustained while in Balad, Iraq, where he underwent irrigation and debridement of an open fibular fracture with fasciotomies. He was subsequently transferred to Germany where he underwent repeat I&D on 22 July. He was then transferred to the local AFB hospital on 26 July, from which he has been transferred for outpatient treatment at Quali-Care Clinic. Patient has returned to the operating room for multiple I&Ds, debridements, and Wound-Evac changes. We discussed with the patient the indications, risks, benefits, and alternatives for this current procedure. The patient desired to proceed with the surgery as planned.

PROCEDURE IN DETAIL: The patient was met in the preoperative holding area where the operative site was confirmed as the left lower extremity and the site was signed by the operating surgeon. Patient was then brought back to the operating room by the anesthesia service. A final time out was held during which time the consent was verified one final time. The patient then received a dose of IV Ancef prior to the start of the procedure. He underwent general endotracheal anesthesia without event. A nonsterile tourniquet was placed on the left upper thigh. He was prepped and draped in the usual sterile fashion. Prior to prepping and draping we had removed his prior Wound-Evac.

We began by removing all the sutures on both the medial and lateral fasciotomy sites. We explored the wounds. The muscle tissue was very healthy, pink, and contractile to the Bovie. No necrotic debris or devitalized tissue was visible on either the medial or lateral fasciotomy sites. We irrigated the wound copiously with several liters of irrigant solution. We then scrubbed the wounds on both the medial and lateral sides with a Hibiclens sponge. We followed that with another look, noting no devitalized tissue remaining. We then completed the irrigation, using a total of 6 L in each wound site.

At this point, we partially closed the medial side using nylon suture both proximally and distally after applying a Wound-Evac sponge to the wound. Again, we got the wound partially closed over the Wound-Evac sponge.

On the lateral side we reapproximated the skin on the distal margin using a running 3-0 nylon suture, but the remainder of the wound was open. Wound-Evac sponge was then applied to this as well. The Wound-Evac

(Continued)

sponges were fixed in place along the margins of the wound with staples. We then secured the Wound-Evac with the occlusive plastic dressing. We bridged the wounds together. We also irrigated out and packed a Wound-Evac sponge into a small wound along the posteromedial aspect of his calf.

After the dressings had been applied, the Wound-Evac was placed to suction. We had great suction and seal. We then applied a short leg posterior splint with a stirrup-type slab splint. This was applied with the bulky Jones cotton for soft tissue rest. The patient tolerated the procedure well. No complications were noted.

POSTOPERATIVE PLAN
Patient's wounds on the medial side may be amenable to primary closure at the next washout. The lateral wound, however, will likely require split-thickness skin grafting. We will plan to take him back to the operating room this coming Tuesday for repeat irrigation and debridement with Wound-Evac change versus possible split-thickness skin grafts.

INTRAVENOUS FLUIDS: 600 mL crystalloid.

ESTIMATED BLOOD LOSS: Minimal.

URINE OUTPUT: Not recorded.

TOURNIQUET TIME: Not used.

COMPLICATIONS: None.

CONDITION: Stable.

_____

Raquel Rodriguez, MD
Orthopedic Surgery

RR:pai
D:7/29/----
T:7/30/----

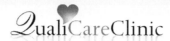

Oromaxillofacial Surgery

Patient Name: David Robert Lepinski   **ID#:** S-9

Date of Operation: 31 July ----   **Age:** 19   **Sex:** Male

PREOPERATIVE DIAGNOSIS
Radiopacity, right body of the mandible.

POSTOPERATIVE DIAGNOSIS
Radiopacity, right body of the mandible.

SURGEON: Leela Pivari, MD

ASSISTANT: Jimmy Dale Jett, RN, Circulating Nurse

ANESTHESIA: General endotracheal.

OPERATION PERFORMED: Surgical exploration and biopsy of radiopacity associated near apex of tooth #28 in the right body of mandible.

MATERIAL FORWARDED TO LABORATORY FOR EXAMINATION: A Moult curette was used to obtain samples of bone, which were submitted for histopathologic analysis.

INDICATIONS: Patient is a 19-year-old airman basic referred to the oromaxillofacial surgery service after routine screening dental x-rays upon induction into the Air Force noted the presence of a radiopaque lesion in his right body of mandible. There was no evidence of cortical expansion associated with this lesion. Patient was brought to the operating room for surgical exploration and determination of lesion.

PROCEDURE IN DETAIL: After proper identification of patient and verification of n.p.o. status, patient was brought to OR 16 where adequate general endotracheal anesthesia was administered via nasal endotracheal intubation. The mouth was thoroughly irrigated with saline, then suctioned. A posterior pharyngeal pack was placed. Then 2% lidocaine with 1:100,000 epinephrine x 1.8 mL, then 0.5% Marcaine with 1:200,000 epinephrine x 1.8 mL were administered into the proposed surgical site to establish hemostasis and prolong anesthesia.

A full-thickness mucoperiosteal flap was reflected via a circular incision extending from the distal of tooth #25 to the mesial of tooth #30. This full-thickness mucoperiosteal flap was reflected, allowing visualization of the right mental nerve, which was isolated and protected during the remainder of this surgical procedure.

A #8 round bur and a rotary handpiece were used to perform corticotomy and surgical exploration of the intramedullary bone between tooth #27 and #28. This site was determined after review of preoperative computed tomography scans showed this area to be in direct location with the radiopacity noted on previous radiographs. Entry into this site approximately 8 mL in depth was accomplished, and there was no soft tissue or evidence of a soft tissue tumor. The roots of teeth #27 and #28 were not violated during this exploration. It was noted at this time that the bone in that area was extremely dense and appeared to have a cortical consistency. A Moult curette was used to obtain samples of this bone, which were submitted for histopathologic analysis with the presumptive diagnosis of idiopathic osteosclerosis.

The site was copiously irrigated with saline. The mucoperiosteal flap was resuspended with interrupted 4-0 chromic sutures. The mouth was thoroughly irrigated, suctioned, and the posterior pharyngeal pack was removed. Patient tolerated the procedure well, was extubated in the operating room, and he was taken to the recovery room in optimal condition. Sponge count verified x2.

(Continued)

ID#: S-9 PAGE 2

ESTIMATED BLOOD LOSS: Minimal.

FLUIDS: 500 mL lactated Ringer's.

URINE OUTPUT: None.

____

Leela Pivari, MD
Oromaxillofacial Surgery

LP:pai
D:7/31/----
T:8/01/----

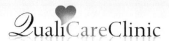

Ophthalmologic Surgery

Patient Name: Marco Anthony Gatti **ID#:** S-10

Date of Operation: 11 Oct ---- **Age:** 66 **Sex:** Male

PREOPERATIVE DIAGNOSIS
Intraocular lens implant.

POSTOPERATIVE DIAGNOSIS
Intraocular lens implant.

SURGEON: Yasmin Naimi, MD

ASSISTANT: Jimmy Dale Jett, RN, Circulating Nurse

ANESTHESIA: MAC administered by Dr. Delaney.

OPERATION PERFORMED: Cataract surgery of left eye.

SPECIMEN REMOVED: Residual lens cortex was removed from the lens capsular bag with the handpiece. Residual material was removed from the eye with an automated handpiece.

PROCEDURE IN DETAIL: The patient was brought into OR 3 and placed under monitored anesthesia control. While under intravenous sedation, 3 mL of retrobulbar block was administered. We used intermittent digital compression placed over the surgical eye and orbit for 5 minutes. After retrobulbar, patient was prepped and draped in the usual sterile fashion. Then 4 iris hooks were draped in sterile fashion. Then a paracentesis port was placed. Viscoat was injected into the right eye, and 4 iris hooks were placed to enlarge the pupil. The globe was then stabilized with the Thornton fixation ring, and the 3 mm phacoblade was used to create a biplanar temporal clear corneal incision into the anterior chamber. The cystitome was used to initiate capsulotomy, and then the Utrata forceps was used to continue curvilinear capsulorrhexis. Balanced salt solution on a blunt cannula was used to hydrodissect the lens. The lens nucleus was then phacoemulsified and aspirated from the eye. Residual lens cortex was removed from the lens capsular bag with the handpiece. Healon was injected into the lens capsular bag. The phacowound was then enlarged with the phacoblade. The IOL was then folded and inserted into the lens capsular bag. Residual material was then removed from the eye with an automated handpiece.

The wounds were hydrated, then integrity was checked and found to be watertight. Patient received 0.5 mL of Ancef and 0.5 mL of dexamethasone. The lid speculum was removed. Maxitrol ointment was applied to the eye, along with pressure patch and Fox shield. The patient was then transferred to the recovery area in stable condition to be discharged after he meets all his criteria. He is to see me in my office tomorrow morning.

PROSTHETIC DEVICES: Intraocular lens placement SN60WF 20.5.

_____
Yasmin Naimi, MD
Ophthalmology

YN:pai
D:10/11/----
T:10/11/----

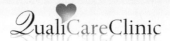

Obstetrics/Gynecology Surgery

Patient Name: Dinah Cash   **ID#:** S-11

Date of Operation: 25 May ----   **Age:** 35   **Sex:** Female

PREOPERATIVE DIAGNOSIS
Intrauterine pregnancy at 8 weeks' estimated gestational age with acute surgical abdomen.

POSTOPERATIVE DIAGNOSIS
Intrauterine pregnancy at 8 weeks' estimated gestational age with acute surgical abdomen.

SURGEON: Tillman Risha, MD

ASSISTANT: Bernard Kester, MD

ANESTHESIA: General endotracheal given by Dr. Delaney.

OPERATIONS PERFORMED
1. Ruptured right distal isthmic ectopic pregnancy (heterotopic).
2. Viable intrauterine pregnancy.

MATERIAL FORWARDED TO LABORATORY FOR EXAMINATION
1. Right ectopic pregnancy.
2. Right fallopian tube.

INDICATIONS: Patient presented to the emergency department with symptomatic hypotension, requiring resuscitation/transfusion with findings of an acute surgical abdomen. Intraabdominal fluid confirmed on FAST exam. Taken emergently to the operating room for an exploratory laparotomy.

FINDINGS: Patient presented to the ED with an acute abdomen and was symptomatic and hypotensive. She was stabilized in the ED and transfusion was initiated. She was taken emergently to the operating room for an exploratory laparotomy. Dr. Kester of general surgery scrubbed in and assisted with the case. There were findings of 2 liters of blood in the abdomen, which was evacuated. Ultimately, active bleeding from a right heterotopic ectopic ruptured pregnancy was identified. The remainder of the abdomen was surgically cleared. Attempt at linear salpingotomy was made, and the ectopic pregnancy was evacuated; however, we were unable to obtain hemostasis. Therefore, a right salpingectomy was then performed, resulting in excellent hemostasis. A total of 6 units PRBCs were given. Otherwise normal uterus, normal ovaries bilaterally, normal left fallopian tube, normal liver and gallbladder, normal spleen, normal vermiform appendix. No pelvic adhesions, no anterior abdominal wall adhesions, no intraoperative complications. Patient was transferred to PACU and subsequently to ICU postoperatively.

Viable intrauterine pregnancy was confirmed with ultrasound postoperatively in the PACU.

PROCEDURE IN DETAIL: Patient presented to the ED with acute-onset abdominal pain and symptomatic hypotension with blood pressure in 70s/40s. Patient was stabilized by the ED team, and blood transfusion was initiated after free fluid in the patient's abdomen was noted on her FAST exam. GYN team was immediately notified secondary to the patient's 8-week gestational age status. A bedside ultrasound was performed, confirming a viable intrauterine pregnancy; however, there was no free fluid in the patient's pelvis, no dilation of the fallopian tubes noted, and she had normal-appearing ovaries on ultrasound. Given the nature of her findings with an acute surgical abdomen, which was rigid with rebound and guarding, free fluid in the abdomen without clear etiology and without known ectopic pregnancy, patient was consented for an emergent exploratory laparotomy.

(Continued)

ID#: S-11   PAGE 2

Patient was taken to the operating room where she was placed under general endotracheal anesthesia without difficulty. Compression devices were placed on her lower extremities and were functioning prior to induction. She was then prepped and draped in the usual sterile fashion in the supine position. A low vertical midline incision was made just above the symphysis up to the level of the umbilicus and carried down through to the underlying fascia, which was incised with scalpel. Kelly clamps were used to identify a window in the peritoneum, tented up, and incised with Metzenbaum scissors. Upon entry into the patient's peritoneum, there was an immediate expulsion of blood and clot from the abdominal cavity.

Peritoneal incision was then extended superiorly and inferiorly. Rapid exploration of the patient's abdomen and pelvis revealed no immediate or obvious source of the bleeding. There was concern for blood in the upper abdomen at this time; therefore, her incision was extended superiorly above the level of the umbilicus in the midline. After extending the superior aspect of the incision, sweep of the upper abdomen revealed approximately 2 liters of blood and clot in the upper abdomen. General surgery staff were scrubbed in, assisting with the case, and after cleaning the clot and free blood in the upper abdomen, inspection of the patient's upper abdomen revealed no active bleeding source with a normal, intact liver, normal spleen, and normal upper abdomen.

Attention was then returned to the patient's pelvis where, after visualization of the patient's pelvis, there was identified a right fallopian tube ectopic pregnancy with a small area of rupture of the fallopian tube in the antimesenteric side of the fallopian tube. Otherwise normal-appearing ovaries bilaterally, normal uterus with no pelvic adhesive disease. Given the location of the ectopic pregnancy and the location of the ovary and fallopian tube outside of the patient's pelvis, this appeared to account for the lack of free fluid in the patient's pelvic cavity. The bleeding appeared to trail along the right paracolic gutter freely.

Following this and the evacuation of the surgical field, a linear salpingostomy was made with electrocautery over the ectopic site, which was then expressed without difficulty. This was sent separately for pathology identification. We were unable to obtain hemostasis of the fallopian tube secondary to continued active bleeding and concern for inability to monitor the resolution of the ectopic, given the patient's current viable intrauterine pregnancy. Decision was made to perform a right partial salpingectomy. This was performed with ligature device transected across near the cornual region out through to the distal isthmic region, incorporating the entire ectopic site. This resulted in excellent hemostasis of the surgical bed.

Following this, continued exploration of the patient's pelvis revealed no other bleeding source. Following this, copious irrigation of the patient's upper abdomen, mesentery, and pelvis was then performed with warm normal saline without difficulty. Following complete irrigation, reinspection of the patient's excision site revealed continued excellent hemostasis.

Attention was then turned to closing the patient's fascia, which was performed with looped 0 PDS in a mass closure-type approach without difficulty. The subcutaneous layers were then copiously irrigated, and the skin was ultimately closed with surgical staples with excellent result. Patient tolerated all procedures well.

Sponge, lap, needle counts were all correct x2. Foley catheter remained in the urinary bladder postoperatively. A total of 6 units PRBCs were transfused both preoperatively and perioperatively. Patient was subsequently transferred to PACU and then to ICU for further observation.

DRAINS: Foley catheter to urinary bladder.

SPONGE COUNT: Correct x2 at end of case.

FLUIDS GIVEN: Intravenous fluids included 4000 mL crystalloid, colloid 500 mL, and transfusion of 6 units packed red blood cells.

(Continued)

ID#: S-11   PAGE 3

URINE OUTPUT: 2500 mL clear urine.

ESTIMATED BLOOD LOSS: 2500 mL.

COMPLICATIONS: No complications at the time of this dictation.

_____

Tillman Risha, MD
Obstetrics/Gynecology

TR:pai
D:5/25/----
T:5/25/----

c: Bernard Kester, MD, General Surgery

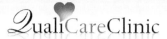

QualiCareClinic

<u>Orthopedic Surgery</u>

Patient Name: Mary Jane Alderman   **ID#:** S-12

Date of Operation: 23 Feb ----   **Age:** 45   **Sex:** Female

PREOPERATIVE DIAGNOSIS
Left shoulder impingement syndrome.

POSTOPERATIVE DIAGNOSIS
Left shoulder impingement syndrome.

SURGEON: Raquel Rodriguez, MD

ASSISTANT: Jack Zullig, MD

ANESTHESIA: General endotracheal by Dr. Avalon.

OPERATIONS PERFORMED
1. Examination under anesthesia.
2. Left shoulder diagnostic arthroscopy.
3. Subacromial decompression.
4. Distal clavicle revision.

SPECIMEN REMOVED: None.

INDICATIONS: This is a 45-year-old female with left shoulder impingement. She is right-hand dominant. She has no history of trauma. The patient has painful and limited range of motion. The patient also has acromioclavicular joint arthritis. The patient had workup done consisting of plain films and MRI, which showed a possible tear of the supraspinatus and possible labral pathology. Acromioclavicular joint arthrosis.

FINDINGS: Diffuse synovitis in the patient's left shoulder. The synovitis does not extend into the biceps. The patient has the labrum intact. There is some fraying anteriorly. No loose bodies in the patient's glenohumeral joint. The patient has no rotator cuff pathology.

PROCEDURE IN DETAIL: During the preoperative visit, the patient's diagnosis, risks, benefits, and adverse effects were discussed with the patient by Dr. Craven. All questions were answered. Informed written and verbal consent were obtained.

On the day of surgery, patient was brought to the anesthesia holding area. The operative surgeon identified and marked the appropriate surgical site. The operative nurse and anesthesia team evaluated the patient. The patient was brought back to the operating suite and transferred to the operating table. She was given preoperative antibiotics by Anesthesia. She was then given general endotracheal anesthesia by Anesthesia. The patient was positioned appropriately on the beach chair.

The patient's left shoulder was examined under anesthesia. She has symmetric passive range of motion compared to the opposite side except for external rotation. With the elbows abducted approximately 90 degrees, the patient has approximately 10 degrees' decrease in external rotation in the left shoulder compared to the right shoulder. Forward flexion and abduction were symmetric to the opposite side, otherwise. Given that the patient's external rotation with the arm at 80 to 90 degrees was decreased, gentle manipulation was done to help release part of that.

The patient's left shoulder was then prepped and draped in the usual sterile fashion. Diagnostic arthroscopy was begun with placing a portal superiorly in the standard fashion. Prior to portal placement, the acromion AC anatomic landmarks were drawn out with a marking pen. A posterior portal approximately 2 fingerbreadths below and 1 fingerbreadth medial to the posterolateral corner of the acromion was made. This was initially

(Continued)

ID#: S-12   PAGE 2

done by injecting 60 mL of fluid into the AC joint. Once the AC joint was distended, next a skin incision was made with an 11 blade. A trocar was then inserted into the joint. Fluid was seen coming out through the trocar; therefore, it was known that we were in the joint. Next a scope was placed through the posterior portal. A diagnostic arthroscopy was begun. The patient was found to have significant synovitis.

Next, under direct visualization an anterior portal was made. This was done by splitting the distance between the coracoid and the anterolateral edge of the acromion. An 18-gauge needle was used. As stated, this was made under direct visualization. Once this portal was made, a yellow trocar was placed into the portal site. A probe was then inserted through this portal, and the diagnostic arthroscopy was begun.

The biceps tendon was visualized. It appeared to be intact. There was noted to be significant synovitis. The inferior and superior edges of the labrum were probed and noted to be intact. The patient's inferior recess had no evidence of loose bodies. The patient's rotator cuff was then evaluated and appeared to be intact. Some mild débridement at the synovium was done with a 4.5 shaver.

Next, attention was turned to the subacromial decompression. The posterior trocar was removed. It was reinserted into the subacromial space. A lateral portal was then made. This was to get into the subacromial space. Once the lateral portal was made, a 4.5 shaver was placed into the subacromial space. The subacromial bursa was débrided. Once adequate débridement had been done, anatomic landmarks inside the joint were identified at the anterolateral corner, the posterolateral corner, and the AP joint. These were visualized. Next an ArthroWand was used to help débride some of the soft tissue. Next a bur was used to do the acromioplasty. The acromioplasty was started at the anterolateral portion, then progressed medially. Once it was determined that an adequate acromioplasty had been done, the attention was then turned to the clavicle.

A distal clavicle incision was done arthroscopically. The distal clavicle joint was identified. Using both the 4.5 shaver and the ArthroWand, the soft tissue was débrided. Next, through the anterior portal the bur was reinserted, and the distal clavicle excision was made. Once it was thought that adequate resection of the distal clavicle had been done, the bur was removed. The anterior incision was slightly extended. Fingertip was used to palpate the acromioclavicular joint. A cross-arm test was done to see if further resection needed to be done. It was determined that more distal clavicle needed to be excised.

Once again the bur was placed through the anterior portal, and more of the distal clavicle was excised. Approximately 1 cm of the distal clavicle was excised. Next the bur was removed. Again the cross-arm test was done, and there was noted no abutment from the distal clavicle and the acromion. Once all this had been completed, the instruments were removed from the shoulder.

The skin was reapproximated anteriorly, since the portal was extended, with horizontal mattress using 3-0 nylon. Arthroscopic portals were closed with a port stitch using 3-0 nylon. Xeroform and a sterile dressing were applied. Sterile dressing consisted of flats and an ABD, both in the axilla and on top of the wound. Hypafix tape was then applied. We injected 40 mg of methylprednisolone and Marcaine into the joint prior to putting on the sterile dressing. The patient tolerated the procedure well and was aroused from her general endotracheal anesthesia.

INTRAVENOUS FLUIDS: 140 mL lactated Ringer's.

ESTIMATED BLOOD LOSS: Less than 10 mL.

TOURNIQUET TIME: Not used.

(Continued)

ID#: S-12   PAGE 3

DISPOSITION: Patient will be taken to the PACU for recovery, then discharged to follow up. Patient is scheduled for physical therapy appointment on 26 Feb, Monday, at 0830 hours. She will be given proper handouts and directions.

_____
Raquel Rodriguez, MD
Orthopedic Surgery

RR:pai
D:2/23/----
T:2/24/----

c: Edward Richard Craven, MD, Orthopedic Shoulder Specialist

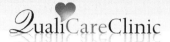

QualiCareClinic

Genitourinary Surgery

Patient Name: John Robin Winston   **ID#:** S-13

Date of Operation: 9 Feb ----   **Age:** 39   **Sex:** Male

PREOPERATIVE DIAGNOSIS
Elective sterility.

POSTOPERATIVE DIAGNOSIS
Elective sterility.

SURGEON: Charles Mendesz, MD

ASSISTANT: Jimmy Dale Jett, RN, Circulating Nurse

ANESTHESIA: General endotracheal by Dr. Avalon.

OPERATION PERFORMED: Bilateral vasovasostomy.

MATERIAL FORWARDED TO LABORATORY FOR EXAMINATION: None.

INDICATIONS: Patient is a 39-year-old male with infertility status post vasectomy in 1996. He has one 10-year-old child by a previous marriage. He was remarried 2 years ago; hence, he desires a reversal of his vasectomy. The risks, benefits, indications, and alternatives of the planned bilateral vasovasostomies were discussed with the patient. Patient understands that there is an approximately 60% chance of patency after the repair as well as a roughly 30% to 40% chance of paternity following repair. All his questions were answered, and he elected to proceed with the procedure as planned.

PROCEDURE IN DETAIL: The patient was met in the holding area where site verification and patient identification were obtained. He was then taken to the operating room where general endotracheal anesthesia was induced by the anesthesia team. Following this, his scrotum was prepped and draped in the usual sterile fashion. Palpation of the scrotum was significant for an easily palpated vasectomy defect on the left, less so on the right.

A midline scrotal incision for approximately 4 cm was made in the median raphe. The left and right testicles were then delivered through the incision. The dartos and associated fascia were bluntly dissected off the testicle and cord using a RayTec. Tethering bands of tissue were taken down by Bovie electrocautery. Care was taken to not enter the tunica vaginalis. Once all the dartos attachments to the testicles and the associated cord were taken down, we first turned our attention to the left vas deferens. The previous vasectomy site was easily identified by the surgical clips, and it was noted to be fairly close to the testicle. A penetrating towel clamp was then placed underneath the vas away from the vessels.

Following this the normal vas, proximal and distal to the vasectomy site, was identified. Using scissors, the area under the vas deferens was sharply dissected. Using a combination of blunt and sharp dissection, the vas deferens was then dissected away from the surrounding tissues. Once adequately isolated, 5-0 PDS stay sutures were placed in the seromuscular portion of the vas, the vas was then transected proximally and distally. The proximal or the abdominal end of the vas cannulated with a 24-French angiocath. Methylene blue was easily injected without resistance. The portions of the vas deferens proximal and distal to the vasectomy defect were then cauterized with Bovie electrocautery in order to prevent an inadvertent anastomosis with these portions. The distal end of the vas was then milked, and a clear liquid was expressed. There was a copious amount of this fluid. The samples were placed on slides and examined under the microscope, where there were found to be copious amounts of nonmotile sperm.

The proximal and distal ends of the vas were then loosely approximated using a 5-0 PDS suture. This was to prevent excessive tension on the repair. The surgical microscope was then brought into position. Using this, 4 full-thickness 9-0 Ethilon nylon sutures were placed, thus approximating the proximal and distal lumina of

(Continued)

ID#: S-13   PAGE 2

the vas deferens. Methylene blue was placed on the cut edge of the vas in order to enhance identification of the lumina prior to the anastomosis.

Once this was completed on the left side, the same procedure was completed on the patient's right side. The results of the microscopic exam were the same bilaterally. Once both sides had been accomplished, 5 mL of fibrin sealant was then placed around the anastomosis on both the right and left sides, sealing the now completed anastomoses. Once this was completed, we prepared to replace the testes within the scrotum. The dartos muscle at the incision was controlled with Allis clamps. Hemostasis was obtained with Bovie electrocautery. The testes were delivered back into their appropriate sides.

Using a running 3-0 Vicryl, the dartos muscle and fascia were closed in the midline. The skin was reapproximated with 3-0 chromic in a running horizontal suture. Dressings consisting of bacitracin fluffs and a scrotal support were applied. The patient tolerated the procedure well, and he was extubated in the operating room. Taken to PACU for recovery.

SPONGE COUNT: Correct at end of case.

FLUIDS: 1200 mL crystalloid.

ESTIMATED BLOOD LOSS: Minimal.

URINE OUTPUT: Not recorded.

COMPLICATIONS: None.

DISPOSITION: Patient will follow up in approximately 1 week for a wound check. He will be scheduled for a semen analysis in 3 months.

_____
Charles Mendesz, MD
Urology Surgery

CM:pai
D:2/9/----
T:2/9/----

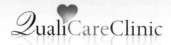

Oromaxillofacial Surgery

Patient Name: Adam Ward   **ID#:** S-14

Date of Operation: 19 Jan ----   **Age:** 52   **Sex:** Male

PREOPERATIVE DIAGNOSIS
Nasal airway obstruction, snoring.

POSTOPERATIVE DIAGNOSIS
Nasal airway obstruction, snoring.

SURGEON: Leela Pivari, MD

ASSISTANT: Anna Maria Iaccarino, RN, Scrub Nurse

ANESTHESIA: General endotracheal by Dr. Delaney.

OPERATIONS PERFORMED
1. Septoplasty with endonasal right spreader graft.
2. Turbinoplasty.
3. Uvulectomy.
4. Radiofrequency ablation of the soft palate.

SPECIMEN REMOVED: None.

INDICATIONS: Patient has had a long history of nasal airway obstruction after nasal trauma 10 years ago. He complains of right greater than left nasal airway obstruction despite maximal medical management. He also complains of snoring. He wishes to proceed with the above procedures, and proper consent has been signed.

PROCEDURE IN DETAIL: The patient was brought into the operating room and placed on the operating room table in supine position. He was intubated, and the bed was turned 90 degrees. His septum was injected with 1% lidocaine with 1:100,000 epinephrine, and 15 mL was used. Afrin-soaked pledgets were placed in the nasal cavity bilaterally. Patient was then prepped and draped in the usual sterile fashion.

A left hemitransfixion incision was made, and a mucoperichondrium mucoperiosteal flap was developed on the left. Using the same incision, the mucoperichondrium mucoperiosteal flap was elevated on the right. The deviated portions of bone and cartilage were then removed. A moderate-sized rent was noted in the floor of the right nasal cavity, but there was no opposing rent. The patient had a slight concavity on the right nasal dorsum onto the middle third, and to address this problem, a septal cartilage graft was placed into the area between the upper lateral cartilage and the septum in the middle third of the nose. The septal flaps were then sutured with 4-0 plain gut on a Keith needle in a quilting fashion. The hemitransfixion incision was closed with 4-0 chromic in a running fashion.

Each inferior turbinate was injected with 1% lidocaine with 1:100,000 epinephrine. The anterior head of the inferior turbinate was incised with a #5 blade, and a Cottle elevator was used to elevate the tissue from the turbinate bone. The microdebrider was then used to microdebride the erectile tissue from the inferior turbinate. The Sayre elevator was used to lateralize the turbinate. A similar procedure was performed on the contralateral inferior turbinate.

Dual splints were placed and fixed to the septum using 2-0 Prolene. A Crowe-Davis mouth gag was then used to retract the oropharynx. The uvula was amputated at its base, and three 3-0 chromic sutures were placed to approximate the anterior and posterior edges of the soft palate. The palatal radiofrequency ablation device was used with 325 joules at this site in the soft palate and 650 joules in the midline.

(Continued)

ID#: S-14   PAGE 2

The patient was then turned over to the Anesthesia Team, and he was recovered from anesthesia, extubated, and brought to the postanesthesia care unit in stable condition. He will be discharged home from PACU once he has met all his criteria.

ESTIMATED BLOOD LOSS: Minimal.

FLUIDS: 1300 mL of crystalloid.

COMPLICATIONS: None.

_____
Leela Pivari, MD
Oromaxillofacial Surgery

LP:pai
D:1/19/----
T:1/20/----

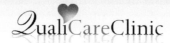

QualiCareClinic

Genitourinary Surgery

Patient Name: Lorenzo D. Renoir　　　　　　　　　　　　　　　　**ID#:** S-15

Date of Operation: 18 Aug ----　　　　　　　**Age:** 72　　　　　　**Sex:** Male

PREOPERATIVE DIAGNOSIS
Elevated prostate-specific antigen (PSA).

POSTOPERATIVE DIAGNOSIS
Elevated PSA.

SURGEON: Charles Mendesz, MD

ASSISTANT: Jimmy Dale Jett, RN, Circulating Nurse

ANESTHESIA: General with MAC by Dr. Delaney.

OPERATION PERFORMED: Transrectal ultrasound biopsy of prostate.

SPECIMEN REMOVED: A total of 13 core biopsies of prostate tissue.

INDICATIONS: The patient is a 72-year-old gentleman with a history of elevated PSA. He has had 2 prior biopsies—10 years or so ago—both of which were benign. His PSA has continued to elevate slightly despite his being on Proscar. He presents for repeat transrectal ultrasound and biopsy of prostate. The patient has been on Coumadin for atrial fibrillation, and he has been taken off that. Preoperative coagulation parameters were noted to be within normal limits. Patient desired the procedure to be done under anesthesia. He understands the risks of misdiagnosed cancer, urinary tract infection, urinary retention, and hematuria.

PROCEDURE IN DETAIL: After correctly identifying the patient in the holding area, he was brought to the operating room. He had received 2 days of oral Levaquin prior to proceeding with the biopsy. After induction of general anesthesia, the patient was placed in the left lateral decubitus position, and transrectal ultrasound was performed.

The patient's prostate volume was approximately 62 cm^3. He had no evidence of extracapsular extension of disease. He had a small intravesical median lobe. No significant hypoechoic or hyperechoic lesions were noted on ultrasound. Patient then underwent a total of 13 core biopsies. He had 3 taken from the left base and 2 from the right and left mid and apex and left base.

Patient tolerated the procedure well and was extubated in the operating room. He was transferred to the recovery room in satisfactory condition. He will receive 1 more day of antibiotics. He will resume his Coumadin 2 days after the procedure. He will follow up with the Coumadin Clinic for further management.

The patient was instructed to call for the results of his biopsy in 7 to 10 days.

_____
Charles Mendesz, MD
Urology Surgery

CM:pai
D:8/18/----
T:8/19/----

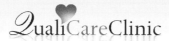

<u>**General Surgery**</u>

Patient Name: Merle Albert Bray   **ID#:** S-16

Date of Operation: 3 Feb ----   **Age:** 33   **Sex:** Male

PREOPERATIVE DIAGNOSIS
Severe gastroesophageal reflux disease.

POSTOPERATIVE DIAGNOSIS
Severe gastroesophageal reflux disease.

SURGEON: James A. McClure Jr, MD

ASSISTANT: Ken Miller, MD

ANESTHESIA: General endotracheal by Dr. Avalon.

OPERATION PERFORMED: Open Nissen fundoplication redo.

SPECIMEN REMOVED: None.

INDICATIONS: This 33-year-old gentleman underwent a laparoscopic Nissen fundoplication 2 years ago with initial improvement in his symptoms, which then recurred after a year. Preoperative workup showed the patient to have a failed graft. Given the patient's age and severity of his reflux disease, it was decided that he would benefit from a redo Nissen fundoplication for control of his gastroesophageal reflux disease.

FINDINGS: There was a sizeable hiatal hernia with adhesions into the pleural cavity between the stomach and the pleura. In addition, the previously performed laparoscopic Nissen fundoplication had fallen apart insofar as the posterior and anterior fundus was no longer sutured together. Instead, they were adherent just posteriorly and anteriorly to the esophagus.

PROCEDURE IN DETAIL: After adequate general anesthesia was obtained, the patient's abdomen was prepped and draped in the usual sterile fashion. A midline incision was created beginning at the xiphoid and extending down to just above the umbilicus. Dissection was carried down through the fascia into the peritoneal cavity using Bovie electrocautery. Thompson retractor was placed. The falciform ligament was ligated between clamps and tied off with suture. The remainder of the falciform ligament was taken down from the liver, and the triangular ligament of the left lobe of the liver was freed up such that we could fold the left lobe of the liver down and out of the way of the esophageal hiatus.

Care was taken to avoid injury to the phrenic vein as well as the left hepatic vein. A retractor was placed to keep the left lobe of the liver out of the dissecting field. The esophagus was then identified, and there was noted to be a moderate amount of adhesions from his prior operative surgery. The scar tissue overlying the gastrohepatic ligament was taken down using Bovie electrocautery. The right crus of the diaphragm was identified and dissected free from surrounding tissue, including the esophagus. A significant amount of scar overlay the esophagus, which was also carefully taken down using Bovie electrocautery. On the left side of the esophagus the patient was noted to have a sizeable hiatal hernia with adhesions to the pleural cavity. This was taken down using Bovie electrocautery with a small defect created within the pleura.

The fundus of the stomach was then freed from adhesions and short gastric was taken. The left crus was dissected free from surrounding tissues, as was the posterior esophagus. Once again a significant amount of scar was encountered. Care was taken to preserve both the anterior and posterior vagi, which were identified and kept along with the esophagus. Once the esophagus was dissected free circumferentially and the fundus was freed up from any scar tissue and adhesions, the esophagus was retracted upward and to the left. The crura of the diaphragm were sutured together in 2 locations using 2-0 Ethibond with pledgets in a horizontal mattress fashion. This was made in a snug fashion.

(Continued)

The posterior wall of the fundus was then wrapped around the esophagus and brought out to the right side. The NO tube was removed and a 60-French bougie placed down into the patient's stomach. Then 2-0 Ethibond suture with pledgets in a horizontal mattress fashion was used to approximate the anterior fundus from the left to the posterior wall of the fundus on the right to create a wrap. The suture was taken to the anterior wall of the esophagus as well. Pledgets were used on both sides. A 1 cm wrap was created longitudinally along the esophagus. Once this was performed, the bougie was removed. The esophagus was then pexed to the crura of the diaphragm anteriorly, posteriorly, and to the left lateral location. This was done with interrupted Ethibond sutures with pledgets. The abdomen was irrigated and hemostasis obtained.

The left lobe of the liver was unfolded and returned to its normal anatomic location. The omentum was placed over the abdominal contents, and the fascia was closed with running looped 0 PDS suture. Subcutaneous tissues were irrigated and the skin closed with staples. Sterile dressing was placed. The patient tolerated the procedure well. He was taken to PACU in good condition.

OF NOTE: Patient had an NG tube replaced after the 60-French bougie was removed, and it was placed within the stomach.

ESTIMATED BLOOD LOSS: 50 mL.

INTRAVENOUS FLUIDS: 3600 mL of crystalloid.

URINE OUTPUT: 110 mL.

_____
James A. McClure Jr, MD
General Surgery

JAM:pai
D:2/3/----
T:2/4/----

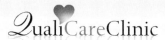
QualiCareClinic

Orthopedic Surgery

Patient Name: Simone Dahl   **ID#:** S-17

Date of Operation: 9 Feb ----   **Age:** 18   **Sex:** Female

PREOPERATIVE DIAGNOSIS
Hallux valgus, right foot.

POSTOPERATIVE DIAGNOSIS
Hallux valgus, right foot.

SURGEON: Gilbert M. Fields, MD

ASSISTANT: Jason Wagner, PA

ANESTHESIA: Local, with intravenous sedation by Dr. Delaney.

OPERATIONS PERFORMED
1. Reverdin-Laird distal metaphyseal osteotomy with screw fixation.
2. Modified McBride bunionectomy, right foot.

SPECIMEN REMOVED: None.

PROCEDURE IN DETAIL: Patient was taken to the operating room and placed on the table in supine position. She was given IV antibiotics as prophylaxis. Local anesthesia was achieved to the area with a 50:50 mixture of 0.5% Marcaine and 1% lidocaine plain. Local hemostasis was achieved with a compression pneumatic tourniquet set at 250 mmHg. Area was then prepped and draped in the usual sterile fashion. After appropriate exsanguination, tourniquet was raised.

Attention was then directed to the first ray whereby dorsal linear incision over the first MTP was performed. All neurovascular structures were cauterized and retracted as necessary. In the intermetatarsal space region, the deep transverse intermetatarsal ligament was transected. This was followed by a lateral arthrotomy, through which the adductor tendon was released at the lateral base of the proximal phalanx. The sesamoid ligament and extensor hallucis brevis tendon were then transected. Incision was then carried over the medial aspect of the joint, whereby an inverted L capsulotomy was performed. The capsule was reflected off the dorsal medial eminence. The exostosis was then resected. The metaphysis was then marked so that the Reverdin-Laird osteotomy could be performed. The triangular wedge was removed, which allowed the distal capital fragment to impact on the metatarsal shaft. The capital fragment was also laterally displaced to close the intermetatarsal angle. This procedure also allowed correction of the proximal articular set angle (PASA). A 1.25 K-wire was introduced to hold the capital fragment while an 18 mm 2.0 cortical screw was used for internal fixation. The K-wire was then removed. The step-off that was created was resected, and then the area was copiously flushed with sterile saline solution.

A medial capsulorrhaphy was then performed to remove redundant capsular tissue. The capsule was then repaired with 2-0 Vicryl. Subcutaneous tissues were closed with 3-0 Vicryl, and skin closure was achieved with 5-0 Vicryl. Betadine-soaked Adaptic, 4 x 8 gauze, 3-inch Kling, and Coban were then used to dress the foot.

The patient tolerated both anesthesia and the procedure went well with no complications. Vital signs were stable. Capillary refill was prompt to all toes.

SPONGE COUNT: Correct. ASA 3, CDC 1.

(Continued)

ID#: S-17   PAGE 2

DRAINS: None.

PROSTHETIC DEVICES: 18 mm 2.0 cortical screw.

COMPLICATIONS: None.

_____
Gilbert M. Fields, MD
Orthopedic Surgery

GMF:pai
D:2/9/----
T:2/9/----

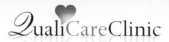

Genitourinary Surgery

Patient Name: David Robert Leo   **ID#:** S-18

Date of Operation: 3 May ----   **Age:** 18 days old   **Sex:** Male

PREOPERATIVE DIAGNOSIS
Possible posterior urethral valves.

POSTOPERATIVE DIAGNOSES
1. Normal urethra.
2. Right partially duplicated renal collecting system with grade 3 unilateral reflux.

SURGEON: Charles Mendesz, MD

ASSISTANT: Jimmy Dale Jett, RN, Circulating Nurse

ANESTHESIA: Sedation and mask ventilation by Dr. Avalon.

OPERATION PERFORMED: Surveillance cystoscopy.

SPECIMEN REMOVED: None.

INDICATIONS: Patient is an 18-day-old premature male infant born at 33 weeks' gestation for a hydramnios seen on prenatal ultrasound. Renal ultrasound and VCUG were performed antenatally with the findings of a partially duplicated right renal collecting system and grade 3 right unilateral vesicoureteral reflux. The voiding portion of the VCUG was suspicious for a possible posterior urethral valve, as reflux was noted, and a dilated posterior urethra was noted. Bilateral renal ultrasound was normal with the left measuring 4.5 cm, the right measuring 4.4 cm. Patient's creatinine was 0.5 prior to VCUG, and after catheterization it dropped down to 0.3. It has remained stable since removal of catheter. We discussed with the patient's family the risks, benefits, alternatives, and indications to diagnostic cystoscopy with possible posterior urethral valve ablation, as this diagnosis was a possibility, although uncertain. The patient's family decided to pursue this procedure for diagnosis. They gave written and verbal consent.

PROCEDURE IN DETAIL: Once proper patient identification and informed consent were obtained, the patient was brought into the operating room and anesthesia provided. The patient was then placed supine frog-legged on the table and prepped and draped in the usual sterile fashion. A 5-French pediatric feeding tube was easily passed into the urinary bladder followed by an 8-French feeding tube with some difficulty. An 8-French cystoscopic sheath, however, was easily passed over the 5-French feeding catheter to allow access to the urethra.

Surveillance cystoscopy was performed, noting mild bladder trabeculation and an orthotopic and normal trigone. The left ureteral orifice was visualized; however, the right was not. The prostatic fossa was not dilated, and there was a normal verumontanum. Upon compression of the bladder, no billowing of posterior urethral valves was noted. The anterior urethra as well was completely normal, and the cystoscopy was terminated. The patient tolerated the procedure well and recovered from his intravenous sedation without problems.

The patient's family was fully informed of the findings at cystoscopy plus the plans for followup, as below.

PLAN: We plan on a renal and bladder ultrasound to be performed in the next 4 to 6 months with a clinic followup after this to evaluate those results. Furthermore, patient should remain on an Amoxil antibiotic prophylaxis for the vesicoureteral reflux. Finally, we shall arrange a repeat VCUG at approximately 1 year of life to evaluate for any resolution of unilateral hydronephrosis. Patient's family was aware and will call to schedule their clinic followup. I have personally ordered the renal and bladder ultrasound through the Hillcrest system.

(Continued)

ID#: S-18   PAGE 2

SPONGE COUNT: Correct at end of case.

COMPLICATIONS: None.

URINE OUTPUT: Not measured.

INTRAVENOUS FLUIDS: 50 mL.

ESTIMATED BLOOD LOSS: Zero.

MEDICATIONS: Amoxil.

_____

Charles Mendesz, MD
Pediatric Urology

CM:pai
D:5/3/----
T:5/4/----

c: Reed Phillips, MD, Pediatrician

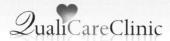
QualiCareClinic

Ear, Nose, and Throat Surgery

Patient Name: Melvin Arney   **ID#:** S-19

Date of Operation: 25 May ----   **Age:** 74   **Sex:** Male

PREOPERATIVE DIAGNOSIS
Supraglottic mass.

POSTOPERATIVE DIAGNOSIS
Supraglottic mass.

SURGEON: Leela Pivari, MD

ASSISTANT: Anna Marie Iaccarino, RN, Scrub Nurse

ANESTHESIA: General endotracheal anesthesia with a 6-0 Armour tube by Dr. Avalon.

OPERATIONS PERFORMED
1. Microdirect laryngoscopy.
2. Supraglottic mass excision.

MATERIAL FORWARDED TO LABORATORY FOR EXAMINATION: Three separate biopsies of the mass lesion were sent to Pathology as specimens.

INDICATIONS: Patient is a 74-year-old African-American male who has complained of 7 months of hoarseness with intermittent hemoptysis, increasing shortness of breath, and the objective feeling that his throat is "closing off." Preoperative workup included a videostroboscopy, which showed an exophytic and papillomatous circular mass obstructing the view of the normal glottis. Preop CT scan showed a supraglottic mass with no other signs of gross disease in the neck. The patient was counseled as to the risks, benefits, and indications of a microdirect laryngoscopy with possible tracheostomy and supraglottic mass excision with possible laser work. The patient desired to proceed with surgery. All questions were answered to the patient's satisfaction.

The patient is on referral from the VA Hospital where he was evaluated by Dr. Lopez and me on Monday, 21 May ----, at which time the patient was found to be resting comfortably with no stridor, no respiratory distress. After we scoped the patient, we referred him to the head & neck clinic for further evaluation and workup. Our evaluation is as above and was concluded in the surgical procedure below.

FINDINGS: Exophytic, papillomatous mass arising from the base of the lingual surface of the epiglottis.

PROCEDURE IN DETAIL: Anesthesia was endotracheal, and the anesthesia service did an awake transoral fiberoptic intubation and used a 6-0 Armour tube.

Patient was identified in the intermediate ICU and his laterality form was signed. Patient was taken to the operating room, placed in the sitting position on the operating table. Anesthesia service gained IV access, an arterial line, and proceeded with a transoral awake fiberoptic intubation assisted by Dr. Avalon with overhead monitored visualization. With the patient intubated, he was put to sleep by anesthesia service. After general endotracheal anesthesia had been achieved, the head of the bed was then lowered into a supine position. The bed had been rotated 90 degrees prior.

At this time, a Lindholm laryngoscope was used to perform the direct laryngoscopy. Of note, the patient was edentulous in the maxillary teeth and had no partials or dentures in his lower teeth. A tooth guard was used to protect the patient's maxillary ridge and laryngoscopy proceeded.

The laryngoscope was put in the vallecula, and the patient was suspended on a mustard stand in the usual sterile fashion. Good visualization of the patient's supraglottic mass was achieved. A 0-degree endoscope was then used

(Continued)

to take pictures of the mass. The mass appeared to be approximately 3 x 3 cm, a circular, pedunculated, exophytic, and papillomatous mass obstructing the view of the normal glottis. A 70-degree scope was then inserted, which afforded visualization of the patient's true vocal cords (which were unaffected by the mass) as well as the anterior commissure (which was unaffected) and the entire scope of the mass itself. The scope was removed.

Attention was turned to the papilloma. Biopsy forceps were then used to take 3 separate biopsies of the lesion, which were sent to pathology as specimens. At this time, a laryngeal blade on the StraightShot microdebrider was used to debride down the mass. This was carried out in a systematic fashion. The tension was used to preserve normal mucosal surfaces of the aryepiglottic folds as well as the false vocal cords. Of note, the papillomatous lesion had a moderate amount of bleeding when it was debrided down to the base near the laryngeal surface of the epiglottis. Epinephrine-soaked pledgets were placed to aid in hemostasis. This slowed down the bleeding well.

At this time, KTP laser with a flexible fiberoptic hand-held piece was inserted. The patient was placed with laser eyewear protection. Everyone in the operating room had correct laser protective eyewear, and the 0.6 mm KTP laser was then used to aid in hemostasis on the remnant lesion, which was at the base of the lingual surface of the epiglottis. This was done to facilitate hemostasis. After good hemostasis had been achieved, the laryngeal microdebrider was then used to complete the mass excision. The microdebrider was removed, and the KTP laser was again used to achieve hemostasis in a broad front along the inferior area of the lingual surfaces of the epiglottis as well as the patient's left aryepiglottic mucosal surface. Hemostasis was found to be good at this time. Some 4 mL of 2% lidocaine was then sprayed with an Angiocath over the patient's glottis to provide anesthesia. The patient was irrigated and suctioned.

At this time the patient was taken off suspension. The laryngoscope was removed. All instruments were removed. The patient was placed in a neutral position. Patient was then turned over to Anesthesia for extubation. He is to recover in the postanesthesia care unit followed by the IJ, then he will be admitted to the ICU with continuous pulse oximetry. If the patient recovers well, the plan is for the patient to be discharged tomorrow morning, postoperative day 1.

The patient was intubated with a 6-0 Armour endotracheal tube at the start of the case. All counts were correct at the close of the case. There were no complications.

SPONGE COUNT: Correct at end of the case.

FLUIDS: 1000 mL crystalloid and 500 mL Hespan.

ESTIMATED BLOOD LOSS: 75 mL.

COMPLICATIONS: None.

_____

Leela Pivari, MD
ENT Clinic

LP:pai
D:5/25/----
T:5/26/----

c: Head & Neck Clinic, Attn: Dr. Lopez

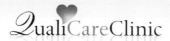

Ophthalmologic Surgery

Patient Name: Mario Bozzi

Date of Operation: 11 July ----

Age: 59

ID#: S-20

Sex: Male

PREOPERATIVE DIAGNOSIS
Temporal arteritis.

POSTOPERATIVE DIAGNOSIS
Temporal arteritis.

SURGEON: Yasmin Naimi, MD

ASSISTANT: Jimmy Dale Jett, RN, Circulating Nurse

ANESTHESIA: Local MAC by Dr. Delaney.

OPERATION PERFORMED: Biopsy of left temporal artery.

MATERIAL FORWARDED TO LABORATORY FOR EXAMINATION: Portion of temporal artery.

PROCEDURE IN DETAIL: After having been properly identified in the preop holding area, the patient was brought to OR 3 and placed under monitored anesthesia control (MAC). At this point a Doppler ultrasound was used to trace the course of the left temporal artery, and a surgical marking pen was used to outline this course.

The temple area was shaved using a standard disposable razor. The skin was then prepped with 5% povidone-iodine and draped in the usual sterile fashion to isolate the left temporal artery. After prepping, local anesthesia consisting of 2% lidocaine with epinephrine was slowly injected through a 25-gauge needle parallel to the artery.

Next, gentle traction was used to pull the skin taut as a #15 blade was used to bisect the skin adjacent to the underlying artery. Small mosquito forceps was used to dissect toward the temporal artery in a subcutaneous plane, at which point the temporal artery was identified. Careful blunt dissection along the side of the vessel was used to expose the artery.

At this point 4-0 silk sutures were used to ligate the exposed temporal artery, 2 sutures on either end, both the proximal and distal ends of the temporal artery. Two small feeder vessels were also ligated using a single 4-0 silk suture.

Next, suture scissors were used to cut the temporal artery in between the distal and proximal ends, where the sutures had been previously placed to ligate the artery. After the artery had been removed, it was measured and determined to be 2.5 cm. It was then placed in formalin for pathologic inspection. General cautery was used to control areas of residual bleeding. Next, two 6-0 Vicryl sutures were used to close the subcutaneous tissue layer. Finally, skin closure was obtained by placing six 6-0 fast-absorbing gut sutures. Bacitracin ophthalmic ointment was applied to the wound, and a 2 x 2 gauze sponge was placed lengthwise over the wound, and a Tegaderm tape was placed over this gauze.

The patient was returned to the postoperative recovery room in stable condition.

FLUIDS: None.

(Continued)

ID#: S-20

ESTIMATED BLOOD LOSS: Minimal.

COMPLICATIONS: None.

DISPOSITION: Stable.

_____
Yasmin Naimi, MD
Ophthalmology

YN:pai
D:7/11/----
T:7/12/----

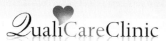

General Surgery Report

Patient Name: Jeremy Crowell   **ID#:** S-21

Date of Operation: 13 June ----   **Age:** 69   **Sex:** Male

PREOPERATIVE DIAGNOSIS
Peritonitis.

POSTOPERATIVE DIAGNOSIS
Perforated diverticulitis.

SURGEON: James A. McClure Jr, MD

ASSISTANT: Bernard Kester, MD

ANESTHESIA: General endotracheal with local by Dr. Delaney.

OPERATIONS PERFORMED
1. Diagnostic laparoscopy.
2. Porter laparotomy.
3. Sigmoid colectomy with Hartmann pouch and end colostomy.

SPECIMEN REMOVED: None.

INDICATIONS: Elderly gentleman with multiple medical problems and abdominal exam concerning for peritonitis and acute abdominal process, requiring operative procedures.

PROCEDURE IN DETAIL: Patient was placed in the supine position in the operating suite. His abdomen was prepped and draped in the usual sterile fashion following general endotracheal intubation by the anesthesia team. Once the patient was intubated, a local anesthesia was infiltrated into the supraumbilical area, and the skin was divided using a knife. The subcutaneous tissues were divided bluntly, and the fascia was elevated using an Allis clamp. The fascia was divided using Bovie cautery, and the abdomen was entered sharply.

Once this was achieved, the Hasson port was placed after an 0 Vicryl had been placed in the fascia. The port was tied in place, and the abdomen was insufflated with CO_2 gas. The abdomen was inspected through two 5 mm working port sites; however, no definite abnormality was seen after a thorough inspection of the gallbladder and appendix and small bowel. Thus the patient was converted to an open procedure for further exploration to explain his severe peritonitis. With thorough manual examination of the bowel, thickening and a perforated region in the sigmoid colon were noted. Thus, it was manually retracted cephalad, and the mesentery was scored. The colon was divided in a disease-free segment, and the mesentery was divided using Endo staplers down to the rectum. Once this had been accomplished, the rectum was cleared circumferentially and divided using the Endo GIA stapler. The ends of the rectum were tagged using 2 very long Prolene sutures, and the abdomen was irrigated thoroughly. No sites of bleeding were noted.

Good hemostasis was noted; thus, the site for the colostomy was selected in the left middle quadrant. The skin was cut using Bovie electrocautery. A cruciate incision was made in the anterior fascia. The muscles were divided between clamps, and the posterior peritoneum was divided using electrocautery. The colon was advanced through the defect, and the fascia was then reapproximated in the midline using running looped PDS sutures. The skin and subcutaneous tissues were irrigated thoroughly and closed with staples. The two 5 mm sites were also closed with staples. The colostomy was then matured using 3-0 Vicryl sutures, bringing the colonic edge to the subdermal region. A colostomy bag was placed. The wounds were viable. The colon was pink. There was no spillage.

(Continued)

ID#: S-21   PAGE 2

Patient tolerated the procedure well. He was extubated in the operating room and was transferred to the intensive care unit for intensive monitoring during his postoperative period.

COMPLICATIONS: None at the time of surgery.

_____

James A. McClure Jr, MD
General Surgery

JAM:pai
D:6/13/----
T:6/14/----

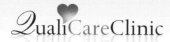

Plastic Surgery Report

Patient Name: Deborah Keith   **ID#:** S-23

Date of Operation: 9 Feb ----   **Age:** 23   **Sex:** Female

PREOPERATIVE DIAGNOSIS
Bilateral nipple inversion (recurrent).

POSTOPERATIVE DIAGNOSIS
Bilateral nipple inversion (recurrent).

SURGEON: Danila R. Fry, MD

ASSISTANT: Jimmy Dale Jett, RN, Circulating Nurse

ANESTHESIA: Local with intravenous sedation by Dr. Avalon.

OPERATION PERFORMED: Correction of bilateral nipple inversion.

SPECIMEN REMOVED: None.

INDICATIONS: This 23-year-old female underwent correction of bilateral nipple inversions 2 years prior at this facility. Since that time the right nipple has retracted somewhat, and the left nipple has retracted nearly completely. She presented to plastic surgery clinic requesting repeat correction of the problem. The proposed procedure as well as the associated risks and benefits were discussed with the patient at length, and questions were answered to her satisfaction. She gave informed consent to proceed.

PROCEDURE IN DETAIL: Patient was brought to the operating room where she was placed on the operating table in supine position. Cardiac monitors were attached, and intravenous sedation was administered. The nipple-areola complex was anesthetized bilaterally with local anesthetic consisting of 1% lidocaine with 1:100,000 epinephrine mixed 1:1 with 0.5% bupivacaine plain. Then 6 mL of anesthetic was injected into the base of each nipple-areola complex for a total of 12 mL. This was allowed to take effect while the patient was prepped and draped in the usual sterile fashion.

The retracted nipple was grasped with forceps and everted enough that a skin hook could be placed into the tip. The skin hook was then used to elevate the nipple out of its fold, so that a 2-0 nylon suture could be placed through its base. With traction on a suture, a stab incision was made at the nipple base with an 11-blade scalpel. Straight iris scissors were then inserted into the incision, into the palpable fibrous bands, which were divided until the nipple was able to stand freely away from the areola with no traction on the traction suture. This was accomplished in an identical fashion on the opposite side.

The stab incision was closed with a single 5-0 fast-absorbing gut suture. A single 0.25-inch Steri-Strip was applied to the incision. The wound was dressed with a sterile gauze 2 x 2. A portion of blue foam egg crate was cut out and fashioned into a splint to prevent compression of the nipple. The retraction suture was passed through the center of the foam splint and taped to the chest wall superiorly on both sides in order to maintain continuous traction during the healing phase. Traction suture will be switched to a 6-o'clock position at 4 days postoperatively. The patient will perform this herself.

She was awakened from the anesthetic and transferred to recovery in good condition. There were no complications at the time of this dictation.

SPONGE COUNT VERIFIED: Correct at end of case.

PROSTHETIC DEVICES: None.

(Continued)

ESTIMATED BLOOD LOSS: Minimal.

INTRAVENOUS FLUIDS: 600 mL crystalloid.

COMPLICATIONS: None.

_____
Danila R. Fry, MD
Plastic Surgery

DRF:pai
D:2/9/----
T:2/9/----

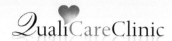

Ear, Nose, and Throat Surgical Report

Patient Name: Lawrence Davis

Date of Operation: 10 March ----

Age: 45

ID#: S-24

Sex: Male

PREOPERATIVE DIAGNOSIS
Nasal airway obstruction, deviated nasal septum.

POSTOPERATIVE DIAGNOSIS
Nasal airway obstruction, deviated nasal septum.

SURGEON: Leela Pivari, MD

ASSISTANT: Jimmy Dale Jett, RN, Circulating Nurse

ANESTHESIA: General endotracheal by Dr. Delaney.

OPERATION PERFORMED: Septoplasty, turbinoplasty, bilateral endonasal batten grafts.

SPECIMEN REMOVED: None.

INDICATIONS: This 45-year-old male has a history of nasal airway obstruction and a deviated nasal septum to the left. He has failed maximum medical therapy.

PROCEDURE IN DETAIL: The patient was taken to the operating room and placed supine on the operating room table. After general anesthesia had been induced, the head of the bed was turned 90 degrees by Anesthesia. At this point, the nasal septum was injected with 1% lidocaine with 1:100,000 epinephrine, a total of 12 mL used. The nose was packed with Afrin-soaked pledgets. The patient was then prepped and draped in the usual sterile fashion for a septoplasty.

On the left side of the nose, a Killian incision was made using a 15 blade. A mucoperichondrial-to-mucoperiosteal flap was elevated using a Freer elevator. A D-knife was used to resect the septal cartilage, being careful to leave a 1 x 1 cm caudal and dorsal strut. The contralateral mucoperichondrial-to-mucoperiosteal flap was elevated. The graft was passed off the field and fashioned into elliptical batten grafts.

At this point the marginal incision was made on the left nostril, and the Converse scissors were used to dissect in a supracondylar plane over the lower lateral cartilage down to the pyriform rim. A small pocket was used to secure the batten graft. The exact same procedure was performed on the right side. The marginal incisions were closed using 5-0 chromic suture in an interrupted fashion.

The inferior turbinates were then injected with 1% lidocaine with 1:100,000 epinephrine. The Killian incision was closed using 4-0 chromic suture in an interrupted fashion. A quilting stitch made of 5-0 plain gut was performed. Next the anterior heads of the inferior turbinate were incised using a 15 blade. A mucoperiosteal flap was elevated, and the bony inferior turbinate was outfractured. The Sayre elevator was used to outfracture the remainder of the turbinate. The exact same procedure was performed on the right side on the inferior turbinate.

The Reuter splints were then secured to the membranous septum using 2-0 black nylon suture, and Telfa splints covered with Bactroban ointment were then placed into the bilateral nasal cavities as well as 2 vestibular splints. The sponge, needle, and instrument counts were all correct at the end of the case. No complications were noted at the end of the case.

(Continued)

ID#: S-24   PAGE 2

The patient was turned over to Anesthesia, where he was extubated and transferred to the PACU in stable condition.

ESTIMATED BLOOD LOSS: Minimal.

COMPLICATIONS: None.

_____
Leela Pivari, MD
ENT Clinic

LP:pai
D:3/10/----
T:3/11/----

QualiCareClinic

Obstetrics/Gynecology Surgery

Patient Name: Leticia Valdez

Date of Operation: 4 June ----

Age: 39

ID#: S-25

Sex: Female

PREOPERATIVE DIAGNOSES
Satisfied parity. Desires permanent surgical sterilization.

POSTOPERATIVE DIAGNOSES
Satisfied parity. Desires permanent surgical sterilization.

SURGEON: Tillman Risha, MD

ASSISTANT: Michael Gerard, DO

ANESTHESIA: Monitored care anesthesia (MAC) with a total of 10 mL of lidocaine without epinephrine injected for a paracervical block by Dr. Avalon.

OPERATION PERFORMED
1. Exam under anesthesia.
2. Diagnostic hysteroscopy with bilateral Essure tubal occlusion device placement.

SPECIMEN REMOVED: None.

FINDINGS: Examination under anesthesia revealed an anteverted uterus, normal in size, shape, and contour, mobile without masses. Hysteroscopy revealed a normal-appearing cavity with ostia visualized bilaterally. At the fundus, the Essure devices were placed in the ostia bilaterally and successfully deployed. An 8-week sized anteverted uterus, normal in size, shape, and contour. Successful bilateral Essure deployment—right with 5 coils, left with 12 coils.

PROCEDURE IN DETAIL: Prior to procedure, patient was counseled extensively on the risks, benefits, and alternatives of permanent sterilization. It was explained to her that the Essure device is absolutely permanent. There is no possibility of reversal after this device has been deployed, no possibility of future pregnancies using any means of assisted reproductive technologies. She understands that this is permanent and desires to proceed with the surgery.

The patient was taken to the operating room and given IV sedation. She was then placed in the high lithotomy position and prepped and draped in the usual sterile fashion. A sterile speculum was then placed, and a single-toothed tenaculum was used to grasp the anterior lip of the cervix. A total of 10 mL lidocaine without epinephrine was injected at the 4-o'clock and 8-o'clock positions for a paracervical block. The Hanks dilators were used to 20 and the Hegar dilators to size 8.

The 8 mm hysteroscope was then advanced into the uterus; the cavity was well visualized, and both ostia were visualized. The Essure device was then advanced through the hysteroscope and the right ostium visualized. The Essure device was then advanced into the right fallopian tube and deployed successfully with a total of 5 coils visible in the uterine cavity. The same procedure was then carried out on the left side. The left ostium was visualized. The Essure device advanced into the fallopian tube and deployed with a total of 12 coils visualized in the uterine cavity. The hysteroscope was then removed. The single-toothed tenaculum was then removed. Hemostasis was noted at the tenaculum sites. The sterile speculum was then removed.

Patient was taken out of the high lithotomy position and taken to the PACU in stable condition. There were no complications. She was discharged to home in stable condition.

PROSTHETIC DEVICE: Essure device.

(Continued)

ID#: S-25

INTRAVENOUS FLUIDS: 500 mL lactated Ringer's.

URINE OUTPUT: Not recorded.

ESTIMATED BLOOD LOSS: Less than 10 mL.

COMPLICATIONS: None.

DISPOSITION: Patient was instructed to continue using contraception for 3 months. She is to return for her hysterosalpingogram at that time, 3 months from now.

Patient was given her Essure card and was instructed to provide that card to any physician who would be planning to perform either further GYN or abdominal procedures on her.

Patient was given the number to the clinic and instructed to follow up for any concerns of infection, increased pain, bleeding. She was instructed to go to the ER for temperature greater than 101 F, severe abdominal pain, and/or heavy bleeding. Plan is for postop followup in 4 weeks.

FINAL DIAGNOSIS is status post hysteroscopy with Essure placement.

_____

Tillman Risha, MD
OB/GYN Surgery

TR:pai
D:6/4/----
T:6/7/----

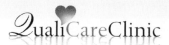

Gastroenterology Surgical Procedure

Patient Name: Evelyn Foote   **ID#:** S-26

Date of Procedure: 10 July ----   **Age:** 19   **Sex:** Female   **DOB:** 20 Aug ----

PREOPERATIVE DIAGNOSIS: Hematochezia.

POSTOPERATIVE DIAGNOSIS: Hematochezia.

SURGEON: Michael Panagides, MD

ASSISTANT: Don Richards, MD

ANESTHESIA: Propofol by Dr. Delaney.

OPERATION PERFORMED: Colonoscopy with biopsy.

MATERIAL FORWARDED TO LABORATORY FOR EXAMINATION: See "findings."

INDICATIONS: This is a 19-year-old female with a history of constipation in the past who presented with recurrent hematochezia despite soft stools. She underwent colonoscopy to rule out polyps, inflammatory bowel disease, and other etiologies for her rectal bleeding. Of note, she has experienced the majority of her rectal bleeding after exertional exercise. She is training heavily for a triathlon.

FINDINGS

1. The entire colonic mucosa had normal mucosal appearance without evidence for colitis, polyps, or other abnormalities.
2. Small lesions consistent with lymphonodular hyperplasia were noted in the patient's cecum and in the terminal ileum.
3. On retroflex view in the rectum, small amounts of scar tissue were noted in the perirectal region that were most consistent with recurrent hemorrhoidal bleeding from constipation.
4. Biopsies were obtained from the terminal ileum as well as other segments of the colon. Further documentation was obtained of the entire colon.

PROCEDURE: History and physical examination performed prior to the procedure. Informed consent outlining risks, benefits, and alternatives to the procedure was obtained prior to procedure having been performed.

After the patient was adequately sedated, the colonoscope was inserted into the rectum. Under direct visualization it was advanced to the terminal ileum. Careful inspection of the colonic mucosa was made as the endoscope was advanced and withdrawn. The quality of the preparation was good. The patient tolerated the procedure well, and there were no complications.

RECOMMENDATIONS

1. Followup biopsies in 2 weeks in outpatient clinic.
2. Patient may be discharged home from Same Day Surgery when awake, tolerating clear liquids, and cleared by Anesthesia.

(Continued)

3. We are going to start Amitiza 24 mcg p.o. b.i.d. to assist with constipation. Will monitor clinical response.
4. Reassured mom that no evidence of inflammatory bowel disease or polyps was seen. Suspect that recurrent bleeding is likely secondary to small hemorrhoids or fissuring at the rectum from previous constipation.

_____

Michael Panagides, MD
Gastroenterology

MP:pai
D:7/10/----
T:7/12/----

c: Linda Galbraith, RN, FNP
    Internal Medicine Clinic

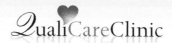

General Surgery Report

Patient Name: Mary Elizabeth Nabb   **ID#:** S-27

Date of Operation: 23 July ----   **Age:** 28   **Sex:** Female

PREOPERATIVE DIAGNOSIS
Acute appendicitis with an 18-week gestation pregnancy.

POSTOPERATIVE DIAGNOSIS
Acute appendicitis with an 18-week gestation pregnancy.

SURGEON: James A. McClure Jr, MD

ASSISTANT: Michael Gerard, DO

ANESTHESIA: General endotracheal by Dr. Avalon.

OPERATION PERFORMED: Laparoscopic appendectomy.

MATERIAL FORWARDED TO LABORATORY FOR EXAMINATION: The appendix was placed in an EndoCatch bag and sent to Pathology.

INDICATIONS: Ms. Nabb is a 28-year-old female with an 18-week pregnancy. She presented with signs and symptoms of acute appendicitis, confirmed by imaging studies. We discussed with her the options, including open appendectomy under local plus laparoscopic appendectomy. As her appendix appeared to be retrocecal, we felt that laparoscopic was best. Questions were answered, patient understood, and she signed her informed consent.

PROCEDURE: After induction of general endotracheal anesthesia, the patient was placed supine and prepped and draped in the usual sterile fashion. A supraumbilical Hasson cannula was placed through the skin incision. The abdomen was then insufflated with gastric pressure to 12 mmHg, and other ports were placed in the right lower quadrant and right upper quadrant. The ileum was grasped. There were adhesions fixing the ileum to the pelvic brim, and these were taken down. The ileum was able to be moved into the upper abdomen. The cecum was rolled toward the midline by incising along the white line of Toldt. The appendix was densely adherent to the underside of the cecum, and the tip of the appendix approximated the liver. The base of the appendix was dissected free of the cecum and stapled with a 45 Endo GIA. The appendix was separated from the pericecal fat and mesentery using the hook electrocautery. The appendix was then completely mobilized off the cecum, and its mesentery was stapled using a 45 Endo GIA stapler.

At this point the appendix was placed in an EndoCatch bag and retrieved through the umbilical port site. All surgical sites were hemostatic. The abdomen was irrigated with saline solution, and the ports were removed. On removing the right lower quadrant port, there was some bleeding from the port site consistent with a branch of the inferior epigastric vessel. The bleeding was controlled with an 0 Vicryl passed through a Carter-Thomason needle driver around the inferior aspect of the wound.

(Continued)

At this point all surgical sites were hemostatic. Ports were removed under direct vision, and the abdominal gas was desufflated. The 12-lumen trocar sites were closed at the fascial level with 0 Vicryl. Skin was closed with a running subcuticular stitch. No complications were observed.

_____
James A. McClure Jr, MD
General Surgery

JAM:pai
D:7/23/----
T:7/24/----

c: Michael Gerard, DO
    OB/GYN Clinic

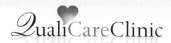

General Surgery Report

Patient Name: Cecilia Gonzalez
Date of Operation: 11 Nov ----   **Age:** 70   **ID#:** S-28
Sex: Female

PREOPERATIVE DIAGNOSIS
Incarcerated femoral hernia, right.

POSTOPERATIVE DIAGNOSIS
Incarcerated femoral hernia, right.

SURGEON: James A. McClure Jr, MD

ASSISTANT: Bernard Kester, MD

ANESTHESIA: General endotracheal by Dr. Delaney.

OPERATIONS PERFORMED
1. Diagnostic laparoscopy.
2. Operative reduction of right femoral hernia.
3. Transabdominal preperitoneal repair using preperitoneal buttressed mesh.

SPECIMEN REMOVED: None.

INDICATIONS: Ms. Gonzalez is a very pleasant 70-year-old lady who had an incarcerated hernia that she had known of for at least a week. She had no obstructive symptoms. CT scan had been obtained in the ED, which determined that there was a loop of bowel in her femoral canal. I discussed with her the fact that this needed to be repaired tonight in order to rule out strangulation. The best way to do this, I felt, was via laparoscopy followed by repair. She understood and signed a written, informed consent.

PROCEDURE: After induction of general endotracheal anesthesia, arms were tucked. Foley catheter was placed. She was prepped and draped in the usual sterile fashion. An infraumbilical incision was made using Hasson technique. The peritoneum was opened sharply and under direct vision. Cannula was inserted. Its presence confirmed by passing laparoscopy, which revealed normal viscera. Patient had a loop of some small intestine that was incarcerated in the right femoral canal. She had no other abdominal wall or groin defects.

Two 5 mm trocars were placed in the left and right sides of the abdomen, respectively, when patient was placed in Trendelenburg position. Using manual traction, the bowel was reduced from the femoral canal. At this point the bowel appeared viable; thus, a transabdominal preperitoneal repair was performed using scissors to take down the peritoneum overlying the right myopectineal orifice. A branch of the inferior epigastric artery was encountered, and this was controlled with clips. The round ligament was separated from the internal ring and divided with clips, freeing up the peritoneum except for where the preperitoneal fat was incarcerated in the femoral canal. Using traction with pressure on the groin, the femoral fat pad was reduced and the peritoneum freed up, exposing Cooper ligament.

(Continued)

ID#: S-28   PAGE 2

At this point a 4 x 6 piece of Prolene soft mesh was inserted into the preperitoneal space. It was doubly clipped to Cooper ligament and clipped anteriorly such that all clips were above the iliopubic tract. At this point the peritoneal flap was then reattached to the abdominal wall using clips. Trocars were removed under direct vision. All surgical sites were hemostatic. Umbilical fascia was closed with Vicryl. Skin was closed with running absorbable subcuticular suture. No complications were observed.

DRAINS: Foley left for drainage.

_____
James A. McClure Jr, MD
General Surgery

JAM:pai
D:11/11/----
T:11/11/----

c: Martha C. Eaton, MD
    Family Practice/Geriatrics

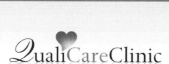

Orthopaedic Surgical Report

Patient Name: Anderson Witten   **ID#:** S-29

Date of Operation: 2 Feb ----   **Age:** 46   **Sex:** Male

PREOPERATIVE DIAGNOSIS
Delayed diagnosis, right Achilles rupture, 3 months' chronicity.

POSTOPERATIVE DIAGNOSIS
Delayed diagnosis, right Achilles rupture, 3 months' chronicity.

SURGEON: Gilbert M. Fields, MD

ASSISTANT: Jack Zullig, MD

ANESTHESIA: General endotracheal by Dr. Avalon.

OPERATION PERFORMED: Debridement with repair of delayed rupture of Achilles tendon using VY advancement, turndown, plantaris weave.

SPECIMEN REMOVED: None.

INDICATIONS: This is an active duty male, 46 years old, who was doing an athletic activity about 3 months ago or so. He felt a pop and had a significant amount of pain in his posterior distal leg, right side. Patient was seen by PCP and diagnosed with an ankle sprain, and he was treated as such.

The patient came to my clinic with continued complaints about 3 months out, and I diagnosed him clinically with a ruptured Achilles tendon, as mentioned. We got an MRI scan followed by an ultrasound, which confirmed this. Throughout the imaging studies, we were able to appreciate the plantaris tendon.

PROCEDURE: After a lengthy discussion with this patient, it was determined that he would benefit from a debridement with an operative repair. On the day of surgery the consents were checked, the site was marked, and patient was brought to the OR. Anesthesia was induced, and the patient was placed prone on the operating room table with all bony prominences well padded. A timeout took place, during which operative site was confirmed. We prepped and draped both legs in the usual sterile fashion.

Next an incision was made on the medial aspect of the Achilles tendon, going through skin and dermal layer on the right side. This was a very lengthy incision, going past the myotendinous junction proximally to the insertion distally. We curved the incision laterally with a gentle curve distally. Care was taken to make full-thickness flaps, keeping the paratenon attached to the skin. This was done by sharply dissecting straight through the paratenon once we identified it. We had to break up a significant amount of adhesions about the area of the previous rupture, as it had scarred in the body's attempt to heal. We were able to free up the tendon in its entire circumference proximally and distally and around the portion that had been damaged by the rupture. We resected an approximately 3.5 cm area of damaged and scarred tendon at the rupture site. Of note, there was a little bit of hematoma in there. The tendon was quite disorganized and damaged. We were able to find decent tendon proximally and decent tendon distally.

Next, Krackow stitches were placed in both ends of each stump. At this point we then did a VY at the cast area. Once all the tendinous bands were released, we used a Krackow stitch on the proximal stump and pulled some, and I was able to gain about 2 cm to 2.5 cm on that. A turndown was made on the distal aspect of the proximal stump, and this was just the most posterior layer of the tendon, leaving the distal portion attached, which we tacked down with some Vicryl sutures. I was then able to fold this over the primary end-to-end repair, which I did for that.

Holding the foot up and checking the tension next to the good leg's ankle tension, we repaired the tendon end-to-end with the Krackow stitches in the core using a little bit more plantar flexion. In other words, just slightly more tension, as I anticipated some relaxation. That was held throughout the repair from that

(Continued)

point forward. The Krackow stitches were tied down, and then the turndown was folded over—so, we had a turndown flap from proximal to distal. That was tacked down as well with Vicryl stitches. Next we did a plantaris weave through the distal stump into the proximal stump, tying it back to itself, leaving its original attachment distally.

The paratenon was then closed carefully, and we were successful in that. Then the skin was closed with no tension. The wound had been copiously irrigated prior to that. Tourniquet was dropped at 100 minutes, and a dorsal slap was placed, pulling the foot into the plantar flexed position. The count was correct at the end of the case. There were no complications.

DISPOSITION: This patient is going to remain nonweightbearing for about 2 weeks. I am going to let him start weightbearing after that with a dorsal blocking splint on, keeping where he is. Each week we will bring it up about 5 degrees. I will let the patient start active and passive therapy and such at about the 6- to 8-week point, depending on how he is doing. Right now I just want his end-to-end repair to heal up pretty nicely.

_____
Gilbert M. Fields, MD
Orthopaedic Surgery

GMF:pai
D:2/2/----
T:2/2/-----

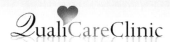

<u>**Orthopaedic Surgical Report**</u>

Patient Name: Anderson Witten   **ID#:** S-30

Date of Operation: 15 March ----   **Age:** 46   **Sex:** Male

PREOPERATIVE DIAGNOSIS
Left Achilles skin breakdown.

POSTOPERATIVE DIAGNOSIS
Left Achilles skin breakdown.

SURGEON: Gilbert M. Fields, MD

ASSISTANT: Jack Zullig, MD

ANESTHESIA: Popliteal block by Dr. Delaney.

OPERATION PERFORMED: Right Achilles incision and drainage.

SPECIMEN REMOVED: None.

INDICATIONS: This is a 46-year-old male, well known to the orthopaedic clinic. He was followed by us after having sustained a chronic Achilles rupture late last year. Patient subsequently was treated with a strengthening procedure as well as an Achilles turndown. He was noted to have some skin breakdown along the edges, and he was subsequently taken back to the operating room approximately 2 weeks after his index procedure on 2 Feb ---- for repeat procedure to consist of pie crusting. After this had been performed, he subsequently had an additional procedure, an additional washout, and he was sent home. Upon return to clinic, patient had what appeared to be wound breakdown along the skin edges. Since that time, patient was admitted to the hospital, placed on IV antibiotics, and presents today for his third I&D of his Achilles tendon.

PROCEDURE: After patient was identified by the nursing team, the anesthesia team, and the surgical team, the surgical site was prepped and marked appropriately by all 3 teams. Patient was then taken back to the operating room where a final timeout was taken to identify the appropriate patient, appropriate time, and appropriate procedure. After this had been done, the patient was prepped and draped in the usual sterile fashion. The wound was irrigated out with 9 liters of normal saline flushed through the wound and using very light curettage.

Finally the patient's wound was débrided thoroughly and several 2-0 nylon sutures were placed, getting the wound edges to appose each other. After this had been completed, a wound V.A.C. was placed over the wound. At this point, the patient was placed in a bulky Jones splint and taken out of the OR and back to the floor.

SPONGE COUNT VERIFIED: Correct x2.

DRAINS: One wound V.A.C.

INTRAVENOUS FLUIDS: 500 mL normal saline.

ESTIMATED BLOOD LOSS: None.

TOURNIQUET TIME: None.

(Continued)

ID#: S-30   PAGE 2

POSTOP PLANS
1. At this time, plans for the patient include a consult with the infectious disease service and followup on his cultures.
2. Will possibly place him on long-term IV antibiotics.
3. Treat him with IV antibiotics until the cultures return. He may need graft coverage in the future.

_____

Gilbert M. Fields, MD
Orthopaedic Surgery

GMF:pai
D:3/15/----
T:3/16/----

c: Beth Brian, MD, Infectious Disease

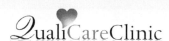

Plastic Surgery Report

Patient Name: Ursula Castro   **ID#:** S-31

Date of Operation: 23 Feb ----   **Age:** 35   **Sex:** Female

PREOPERATIVE DIAGNOSIS
Symptomatic macromastia, redundant abdominal wall skin and fat.

POSTOPERATIVE DIAGNOSIS
Symptomatic macromastia, redundant abdominal wall skin and fat.

SURGEON: Danila R. Fry, MD

ASSISTANT: Anna Marie Iaccarino, Scrub Nurse

ANESTHESIA: General endotracheal by Dr. Avalon.

OPERATIONS PERFORMED
(1) Bilateral breast reductions. (2) Abdominoplasty.

MATERIAL FORWARDED TO THE LABORATORY FOR EXAMINATION
(1) Right and left breast tissue. (2) Abdominal wall skin and fat.

INDICATIONS: Patient is a 35-year-old woman who had been evaluated in the plastic surgery clinic for complaints of neck, back, and shoulder pain for several years. The patient complained of large, ptotic breasts and pain in her shoulders secondary to the bra strap, pain in her upper back, neck, and shoulder. The patient was evaluated and noted to have large, ptotic breasts. She was felt to be a good candidate for breast reduction surgery. The surgery and its indications, alternatives, risks, and potential complications were discussed with the patient. After a thorough discussion, she elected to proceed.

Additionally, Ms. Castro complained of loose skin and fatty tissue on her lower abdomen since the delivery of her last baby. The patient has had prior cesarean section deliveries of 2 children, and she had noted an overhang of skin above the incision. The patient's abdomen was evaluated. She was noted to have redundant abdominal wall skin and fat amenable to abdominoplasty surgery. The procedure, its indications, alternatives, risks, and potential complications were discussed. After a thorough discussion, she elected to proceed.

PROCEDURE IN DETAIL: After informed consent and proper identification, the patient was transferred into the operating room, placed on the operating room table in a supine position. Appropriate monitoring equipment was connected to the patient by the anesthesiologist. General endotracheal anesthetic was induced by the anesthesiologist, and when deemed adequate, the patient was prepped and draped in the usual sterile fashion. Patient had been marked while awake and upright for the Wise-type pattern inferior pedicle-type breast reduction. Additionally, her abdomen had been marked for abdominoplasty procedure.

The breast tissues were infiltrated with a total of 40 mL of a local anesthetic solution injected into each breast. The local anesthetic consisted of 0.25% lidocaine with epinephrine 1:400,000. The operation was begun by identifying the nipple-areola complex and circumscribing it with a 42 mm cookie cutter. The nipple-areola complex was then circumscribed with a 2 cm border, which was deepithelialized sharply with a scalpel blade. The planned incision lines were then incised with a scalpel and flaps of skin and breast tissue elevated in the medial, lateral, and cranial aspects of the breast. After elevating the flaps, attention was directed to removal of breast tissue. Tissue was then removed from the medial and lateral aspects of the breast, preserving the inferior pedicle. The majority of breast tissue removed came from the lateral aspect of the breast. Skin was then removed from the remaining breast tissue. The wounds were then copiously irrigated and inspected for hemostasis. Small bleeding points were identified and cauterized with electrocautery. Skin staples were then used to approximate the cut skin edges, and the patient was placed in an upright position. She was inspected for symmetry and size match. Symmetry and size match were noted to be good.

(Continued)

ID#: S-31   PAGE 2

Attention was directed toward placement of the nipple-areola complex. A location 47 mm from the inframammary incision was identified for the caudal border of the nipple-areola complex. The location was marked with a 38 mm cookie cutter. The patient was returned to a supine position and attention directed toward wound closure. The incisions were repaired in 2 layers with deep dermal sutures of 3-0 Monocryl and a running subcuticular suture of 3-0 Monocryl and Steri-Strips. After repair of the vertical and horizontal incisions, the nipple-areola complex was re-marked with a 38 mm cookie cutter. A button of skin and breast tissue was removed to allow delivery of the nipple-areola complex. The nipple-areola complex was delivered through the hole and sutured in place in 2 layers with deep dermal sutures of 3-0 Monocryl and a running subcuticular suture of 3-0 Monocryl and Steri-Strips. Total weight of tissue removed from the right breast was 306 g and from the left was 168 g. Breasts were dressed with sterile gauze.

Attention was directed toward performing the abdominoplasty surgery. The abdominoplasty was begun by identifying the previously marked incision lines. The skin was incised with a scalpel blade, and electrocautery was used to incise through the subcutaneous tissues down to the level of the abdominal wall fascia. The skin and subcutaneous tissues were elevated from the abdominal wall fascia to the level of the umbilicus. The umbilicus was circumscribed with a scalpel blade and freed from the flap, leaving it adherent to the abdominal wall musculature. Dissection continued superficial to the abdominal wall fascia, extending up to the caudal margin and xiphoid process. The wound was then copiously irrigated and inspected for hemostasis. Small bleeding points were cauterized with the electrocautery.

Attention was then directed to performing a plication of the rectus abdominis fascia. Adson forceps was used to approximate the anterior rectus sheath to gain an estimate of the extent of possible plication. Interrupted sutures of 0 Ethibond were placed in an interrupted figure-of-8 fashion to imbricate the anterior rectus sheath. This resulted in an improvement of the overall tone of the abdominal wall musculature.

Attention was then directed to excising the excess abdominal wall skin and fat. The previously estimated tissue was confirmed and excised sharply with the electrocautery. The incisions were approximated with skin staples and the location of the umbilicus identified. A V-shaped incision was placed at the corresponding location in the midline with a scalpel blade. A button of fatty tissue was removed deep to the incision to allow delivery of the umbilicus. The umbilicus was incised on its cranial aspect to create a heart-shaped umbilicus, which would be inset into the V-shaped incision. A Marcaine pain catheter was placed through the skin and secured in the midline with loose sutures of 4-0 Monocryl. Two 7 mm Blake drains were placed, exiting the pubic hair region.

The incisions were repaired in 3 layers. Interrupted sutures of 3-0 PDS were used to approximate the Scarpa fascia. The skin was repaired with deep dermal sutures of 3-0 Monocryl and a running subcuticular suture of 3-0 Monocryl and Steri-Strips. The umbilicus was inset with deep dermal sutures of 3-0 Monocryl and a running suture of 5-0 Prolene. The pain catheter was connected to a Marcaine reservoir filled with 0.25% Marcaine to infuse at 2 mL/h.

The final dressing on the wound was half-inch Steri-Strips and sterile gauze followed by an abdominal binder. The operation was performed without complication, and the patient tolerated the procedure well. She was transferred to the recovery room, awake, extubated, and in good condition.

ESTIMATED BLOOD LOSS: 100 mL.

COMPLICATIONS: None.

_____
Danila R. Fry, MD
Plastic Surgery

DRF:pai
D:2/23/----
T:2/24/----

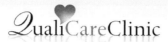

General Surgery Report

Patient Name: Thomas A. Clegg   **ID#:** S-32

Date of Operation: 15 March ----   **Age:** 79   **Sex:** Male

PREOPERATIVE DIAGNOSIS
History of supraglottic laryngeal squamous cell cancer with probable recurrence and near-obstructing esophageal mass.

POSTOPERATIVE DIAGNOSIS
History of supraglottic laryngeal squamous cell cancer with probable recurrence and near-obstructing esophageal mass.

SURGEON: James A. McClure Jr, MD

ASSISTANT: Don Richards, MD

ANESTHESIA: General endotracheal by Chuck Delaney, MD

OPERATIONS PERFORMED
1. Placement of a feeding catheter jejunostomy.
2. Placement of a Port-A-Cath.

SPECIMEN REMOVED: None.

INDICATIONS: Col. Clegg is a 79-year-old male with a history of supraglottic laryngeal cancer back in 1990, squamous cell. The patient has had a probable recurrence with extension into the esophagus, as shown by a recent EGD that showed a near-obstructing mass in the proximal esophagus.

COMPLICATIONS: None.

ESTIMATED BLOOD LOSS: Less than 10 mL.

CONDITION: Stable.

PROCEDURE IN DETAIL

Procedure #1: After informed consent was obtained and Col. Clegg had all his questions and concerns addressed, he was taken back to the operating room and placed supine on the operating table. Next general endotracheal anesthesia was induced without complication. The patient's abdomen and pelvis were then prepped and draped in the usual sterile fashion. A 15-blade scalpel was used to make an approximately 4 cm to 5 cm incision, starting just above the umbilicus and extending just below the umbilicus.

Next electrocautery was used to extend the incision down to the level of the fascia. The fascia was opened with electrocautery. The peritoneum was grasped and opened sharply, and the abdomen was entered under direct vision. Exploration of the abdomen was done. The abdomen was grossly normal. The ligament of Treitz was identified. The small intestine was run from the ligament of Treitz to the cecum. No gross abnormalities were appreciated on exam.

Next the ligament of Treitz was again identified and we went approximately 40 cm distal to the ligament of Treitz, which was our site of feeding catheter jejunostomy. Next a 3-0 silk suture was placed at our site where our feeding catheter jejunostomy (FCJ) tube was to be inserted in a pursestring fashion. The bowel was opened using electrocautery. The FCJ tube was inserted distally into the jejunum. The pursestring suture was then tied down to secure the tube in place.

(Continued)

ID#: S-32   PAGE 2

We chose a site in the left upper quadrant where the FCJ would come out of the skin. Electrocautery was used to make a 5 mm incision in the skin, and a tonsil clamp was used to enter the abdomen under direct vision without intraabdominal injury. The FCJ tube was then taken out of the abdominal wall. The jejunum was then secured in Stamm fashion to the anterior abdominal wall with 2-0 silk sutures. Four 2-0 silk sutures were used to secure the jejunum to the anterior abdominal wall in four quadrants. This brought the jejunum up to the anterior abdominal wall very nicely and secure. In addition, one proximal 2-0 silk suture and one distal 2-0 suture were used to secure the jejunum to the anterior abdominal wall. Next the FCJ was secured in place and noted to flush easily. The abdomen was then again inspected and noted to be hemostatic. We proceeded with closure of the fascia.

The fascia was then closed with 1-0 PDS in a running fashion. Subcutaneous tissue was then irrigated out, and the skin was closed with staples. Sterile dressings were placed over the wound, and the FCJ was secured in place with a dressing and tape.

Procedure #2: The patient's drapes were completely taken down, and the patient's left chest and arm were again prepped and draped in the usual sterile fashion. New instruments were used for the second procedure. After the patient had been reprepped and draped, he was placed in Trendelenburg position. We then used the finder needle to enter the left subclavian vein without difficulty. This drew back dark blood that was nonpulsatile. We then advanced the wire in standard Seldinger fashion. C-arm was brought in, and it confirmed that the wire was in the superior vena cava.

Next we secured the wire to the drape and proceeded with making our subcutaneous cavity for placement of the Port-A-Cath. A 2 cm incision was made with a 15-blade scalpel approximately 3 to 4 cm below the needle stick site. Next a pocket was made by elevating the skin with skin hooks. Electrocautery was used to make a pocket approximately 2 x 2 cm. This was adequate space in which to put the Port-A-Cath. We then used the tunnel catheter to connect the pocket with the initial needle stick sites. The dilator and sheath were then placed over the wire and inserted into the subclavian vein down into the superior vena cava under direct vision with radiologic confirmation.

Next the catheter was placed in the sheath, and the sheath was peeled back with minimal difficulty. The catheter was then confirmed with the C-arm and noted to be slightly distal, and the catheter was pulled back approximately 3 cm to be at the junction between the SVC and the atrium. We then secured the catheter to the port and put the cap on and screwed it down tightly. The catheter was then checked, and it drew back dark blood and flushed with no problems. The Port-A-Cath was then inserted into the pocket, and it was sewn in place with 2-0 Prolene suture. Scarpa fascia was then closed with a 3-0 Vicryl suture, the skin was closed with 4-0 Monocryl in interrupted fashion, and Dermabond was placed.

In addition, the 5 mm incision from the site of the needle stick was also closed with a 4-0 Monocryl in a simple, interrupted fashion, and Dermabond was placed over the wound. At the end of the case the port was again checked, and it drew back blood without difficulty. It was flushed with 1 mL of 1:1000 heparin solution.

At the end of the case, the patient was awakened. He tolerated the procedure well. There were no complications. He was transferred to the PACU in stable condition.

_____

James A. McClure Jr, MD
General Surgery

JAM:pai
D:3/16/----
T:3/16/----

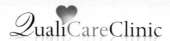

Genitourinary Surgery Report

Patient Name: Beldon Kays   **ID#:** S-33

Date of Operation: 29 Sept ----   **Age:** 46   **Sex:** Male

PREOPERATIVE DIAGNOSIS
Penile fracture.

POSTOPERATIVE DIAGNOSIS
Penile fracture, urethral disruption.

SURGEON: Charles Mendesz, MD

ASSISTANT: Jimmy Dale Jett, Circulating Nurse

ANESTHESIA: General endotracheal.

OPERATIONS PERFORMED
1. Retrograde urethrogram.
2. Penile exploration.
3. Repair of bilateral ventral corporal defect/penile fracture.
4. Repair of urethral laceration/disruption.
5. Circumcision.

SPECIMEN REMOVED: Foreskin.

INDICATIONS: Patient is a 46-year-old male who presented to the ED after sudden painful penile detumescence during intercourse approximately 4 hours prior to evaluation today. He was noted to have blood at his meatus immediately after the intercourse and as well was noted to have blood at the meatus initially in the clinic. Patient was able to void with initial gross hematuria that cleared.

On examination, he had severe penile ecchymosis and edema confined to Buck fascia consistent with penile fracture. Because of the blood at the meatus, there was a great concern for urethral disruption as well, and it was recommended to the patient that he undergo emergent retrograde urethrogram with penile exploration and repair of any defects. The possible injuries to the penile shaft and penile urethra were explained in detail to the patient as well as his risks of long-term penile curvature and impotence, risk of penile or urethral injury, risk of recurrent urethral stricture, risk of abscess or infection, as well as anesthesia risks. These were all explained to the patient in great detail, and he appeared to understand and wished to proceed.

PROCEDURE IN DETAIL: After adequate general anesthesia, the patient was placed in the supine position. His genitalia were initially prepped briefly for the retrograde urethrogram. A retrograde urethrogram was performed using approximately 20 mL of contrast with a C-arm fluoroscopy. There appeared to be a partial disruption in the anterior urethra, approximately in the midshaft of the penile urethra. Some tortuosity and some significant extravasation were seen; however, there was a clear disruption that was obviously a partial disruption in the midpenile urethra.

At this point patient was shaved, prepped, and draped in the usual sterile fashion. A circumcision incision was made in the severely edematous and ecchymotic distal foreskin—performed approximately 1 cm proximal to the glans. A second circumferential incision was made in the outer foreskin, and the sleeve of excess edematous foreskin was excised using sharp and cautery dissection. The penile skin was then degloved down to the base of the penis circumferentially. Prior to this, a Foley catheter had been gently placed with no resistance. It was packed into the bladder, and 600 mL of clear urine was immediately evacuated from the bladder. The balloon was inflated with 10 mL of water.

(Continued)

ID#: S-33   PAGE 2

During the degloving of the penis, a significant hematoma and ecchymoses were noted from the ventral aspect, tracking over to the left side as well. After careful inspection, there was a significant tear and disruption in the ventral urethra, approximately 270 degrees in circumference, with the dorsal plate of the urethra intact. The Foley catheter could be seen going through the urethra at this point. After meticulous dissection, including dissection down to Buck fascia and down to the base of the penis, 2 bleeding corporal defects were noted ventrally. These defects were the penile fracture that had occurred during his intercourse earlier today. They were adjacent to the urethral disruption of the ventral midportion of the penile urethra. It appeared that the corporal defects and the urethral tear were at the exact same level. The corporal defects were then isolated and closed using figure-of-8 2-0 PDS sutures.

At this point, the urethral defect was inspected and the urethra was isolated proximal and distal to the defect. Because of the appearance of a corporal involvement posterior to the tear, the urethra was transected at this level, and the edges of the urethral disruption were carefully trimmed, taking a minimal amount of tissue. At this point, there was a moderate erection that was preventing a tension-free anastomosis, and the corpus was irrigated with 1 mL of dilute phenylephrine solution with immediate detumescence without complication. The urethra was then carefully mobilized proximally about 3 to 4 cm and distally about 1 to 2 cm with excellent mobilization of the proximal and distal urethra, which could then be brought together without tension. The distal end was spatulated at the ventral portion with the urethral tear. It was noted to show a weakness in the wall of the urethra.

An anastomosis was then performed with 5-0 PDS sutures in a full-thickness mucosa in interrupted fashion. Approximately 10 to 12 interrupted 5-0 PDS sutures were placed circumferentially and tied on the outer surface of the urethra. In this fashion, the urethral anastomosis was completed and appeared to be an excellent, watertight anastomosis with no tension. A small amount of bleeding was noted, which was noted dorsal to the urethral anastomosis. Hemostasis was obtained with figure-of-8 4-0 PDS sutures. At this point, there was a small amount of bleeding noted from the dorsal anastomosis that was minimal at most. Some 2 mL of Tisseel fibrin glue was injected around the anastomosis, and complete hemostasis was obtained. The anastomosis was sealed as well.

Another figure-of-8 plicating suture was performed in the area of the bilateral corporal disruption to take some pressure off the ventral aspect of the anastomosis. A second layer was closed over the urethral anastomosis of the dartos fascia circumferentially using interrupted 3-0 Vicryl sutures. The wound was irrigated, and the skin was closed using interrupted 3-0 chromic sutures. Sterile penile dressing was put into position.

Of note, the Foley catheter was replaced during the urethral anastomosis prior to completing the ventral suture placements. Foley catheter was draining clear urine at the end of the procedure. Patient had no surgical complications. He was noted to have urethral disruption, as noted, from his trauma. Both corporal disruptions and the urethral disruption were repaired, as noted. At the end of the procedure, the patient was awakened in the operating room without complication. He appeared to tolerate the procedure well and was transferred to PACU in stable condition.

COMPLICATIONS: No surgical complications at the time of this dictation.

Charles Mendesz, MD
Urology Surgery

CM:pai
D:9/29/----
T:9/30/----

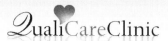

Orthopedic Surgery Report

Patient Name: Jerry Graham   **ID#:** S-34
Date of Operation: 20 Apr ----   **Age:** 57   **Sex:** Male

PREOPERATIVE DIAGNOSIS
Left arm amputation, status post successful reimplantation.

POSTOPERATIVE DIAGNOSIS
Left arm amputation, status post successful reimplantation.

SURGEON: Raquel Rodriguez, MD

ASSISTANT: Mack Stolga, MD

ANESTHESIA: General endotracheal by Carl Erickson Avalon, MD.

OPERATION PERFORMED: Left total elbow arthroplasty.

SPECIMEN REMOVED: None.

INDICATIONS: Mr. Graham is a 57-year-old male who sustained a left arm traumatic amputation. The patient was successfully replanted (reimplanted). The patient has demonstrated excellent soft tissue healing as well as some return of nerve function. The treatment options have been discussed with the patient, and he has subsequently elected for a left total elbow arthroplasty.

PROSTHETIC DEVICES: Coonrad/Morrey total elbow system with a small, 6-inch humeral component and a small, 3-inch ulnar component.

PROCEDURE IN DETAIL: The patient was identified, brought to the operating room, placed supine on the operating table. Preoperative antibiotics were given. General endotracheal anesthesia was obtained. The patient was then placed in the right lateral decubitus position with all areas well padded. The left arm was then placed over an elbow holder, which was well padded as well. The left upper extremity was then prepped and draped in the usual sterile fashion. A sterile tourniquet was placed. Extremity was exsanguinated and tourniquet inflated to 250 mmHg.

Using a posterior approach to the elbow with careful attention to protect the skin flaps, careful dissection was made through the skin and subcutaneous tissue with hemostasis obtained with bipolar cautery. The triceps fascia and tendon were identified. Careful flaps were elevated, both medially and laterally. A triceps-splitting approach was used to approach the elbow. The antibiotic cement spacer was identified. All soft tissue was removed from the distal tip of the olecranon. The lateral collateral ligament insertion was then elevated to expose the radial head. A radial head excision was then performed with a microsagittal saw. The radial head that was excised was used for bone graft for the anterior flange portion of the total elbow system. All soft tissue was then removed from the elbow capsule. The distal humerus was then prepared. Sequential reaming was performed up to 10.5 mm. Sequential broaching was then performed for a 6-inch, small humeral component. The anterior capsule was released anteriorly for a long flange. Once this was accomplished, the wound was then copiously irrigated with normal saline solution.

Attention was then placed to the ulna. The tip of the olecranon was removed with a small microsagittal saw. A bur was used to enter the medullary canal. The canal was identified with small Rush awls. Sequential broaching was then performed up to a 3-inch, small ulnar component. A trial reduction was then performed with a 6-inch, small humeral component and a 3-inch, small ulnar component. Slight lack of extension was noted, approximately 20 to 30 degrees. Skeletal shortening was then performed on the distal humerus, approximately 5 to 7 mm. Again the trial components were placed. Near full extension was noted. The canals were prepared and irrigated with normal saline solution. Cement was then prepared, which was impregnated with gentamicin as well as tobramycin, 1 g. The Coonrad/Morrey small, 6-inch humeral component as well as the small, 3-inch ulnar

(Continued)

component were then cemented into position. The bushing was placed. The elbow was held in full extension until the cement hardened. Good extension and flexion were noted in the operating room. Bone grafting was done in the anterior flange with the radial head, which was resected.

Again, the wound was copiously irrigated with normal saline solution. The triceps fascia and tendon were closed with #2 FiberWire with a locking whip stitch. Three bone tunnels were then created in the proximal ulna and olecranon. The triceps insertion was then repaired with #2 FiberWire to bone. A medium Hemovac was placed. Subcutaneous layer was closed with 2-0 Vicryl suture in interrupted fashion. The skin was closed with 3-0 nylon suture. Sterile dressings were placed. The patient was splinted in full extension with an anterior splint. Awakened from general endotracheal anesthesia, the patient was taken to recovery in stable condition.

_____

Raquel Rodriguez, MD
Orthopedic Surgery

RR:pai
D:2/7/----
T:2/8/----

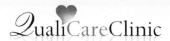

General Surgery Report

Patient Name: Peter Mwongi   **ID#:** S-36

Date of Operation: 16 Dec ----   **Age:** 26   **Sex:** Male

PREOPERATIVE DIAGNOSIS
Recurrent left inguinal hernia.

POSTOPERATIVE DIAGNOSIS
Recurrent left indirect inguinal hernia.

SURGEON: James A. McClure Jr, MD

ASSISTANT: Charles Mendesz, MD

ANESTHESIA: General endotracheal by Carl Erickson Avalon, MD

OPERATIONS PERFORMED
1. Left groin exploration.
2. Repair of left recurrent indirect inguinal hernia with mesh plug.
3. Circumcision by urology service (to be dictated separately from these procedures).

MATERIAL FORWARDED TO LABORATORY FOR EXAMINATION: None.

FINDINGS: A 2 mm aperture at the internal ring with recurrent indirect inguinal hernia. No evidence of direct inguinal hernia.

PROCEDURE IN DETAIL: Mr. Mwongi, a native of Kenya, came to the operating room after having given informed consent. He was anesthetized in the supine position. He was prepped and draped in the usual sterile fashion. Careful manual palpation of the ordinary, expected external landmarks was performed, and we instilled 10 mL of 0.5% Marcaine without epinephrine in an ilioinguinal nerve block 1 cm inferior and medial to the anterior-superior iliac spine. We then infiltrated another 2 mL along our line of incision. We used his previous incision to enter the groin.

We made a 5 cm long incision in the old scar with scalpel, then used careful cautery dissection, elevating the skin edges with Addison forceps to enter down into the subcutaneous tissues. As the patient was relatively slim and asthenic in body habitus, we dissected very slowly and carefully, pausing to carefully palpate and reidentify landmarks. This was necessary because the field of operation was extensively scarred from his two prior hernia surgeries. The scar was not thin and wispy; it was solid and rubbery.

We were able to dissect down to the internal ring by palpation without injury to the cord structures, then carefully dissect out the inferior edge of the inguinal ligament, after which we entered the inguinal canal by opening the external oblique with cautery and forceps. Then we elevated the inferior edge of the external oblique on Allis clamps and dissected the cord structures off it with gentle DeBakey and cautery dissection. We followed the shelving edge of the inguinal ligament all the way lateral to the internal ring. We then came back around superolaterally and dissected the cord free from the canal in a similar fashion, revealing the internal oblique aponeurosis. Again, this was extensively scarred.

Along the midportion of our superior dissection on the actual internal oblique aponeurosis, a small, pulsatile artery began to bleed. This was dissected out, identified, and transfixed with two separate figure-of-8 3-0 Vicryl suture ligatures, which resulted in good hemostasis. This did not appear to be in any way part of the cord structure—although with the extensive distortion and scarring, it is impossible to say whether or not this was one of the original cord structures from his first surgery. We had encircled the cord with a Penrose drain, and we were

(Continued)

able to identify the vas deferens and two vascular structures in the cord. We did not dissect or skeletonize the cord further, as it was relatively thin and atretic. We were able to follow the cord all the way to the internal ring and identify no other sac protruding along the cord.

In the direct space, careful palpation identified no direct defect; in fact, the internal oblique appeared to have been pulled down and sutured to Cooper ligament or at least the inferior edge of the internal oblique. It was a solid, intact closure in the direct space. We irrigated and suctioned. We found that we had good hemostasis.

We then chose to close the direct hernia defect by inserting a mesh plug. We used a small PerFix Prolene plug, which we made even smaller by cutting off the internal layer of petals, leaving the external layer of petals. This fit easily into the defect without providing undue compression upon the cord structures. We sutured it into place with a series of five interrupted 0 Ethibond sutures, suturing inferiorly to shelving edge of the inguinal ligament, laterally to same, and then superomedially to the internal oblique aponeurosis. We then palpated the cord. It was intact and did not appear to be compressed. We were able to place a Kelly clamp in between the cord and the mesh; however, we were unable to place a finger in the defect.

We irrigated and inspected. We had good hemostasis. We closed the scarred and distorted external oblique aponeurosis, carefully taking small bites of the tissues in long travels with a 2-0 Vicryl suture to minimize the possibility of nerve injury. After this was done, we irrigated and inspected subcutaneous tissues. These were also clean and dry, so we closed the skin with a series of interrupted deep dermal 3-0 Vicryl sutures and a running intradermal 4-0 Monocryl suture. We applied Dermabond to the wounds, then called Dr. Mendesz. The patient tolerated this portion of the operative procedure well.

The patient was released intraoperatively to the urology service. Dr. Mendesz came in to perform the patient's concurrent circumcision, after which the patient will be sent to recovery.

SPONGE COUNT VERIFIED: Correct x2 at end of procedure.

ESTIMATED BLOOD LOSS: Less than 50 mL.

INTRAOPERATIVE FLUIDS: 1 L.

COMPLICATIONS: None.

_____

James A. McClure Jr, MD
General Surgery

JAM:pai
D:12/16/----
T:12/16/----

c: Charles Mendesz, MD, Urology

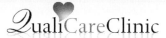

Orthopaedic Surgery Report

Patient Name: Gianpalo Bussappo   **ID#:** S-37

Date of Operation: 21 Feb ----   **Age:** 82   **Sex:** Male

PREOPERATIVE DIAGNOSIS
Right hip arthritis.

POSTOPERATIVE DIAGNOSIS
Right hip arthritis.

SURGEON: Gilbert M. Fields, MD

ASSISTANT: Jesse D. Smith, MD

ANESTHESIA: General endotracheal by Dr. Delaney.

OPERATION PERFORMED: Right total hip arthroplasty.

SPECIMEN REMOVED: None.

INDICATIONS: Mr. Bussappo, an 82-year-old Italian male, has had increasing pain and right hip degenerative changes for several months. He has finally reached the point where he wants to proceed with a total hip replacement after failing conservative therapy. The risks, benefits, alternatives, indications, including the risk of pain, bleeding, infection, dislocation, limp, loss of function, damage to adjacent structures, need for revision, implant loosening, DVT, and loss of limb or life were discussed with him. Patient agreed to proceed with surgery.

DRAIN: Stryker reinfusable drain.

PROSTHETIC DEVICES
1. Implants consisted of a DePuy Pinnacle 56 mm acetabular cup.
2. S-ROM 36 mm +6 metal-on-metal femoral head.
3. 36 x 56 mm metal inserts.
4. 20 x 15 x 165 with a 36 standard neck and a +A lateral offset S-ROM femoral stem and a D-large ZTT proximal sleeve.

IV FLUIDS: 2200 mL crystalloid and 500 mL colloid.

ESTIMATED BLOOD LOSS: 500 mL.

URINE OUTPUT: 400 mL.

SPONGE COUNT VERIFIED: Correct at end of case.

PROCEDURE IN DETAIL: Patient was identified in the holding area by the operative team. The correct surgical site was marked, patient was taken to the lock room where an epidural was placed. He was then brought back to the OR where he underwent induction of general anesthesia and intubation without difficulty. A Foley catheter was placed. He did receive Ancef and some myosin prior to the procedure starting. He was placed in a lateral position on the pegboard and secured in place using pegs. All his prominences were padded appropriately. The right lower extremity was then prepped and draped in the usual sterile fashion.

An approximately 15 mm incision was made and extended over the greater trochanter. The incision was carried down through skin and subcutaneous tissue to the level of the IT band. The IT band was split in line with the incision. Hemostasis was obtained during this dissection. The Charnley retractor was placed, and the abductors were

(Continued)

removed as a sleeve along with some of the vastus lateralis. Capsulectomy was performed after pulling back the abductors. The femoral head and neck were exposed. The standard transverse cut was made at the inferior portion of the femoral head and then extending vertically up into the pyriform fossa. The head was removed without difficulty. The acetabulum was inspected, and soft tissue was débrided.

We began reaming with a size 46 reamer until we had reached the medial wall, then progressively reamed up starting at the position of the right cup, until we reached a size 56. We trialed, and we were happy with the trial. We then implanted the acetabular cup with a good fit. No screws were placed. The trial liner was then placed.

We then turned our attention to the femur. Using the box cutter, we cut the lateral portion and the medial portion of the greater trochanter. We then reamed up to a size 15 for the stem. We then used the miller to ream out the calcar portion and trialed with the sleeves and found that a 20-D large was the best fit. It did sit up slightly prominently, but the B recessed too far into the bone, so we decided to go with the D large. This was left in, and then we trialed with a +6 stem, and we were happy with our trial. We had no chuck. Leg lengths were equal, and there was no dislocation with full adduction and internal rotation or with extension and abduction and external rotation.

Following this, the trial implants were removed. Everything was irrigated thoroughly with normal saline. The sleeve was placed, and the stem was implanted with neutral version. We then again trialed with this in place, and we were happy with our trial. The head was placed on. The metal liner was placed and the head was reduced without difficulty. The abductors were closed with No. 1 Ethibond through drill holes. Vastus lateralis was also closed with No. 1 Ethibond. Stryker infusion drain was placed. The tensor fascia lata was closed with 0 Vicryl. Skin was closed with 3-0 Vicryl and 3-0 Monocryl. Dressing consisted of Steri-Strips, Xeroform dressing flats, and foam tape. Patient was awakened from anesthesia without difficulty and taken to the PACU for recovery.

POSTOPERATIVE PLAN will be for the patient to be partial weightbearing for 6 weeks. He will be seen by Physical Therapy. He will be on DVT prophylaxis for 2 to 3 weeks.

Gilbert M. Fields, MD
Orthopaedic Surgery

GMF:pai
D:2/21/----
T:2/22/----

c: Michael Barker, MD, Physical Medicine & Rehabilitation

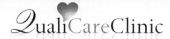

Obstetrics/Gynecology Surgery

Patient Name: Ladonna Young

Date of Operation: 2 May ----

Age: 22

ID#: S-38

Sex: Female

PREOPERATIVE DIAGNOSIS
Intrauterine fetal demise at 15 weeks.

POSTOPERATIVE DIAGNOSIS
Intrauterine fetal demise at 15 weeks.

SURGEON: Tillman Risha, MD

ASSISTANT: Jimmy Dale Jett, RN, Circulating Nurse

ANESTHESIA: General endotracheal by Chuck Delaney.

OPERATIONS PERFORMED
1. Amniocentesis.
2. Dilation and evacuation.

MATERIAL FORWARDED TO LABORATORY FOR EXAMINATION
1. Placenta and amniotic fluid.
2. Contents of uterus/products of conception.

FINDINGS: Approximately 15-week intrauterine fetal demise (IUFD). Amniocentesis was performed with return of 8 mL of serosanguinous fluid. Laminaria were removed. Cervix was dilated to #15 using Hegar dilators after a paracervical block had been placed. Suction curetting #14 was used. Sopher forceps was used to remove the calvaria. Copious tissue return. Ultrasound showed thin endometrial stripe. Sharp curetting showed good cry throughout. All fetal parts accounted for.

SPONGE COUNT VERIFIED: Correct at end of case.

ESTIMATED BLOOD LOSS: 100 mL.

URINE OUTPUT: 100 mL.

INTRAVENOUS FLUIDS: 1300 mL.

PROCEDURE IN DETAIL After consent had been obtained, patient was taken to the operating room where general endotracheal anesthesia was found to be adequate. She was initially placed in the supine position. An ultrasound was performed, and a pocket of fluid was found. The abdomen was prepped with iodine solution. Amniocentesis was then performed without complication with the return of 8 mL of serosanguinous fluid.

Patient was then prepped and draped in the usual sterile fashion in the high dorsal lithotomy position. A speculum was placed in the patient's vagina, and a paracervical Bucky. The four laminaria previously placed were then removed. Then 1% lidocaine without epinephrine was used. Cervix was then dilated up to a #15 using Hegar dilators. A 14-French suction curette was then used to evacuate copious amounts of tissue from the uterus. Sopher forceps was then used under ultrasound guidance to crush and then remove the calvaria. Sharp curetting was then used until good cry was noted throughout. Ultrasound revealed a thin endometrial stripe.

(Continued)

All instruments were removed from the patient's vagina. Excellent hemostasis was noted. The contents of the vacuum were then removed, and all fetal body parts were accounted for. Patient tolerated the procedure well. Sponge, lap, and needle counts were correct at the end of the procedure. Patient was taken to the recovery room in stable condition.

_____
Tillman Risha, MD
Obstetrics/Gynecology

TR:pai
D:5/2/----
T:5/3/----

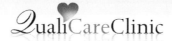

Genitourinary Surgery Report

Patient Name: Rosemary Reyna   **ID#:** S-39

Date of Operation: 21 April ----   **Age:** 27   **Sex:** Female

PREOPERATIVE DIAGNOSIS
Right ureteral lithiasis.

POSTOPERATIVE DIAGNOSIS
Right ureteral lithiasis.

SURGEON: Charles Mendesz, MD

ASSISTANT: Anna Marie Iaccarino, Scrub Nurse

ANESTHESIA: General endotracheal by Dr. Chuck Delaney.

OPERATIONS PERFORMED
1. Cystourethroscopy under anesthesia.
2. Right semirigid ureteroscopy with basket stone extraction.
3. Right double-J ureteral stent placement.

MATERIAL FORWARDED TO LABORATORY FOR EXAMINATION: Stone.

INDICATIONS: Rosemary Reyna is a 27-year-old female who failed a trial of spontaneous stone passage of a 3.5 mm distal right ureteral stone of greater than 4 weeks. Pain of this stone was lifestyle limiting and causing her to miss work. She was counseled regarding the nature of her disease, including the risks, alternatives, and benefits of therapy. She elected to proceed to the operating room for stone removal.

DRAINS: 6-French by 24 cm right double-J ureteral stent.

FLUIDS: 1000 mL lactated Ringer's.

ESTIMATED BLOOD LOSS: None.

URINE OUTPUT: Not measured.

TOTAL LITHOTOMY TIME: 20 minutes.

PROCEDURE IN DETAIL: This patient was correctly identified, site had been signed, and verification had been performed. The patient was given preoperative antibiotics in the holding area. She was then transported to the cystoscopy suite where she was placed upon the operating room table. General anesthesia was induced by anesthesia service. She was placed in lithotomy position, and her genitalia were prepped and draped in the usual sterile fashion. A 22-French rigid cystoscope was passed into the bladder. The urinary bladder was systematically surveyed using both 7-degree and 12-degree lenses. The bilateral ureteral orifices were orthotopic and had clear efflux. No stones, tumors, or other abnormalities were noted in the urinary bladder.

A 0.035 Sensor Glidewire was passed into the right ureteral orifice and up into the right renal pelvis under fluoroscopic visualization. The bladder was drained, and the cystoscope was removed. A 7-French semirigid ureteroscope was then selected and passed alongside the wire into the distal right ureter. This portion of the ureter was very tight and had significant ureteral spasm. Therefore, the scope was removed and a 4 cm 15-French balloon dilating catheter was passed over the wire into the distal right ureter under fluoroscopic visualization. The distal ureter was balloon dilated for approximately 1 minute.

The balloon was deflated and the catheter was removed, maintaining the wire in position. The ureteroscope was then passed alongside the wire again, and in the distal ureter a stone could be visualized on both

(Continued)

ID#: S-39   PAGE 2

fluorography and ureteroscopy approximately 2.5 cm proximal to the bladder in the right ureter. The Sensor wire was exchanged for a 0.035 Glidewire in order to facilitate passage of the scope beyond the stone. The stone was dislodged and maintained in vision. A 2.4-French nitinol stone basket was used to grasp the stone. The stone was removed intact and passed off the table as a specimen. A 6-French by 24 cm right double-J ureteral stent was placed in standard fashion under fluoroscopic visualization.

After the stent was placed, a cystoscope was again passed into the bladder. The bladder was inspected and an appropriate coil was seen in the bladder. The bladder was drained, and a **B&O** suppository was inserted in the rectum. Patient tolerated the procedure well.

Upon attempting to extubate the patient, Anesthesia noted that her peripheral oxygen saturations had dropped to 70%, and she was demonstrated to be tachycardic into the 120s. The patient was extubated successfully without difficulty, and her saturations promptly rose to 100% with supplemental oxygen. The patient was transported to PACU in stable condition; however, in the PACU she remained subjectively short of breath and had mild tachycardia in the low 100s. She had an intermittent need for supplemental oxygen. The patient was closely observed, and a duplex ultrasound was negative for deep vein thrombosis. A CT angiogram of the chest was negative for pulmonary embolus. The patient was admitted for overnight observation and did well.

DISPOSITION: Patient will follow up in Dr. Mendesz's urology clinic in 1 week, and she is to see her PCP for a complete physical exam as soon as possible—refer to cardiology and/or vascular services if necessary.

Charles Mendesz, MD
Urology Surgery

CM:pai
D:4/21/----
T:4/22/----

c: Linda Galbraith, RN, FNP
    Internal Medicine Clinic

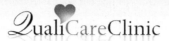

Ear, Nose, and Throat Surgery Report

Patient Name: Katrinka Thomas   **ID#:** S-40

Date of Operation: 8 Sept ----   **Age:** 39   **Sex:** Female

PREOPERATIVE DIAGNOSES

1. Nasal airway obstruction.
2. Inferior turbinate hypertrophy.

POSTOPERATIVE DIAGNOSES

1. Nasal airway obstruction.
2. Inferior turbinate hypertrophy.

SURGEON: Leela Pivari, MD

ASSISTANT: Danila R. Fry, MD

ANESTHESIA: General endotracheal.

OPERATIONS PERFORMED

1. Open septal rhinoplasty.
2. Inferior turbinate lateralization, bilateral.

SPECIMEN REMOVED: None.

INDICATIONS: Patient is a 39-year-old female with a history of nasal airway obstruction who, upon evaluation, was noted to have septum that was in the midline. However, she was noted to have severe supraalar pinching causing internal valve collapse. Patient was also concerned about a slight dorsal hump, which she wanted to address. She was consented for the above procedures. Dr. Fry of plastic surgery will assist with the procedures.

PROCEDURE IN DETAIL Patient was taken from the preop area to the operating room and placed supine. She underwent general endotracheal. Once adequate general anesthesia was achieved, the bilateral nasal cavity was packed with Afrin-soaked pledgets. After allowing adequate time for decongestion, 1% lidocaine with 1:100,000 epinephrine was infiltrated throughout the external and internal nose. After allowing adequate time for vasoconstriction, the nose and face were prepped and draped in the usual sterile fashion.

A No. 15 blade was then used to make an incision in the standard Killian fashion to address the septum and harvest septal cartilage. Mucoperichondrial flaps were then elevated on the left side of the nose and then taken back over the bone. Collagen was then excised for grafting purposes, leaving 15 mm of the dorsal strut and 15 mm of the caudal strut. Once the cartilage was removed, bone was noted to be in the midline, so no bony septum was excised.

Attention was then turned to the external rhinoplasty approach. An 11 blade was used to make an inverted "V" midcolumellar incision. This was connected to the marginal incision with a 15 blade bilaterally. The skin and soft tissue envelope was then elevated up off the nasal tip and the nasal dorsum. It was noted that the patient had significant internal curvature of her lateral crura. Therefore, the lateral crura were elevated off the vestibular skin bilaterally. The collagen that had been harvested from the septum was then placed as lateral crural extension grafts bilaterally. They were then secured with 5-0 PDS and then placed into precise pockets bilaterally.

Attention was then turned to the cartilaginous and bony hump, where a 15 blade was used to reduce the size of the cartilaginous hump. The Rubin osteotome was then used to reduce the size of the bony hump. The irregular edges of the bony dorsum were then rasped so that the dorsum was smooth. A columellar strut was then fashioned between the medial crura using the septal cartilage. Using the cartilaginous hump cartilage, a crushed

(Continued)

ID#: S-40

piece of cartilage was put in the infratip lobule just to smooth out the infratip lobule. Then 6-0 clear nylon sutures were used to do an interdermal suture as well as intradermal sutures. The midcolumella incision was then closed with 6-0 PDS suture. The skin was closed with 7-0 black nylon suture. The marginal incisions were closed with 5-0 Vicryl suture. At this point, the Sayre elevator was used to lateralize the inferior turbinates to maximize the size of her nasal cavity. Telfa packing was placed into the nasal cavities bilaterally. Vestibular splints were then placed, which were fashioned from 0.25 mm Reuter splints. Mastisol, Telfa, Steri-Strips, and then a Dermoplast splint were placed on the dorsum. A mustache dressing was then placed.

Patient was then awakened, extubated, and taken back to the PACU, having tolerated the procedure well without complications.

_____

Leela Pivari, MD
ENT Clinic

LP:pai
D:9/8/----
T:9/9/----

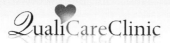

General Surgery Report

Patient Name: Carol Gallanthen   **ID#:** S-42
Date of Operation: 22 Feb ----   **Age:** 43   **Sex:** Female

PREOPERATIVE DIAGNOSES
1. Obstructive defecation syndrome, rectocele, enterocele. History of fecal incontinence.
2. Previous stomal hernia with possible reherniation, status post mesh repair.
3. Posterior vaginal vault prolapse.
4. Status post sphincteroplasty.

POSTOPERATIVE DIAGNOSES
1. Obstructive defecation syndrome due to rectal stricture and redundant sigmoid.
2. Posterior vaginal vault prolapse.
3. Stomal hernia.

SURGEON: James A. McClure Jr, MD

ASSISTANTS: Bernard Kester, MD, and Charles Mendesz, MD

ANESTHESIA: General endotracheal and epidural catheter.

OPERATIONS PERFORMED
1. Lysis of adhesions x3 hours.
2. Sigmoid resection.
3. Abdominosacral colpopexy of the posterior vaginal wall.
4. Cystoscopy.
5. Rigid proctoscopy.
6. Mobilization of the splenic flexure.

MATERIAL FORWARDED TO LABORATORY FOR EXAMINATION: Sigmoid colon and rectum.

INDICATIONS: Patient is a 47-year-old white female who has a complicated history due to an obstetric injury requiring a suture repair some 12 years ago that healed poorly after surgery. She developed an abscess in the wound and required multiple debridements, eventually healing by secondary intention of her perineal wound. It was felt at that time that she had a latex allergy, which most likely explained her failure to properly heal her surgical incision. Subsequently, she underwent redo suture plasty by a doctor at Forrest General. Since that time the patient has developed severe obstructive defecation combined with fecal incontinence at times. From her preoperative workup, it was noted that she had a large rectocele and poor posterior vaginal wall support. On her defecography, it seemed that there was a large enterocele that obstructed her rectum with Valsalva maneuver. Her incontinence is attributed to the collection of stool within a large rectocele while she is making attempts to defecate. Patient has also had herniation at her previous stoma site in the right lower quadrant, and this has been repaired with laparoscopic mesh placement. Patient has significant right lower quadrant abdominal pain, which is most likely due to reherniation or adhesive loops of bowel in the right lower quadrant. Patient was brought to the operating room for lysis of adhesions and possible repair of right lower quadrant hernia, sigmoid resection and rectopexy, in addition to abdominosacral colpopexy for vaginal wall support, and to obliterate cul-de-sac in order to prevent further obstructive defecation.

PROCEDURE IN DETAIL: After obtaining informed consent, the patient was brought to the operating room where an epidural catheter was placed by the anesthesia team. Patient was then placed in supine position while oral endotracheal was performed. The patient was then placed in the low lithotomy position and prepped and

(Continued)

draped in the usual sterile fashion. Patient's lower midline abdominal incision was reentered, and the dissection was carried down to the midline fascia using Bovie electrocautery. The fascia was entered sharply with scalpel at the superior-most portion of the wound where adhesions would most likely be at a minimum.

The abdomen was entered cautiously, and adhesions were taken down by sharp dissection using Metzenbaum scissors. Extensive omental adhesions to the right lower quadrant were enmeshed all along the midline incision. Once dissection was carried out to the lateral margins of the mesh, here it was found that several loops of small bowel were adherent to the laparoscopic tacks, which were placed to hold the mesh in place. These adhesions were carefully taken down, and several small serosal tears were repaired with 3-0 Vicryl sutures in Lembert fashion. Once the adhesions were successfully dissected, then the Bookwalter retractor was set up, and the entire omentum and small bowel were placed into the upper abdomen and held in place with the Bookwalter retractor.

Next, attention was focused on the sigmoid colon. The sigmoid appeared to be redundant with 2 to 3 turns that were causing some kinking of the sigmoid from scar tissue. This scarring is most likely due to previous episodes of diverticulitis, as it was in the sigmoid colon, and it was typical of diverticular disease. The sigmoid colon was effectively blocking the pelvic inlet, so it was presumed that the patient did not suffer from an enterocele but that the sigmoid colon itself was causing obstruction of the rectum with attempts at defecation. The sigmoid colon was completely dissected away from the lateral pelvic sidewall, and the adhesive scar tissue was dissected as well. It was found at this time that just distal to the rectosigmoid junction there was an area of stricture in the rectum where the rectum was adherent to the vaginal apex. This area was dissected carefully as the rectum was taken off the vagina with Bovie electrocautery. As the dissection of the rectum continued laterally, special care was taken to identify the ureters on both sides and confirm that they were uninjured during the dissection. The hypogastric neural plexus was also preserved throughout the dissection. The rectum was then dissected posteriorly, posterior to the mesorectal fascia. This was carried down within several centimeters of the perineal body. Dissection of the vagina continued down using sharp dissection as distally as was possible. This took us within 1 cm of the perineal body. A site was chosen on the rectum for division with a GIA stapler so that dissection and mesh placement down to the pelvis could proceed unimpeded. The rectum was divided, and then the sigmoid colon was tucked into the upper abdomen with the small bowel. Next the abdomen and pelvis were copiously irrigated and checked for hemostasis.

At this point Dr. Kester took over control of the case and performed his abdominosacral colpopexy. With an EEA sizer in the vagina, the posterior vaginal wall was completely dissected away from the rectum until dissection was adequate to place his stay sutures for the mesh placement. Sacral promontory was dissected down to the middle sacral vessels, and a site was chosen for placement of two 1-0 Ethibond sutures as stay sutures for this sacral portion of the fixation. Next, as rectovaginal exam was being performed by Dr. McClure, Dr. Kester proceeded to place 3 rows of 2-0 PDS suture along the posterior wall of the vagina. These were placed in the middle, left lateral, and right lateral positions down the back wall of the vagina with the distal-most row being within 2 cm of the perineal body. Next, soft Prolene mesh was trimmed to fit the shape of the posterior wall of the vagina with adequate length to reach the sacral promontory. The mesh was fixed onto the posterior wall of the vagina with the previously placed PDS sutures, then brought around the right side of the rectum and fixed to the sacrum with the previously placed Ethibond sutures. There was adequate peritoneal coverage for the mesh so that it would not be in contact with the rectum.

Dr. Mendesz then took over, turning the attention to performing a cystoscopy to confirm that the urinary bladder was without injury and that indigo carmine was seen excreted from both ureteral orifices. After confirmation of normal anatomy, the case was returned to Dr. McClure.

Next, the splenic flexure of the colon was mobilized using Bovie electrocautery to obtain adequate length to make the anastomosis. The descending colon was then divided in an area of soft, pliable bowel. The staple line was removed from the proximal margin of the resection, and a pursestring suture was placed using 2-0 Prolene.

(Continued)

ID#: S-42   PAGE 3

The anvil of the 31 mm EEA stapler was placed within the proximal margin of the resection, and the pursestring suture was tied down. An additional 3-0 Vicryl pursestring suture was placed to hold the anvil in place.

Next, the EEA stapler was passed into the rectum, but the stapler was unable to be passed to the end of the rectum due to the previously mentioned area of stricturing. Stapler was removed, and attention was returned to the abdomen so that the lower resection of the rectum could be performed. A TA stapler was used to divide across midrectum so that the strictured portion of the rectum was removed. Next, the 31 mm EEA stapler was again passed into the rectum, and this time it was passed without difficulty. The spike was extended through the rectal staple line, and then the anvil was brought down onto the stapler. The stapler was closed and fired. The anastomosis was reinforced with 3-0 Vicryl Lembert sutures. Then the anastomosis was tested for leaks. The proximal colon was occluded between fingers, and then proctoscope was inserted into the rectum. The colorectal anastomosis was insufflated under the abdominal fluid. No bubbles were seen, and insufflation was passed out the anus at the time of the proctoscopic test. The gas was removed from the rectum via the proctoscope, and the pelvis was again copiously irrigated and checked for hemostasis.

Next, the pelvic drain was placed just proximal to the colorectal anastomosis and brought out through the left lower quadrant. It was a 10 flat JP drain that was intended just to remove any fluid collections that occur near the anastomosis. The omentum was brought down to protect the anastomosis from the mesh and also to separate the anastomosis from the pelvic drain. Next, the abdominal wall was again inspected to determine the need for removing the previously placed mesh. It was found that the mesh was completely peritonealized, and after removing the tacks that were adherent to the small bowel, there were really no other tacks that needed to be removed. As there was no hernia recurrence at the right lower quadrant, the mesh was left in place. Decision was made to close the abdomen.

Two sheets of Seprafilm were placed under the midline fascia. Fascia was closed with #1 PDS suture. Skin edges were reapproximated with skin staples, and a sterile dressing was applied. The left lower quadrant drain was sutured in place with 2-0 nylon suture. Patient was recovered from general endotracheal anesthesia and transported to the recovery room in stable condition.

The operation and operative findings were discussed immediately following the procedure with the patient's spouse and other family members present.

DRAINS: Single 10 flat JP in the pelvis.

ESTIMATED BLOOD LOSS: 600 mL.

URINE OUTPUT: 600 mL.

FLUIDS: Crystalloid 5900 mL, colloid 1500 mL.

BLOOD TRANSFUSION: One unit packed red blood cells.

James A. McClure Jr, MD
General Surgery

JAM:pai
D:2/23/----
T:2/24/----

c: Charles Mendesz, MD, Urology Surgery
    Bernard Kester, MD, General Surgery

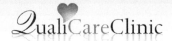

Orthopedic Surgery Report

Patient Name: Lightbourne Byfield   **ID#:** S-43

Date of Operation: 7 Oct ----   **Age:** 55   **Sex:** Male

PREOPERATIVE DIAGNOSIS
Left knee degenerative arthritis.

POSTOPERATIVE DIAGNOSIS
Left knee degenerative arthritis.

SURGEON: Gilbert M. Fields, MD

ASSISTANT: David Castillo, MD

ANESTHESIA: Epidural performed by Dr. Avalon.

OPERATION PERFORMED: Left total knee arthroplasty.

INDICATIONS: Mr. Byfield, a native of Jamaica, who has been followed in the orthopedic clinic, has had pain with his knee for quite some time, and has had x-rays exhibiting degenerative changes in his knee in the medial compartment. He has had significant pain, and he failed conservative treatment. He has been unable to tolerate things without activity restriction. Steroid injection and viscus supplementation has not achieved relief for him. He has had no significant findings in his knee other than the degenerative changes. For the above reasons, patient requested we go ahead with knee arthroplasty. He does have multiple medical problems, but prior to his procedure he was evaluated thoroughly by Internal Medicine. He has a Greenfield filter in place because of a history of DVT. He was on Coumadin, which he stopped prior to the procedure in adequate time to resume a normal INR. He has had MS with no flares for 10 years. He has a history of chronic obstructive pulmonary disease. On his left side, his involved side, he has a history of an old tibial fracture that did complicate the alignment because we had to base our alignment off the proximal tibia alone. However, we were very well aware of and prepared for this when the procedure started.

PROSTHETIC DEVICES: Implants include a Zimmer NexGen knee. The tibial component was a size 6 stemmed component. The femoral component was a size F. The poly was a 12 mm. The patellar reamer was a 41 mm reamer. The Ollier implant was 35 mm diameter, 9 mm thickness.

PROCEDURE IN DETAIL: Patient was brought to the operating room after his Ancef had been instilled. He was prepped and draped in the usual sterile fashion. Our standard medial parapatellar incision was used. We dissected it and excised our tissues to visualize our joint well. After we had excellent visualization of our joint, we made our tibial cut first. The tibial cut was resected based off the deficient side. A 2 mm resection was based off the medial side, and the alignment was based off the anterior tibial press proximally. We did not want to align him based on his foot because he has a distal angulation, which he has tolerated well for many years. If we turned him back, this would cause him further problems. We then verified that our cut was well aligned using the long alignment guide.

We then turned our attention to his femur. The femoral sizer was placed into the hole. We visualized that this was a size F femur. Based on that size, we then placed the distal femoral cutter on. A standard distal cut was made, and this was at 6 degrees of valgus. The cuts were then measured using 10 mm and 12 mm blocks, and we found that we had a square space, and the soft tissues were well aligned and required no releases. Based on these 2 cuts, we then placed our size F 4-in-1 cutter. Using this cutter with 1 pin into the anterior tibia, we positioned it using the tensioner. The tensioner device was turned off the posterior condyles to 40 mm on each side. This approximated a square box. We turned our anterior 4-in-1 cutter to align and make a perfectly square box in 90 degrees of flexion and pinned this in place. This was approximately 3 degrees of external rotation and seemed very appropriate.

(Continued)

ID#: S-43   PAGE 2

We then made our 4 cuts and notched for our groove as well as making our log holes on the femur. The femoral notch cutter for the posterior stabilizing device was then placed. This box was cut cautiously, and there were no notches made. We then finished our tibia using the size 6 tray. The size 6 tray fit well, and it was aligned off the tibial tubercle to be central. It was placed in a slight amount of external rotation. Then we placed our trial implants and turned our attention to the patella. The patella took us some time because after we reamed down to 14 mm of remaining thickness, we placed the buttons, and a 35 mm button was used. However, it was into very hard, corticated bone in one location. This drill hole took us quite some time to get into perfect position. Eventually, by putting the drill into a drill instead of into a reamer, we were able to drill this hole sufficiently. We found the patellar implant set perfectly. This took approximately 10 or 15 minutes, slowing us down.

We then mixed cement, washed the joint thoroughly with sterile saline, removed all loose soft tissues, and prepared the implants on the back table. Cement was applied to both the implants and to the tibia. The tibia was tamped into place. All excess cement was removed. We then implanted the femoral implant. Cement was placed into the plug holes and excellent alignment was achieved. This was tamped down into place and was visualized to be down in all locations. Excess cement was removed.

We then put our patella in place using a patellar clamp, clamping it down and holding it in position during the cement hardening process. This all was achieved easily, and we placed the 12 mm trial spacer in place until the cement had hardened. After it had hardened on the back table, we removed the spacer. During this time we were irrigating the knee with sterile saline. Spacer was removed, and a 12 mm poly was inserted. Once again our stability was excellent, and our range of motion was outstanding—from 0 to 125 degrees. The wound was further irrigated and closed over a drain using 2-0 Vicryl and a subcuticular 4-0 Vicryl running. Steri-Strips were placed.

The patient was placed into a postop dressing and taken to recovery in good condition. He was awake during the entire procedure with epidural anesthesia. There were no complications.

ESTIMATED BLOOD LOSS: None.

TOURNIQUET TIME: 120 minutes.

Gilbert M. Fields, MD
Orthopedic Surgery

GMF:pai
D:10/8/----
T: 10/9/----

QualiCareClinic

Ear, Nose, and Throat Surgical Report

Patient Name: George Whiting   **ID#:** S-44

Date of Operation: 26 Jan ----   **Age:** 36   **Sex:** Male

PREOPERATIVE DIAGNOSIS
Symptoms of chronic sinusitis.

POSTOPERATIVE DIAGNOSIS
Symptoms of chronic sinusitis.

SURGEON: Leela Pivari, MD

ASSISTANT: Anna Maria Iaccarino, RN, Scrub Nurse

ANESTHESIA: General endotracheal.

OPERATIONS PERFORMED
1. Functional endoscopic sinus surgery with anterior posterior ethmoidectomy, sphenoidotomy, and maxillary antrostomy on the right.
2. Anterior posterior ethmoidectomy, sphenoidotomy, and maxillary antrostomy on the left.

MATERIAL FORWARDED TO LABORATORY FOR EXAMINATION
(1) Inspissated mucus. (2) Contents of the left sphenoid sinus.

INDICATIONS: The patient has a history of sinus surgery in the past. He presents again with the symptoms of chronic sinusitis and a CT scan of the sinuses that is consistent with his history of allergic fungal sinusitis.

PROCEDURE IN DETAIL: Patient was brought to the operating room and placed on the operating table in supine position. He was intubated, and the bed was turned 180 degrees. Afrin-soaked pledgets were placed in bilateral nasal cavities. He was then prepped and draped in the usual sterile fashion. Then 1% lidocaine with 1:100,000 epinephrine was injected into the axilla of the middle turbinate on the right. Some 7 mL was used. The middle turbinate was then medialized using a Freer.

A microdebrider was used to remove polypoid tissue from the region of the maxillary antrostomy, which had been made previously. There was a portion of the maxillary antrostomy that was still stenotic with a scar band. This scar band was taken down with a Tru-Cut forceps and then a microdebrider. InstaTrak guidance was utilized during the case. Then straight suction, using InstaTrak guidance, was used to define the various landmarks. Care was taken to remove polypoid tissue and debris and diseased air cells, leaving a layer of air cells along the lamina papyracea through most of its course and along the skull base.

Dissection was carried down to the base of the sphenoid. The sphenoid was entered using InstaTrak-guided straight suction. Tru-Cut forceps was used to widen the sphenoidotomy. A similar procedure was performed on the contralateral side—again with microdebridement of polypoid tissue. Once the base of the sphenoid was reached, it was entered once again with the straight suction. In the sphenoid sinus it was discovered that there was inspissated mucus, potentially consistent with an allergic form of sinusitis. This was removed, and the sphenoid sinus was visualized as empty of debris. The frontal sinus outflow tract was also addressed, using the microdebrider at the frontal recess to remove polypoid tissue.

(Continued)

ID#: S-44

Once adequate dissection had been completed on each side, the patient was turned back over to the anesthesia team. He was extubated and brought to the PACU from which he will be discharged home following discharge protocol.

ESTIMATED BLOOD LOSS: Minimal.

FLUIDS: 1500 mL crystalloid.

_____

Leela Pivari, MD
ENT Clinic

LP:pai
D:1/26/----
T:1/27/----

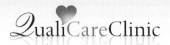

General Surgery Report

Patient Name: Charles "Chuck" Nash   **ID#:** S-45

Date of Operation: 23 Sept ----   **Age:** 42   **Sex:** Male

PREOPERATIVE DIAGNOSIS
Left inguinal hernia.

POSTOPERATIVE DIAGNOSIS
Direct left inguinal hernia.

SURGEON: James A. McClure Jr, MD

ASSISTANT: Jimmy Dale Jett, RN, Circulating Nurse

ANESTHESIA: General endotracheal by Dr. Delaney.

OPERATION PERFORMED: Open left inguinal herniorrhaphy with mesh repair.

SPECIMEN REMOVED: None.

INDICATIONS: Mr. Nash is an active-duty Colonel who had presented to my general surgery clinic with complaints of pain and a bulge in his left groin. On examination, the patient was given a diagnosis of left inguinal hernia. Risks and benefits of operative repair were discussed with the patient. Patient considered and then consented freely to having the procedure performed.

PROCEDURE IN DETAIL: Patient was brought to the operating room on 23 Sept and placed in supine position. At this point general endotracheal anesthesia was administered in an excellent fashion. The patient's left groin was then prepped and draped in the usual sterile fashion. The procedure was begun by making an approximately 4 cm incision about two-thirds of the way between the anterior and superior iliac spine at the pubic tubercle. This incision was carried through the skin and subcutaneous tissues and down to the level of the external abdominal oblique fascia. This fascia was then incised and opened through the external ring and then slightly lateral toward the internal ring.

At this point the spermatic cord was easily identified and freed from the external oblique superiorly as well as the wall of the inguinal canal. After complete circumferential control was obtained, a Penrose drain was placed around the spermatic cord. All the important structures, including the vas deferens and the pampiniform plexus, were identified. At this point it was easily seen that the patient had a very large, direct hernia. Dissection was continued laterally toward the internal ring where we did see the inferior epigastric vessels. No evidence of an indirect hernia could be seen.

At this point a decision was made to repair the hernia with the Prolene hernia system mesh. The preperitoneal space was carefully dissected bluntly using finger dissection through the internal ring. Once this was performed, the Prolene hernia system mesh was inserted into the preperitoneal space. Then the anterior component of the mesh was tacked medially to the pubic tubercle with 2-0 Vicryl stitch, then superiorly along the internal oblique aponeurosis. The lateral tail was tucked under the external oblique. The internal ring was recreated by making a small incision into the mesh, placing this around the cord, and then fixing this to the shelving edge of the inguinal ligament.

At this point hemostasis was assured. The external oblique was then reapproximated using 3-0 Vicryl running stitch. Approximately 10 mL Marcaine was then injected into the fascia and the muscle. Then the deep layers of the subcutaneous tissue and Scarpa fascia were closed using interrupted 3-0 Vicryl sutures. Once again, 10 mL Marcaine was placed in the subcutaneous tissues. Several deep dermal interrupted 3-0 Vicryls were

(Continued)

ID#: S-45 PAGE 2

used to reapproximate the dermis, and the skin was reapproximated using a 4-0 running Monocryl suture in a subcuticular fashion. Steri-Strips were applied. Sterile dressings were applied.

At the end of the case, all sponge and needle counts were correct. Patient was recovered from his anesthesia and sent to PAR for postoperative care. No complications at the time of this dictation.

_____

James A. McClure Jr, MD
General Surgery

JAM:pai
D:9/23/----
T:9/24/----

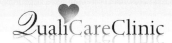

Orthopedic Surgical Report

Patient Name: Tina Jane Wolfe   **ID#:** S-46

Date of Operation: 27 Oct ----   Age: 68   **Sex:** Female

PREOPERATIVE DIAGNOSIS
Left distal radius fracture.

POSTOPERATIVE DIAGNOSIS
Left distal radius fracture.

SURGEON: Raquel Rodriguez, MD

ASSISTANT: Jack Zullig, MD

ANESTHESIA: LMA by Dr. Delaney.

OPERATION PERFORMED: Open reduction, internal fixation of left distal radius fracture with dorsal bone grafting with allograft.

SPECIMEN REMOVED: None.

INDICATIONS: The patient is a 68-year-old right-hand dominant white female who fell a week ago on 21 Oct, sustaining a left distal radius fracture. She initially was placed in a splint and brought back for operative fixation. Indications, risks, benefits, and alternatives to fixation were discussed with the patient, and all questions were answered. She freely gave her consent to proceed.

TOURNIQUET TIME: 87 minutes.

FLUIDS IN: 1.6 L crystalloid.

ESTIMATED BLOOD LOSS: 70 mL.

URINE OUTPUT: Not measured.

COMPLICATIONS: There were no complications.

PROCEDURE IN DETAIL: The patient was met in the preoperative holding area where the operative extremity was initialed and the appropriate paperwork was completed. The patient received Ancef 1 gram IV preoperatively, and she was taken back to the operating room where LMA was administered by the anesthesia team. Left upper extremity was placed on a hand table. A nonsterile tourniquet was placed on the left upper extremity. The patient was then prepped and draped in the usual sterile fashion.

An approximately 10 cm incision was made over the flexor carpi radialis. The incision was taken down through the skin and subcutaneous tissue until the FCR tendon was seen. We incised through the FCR sheath, and the FCR tendon was then retracted. We went through the floor of the FCR. Prior to starting the procedure the extremity had been exsanguinated, and the tourniquet had been elevated. After we went through the FCR sheath, the flexor pollicis longus (FPL) was bluntly dissected out of the way.

The fracture was seen, and the perimeter coordinators were largely disrupted. It was noted that she had a significantly comminuted fracture. We exposed distally as well in order to get into the intraarticular space to ensure that we got good articular reduction. Again, she was significantly comminuted, especially with dorsal comminution. She also had coronal as well as sagittal fracture lines interarticularly. She had significant displacement of the styloid.

We then reduced the coronal fracture line, and the volar piece was again matched up with the dorsal piece. We used 0.045 K-wires to secure these fragments. The styloid piece was then liberated from the brachioradialis tendon so we could get better mobilization of this fragment. It was then also reduced to the remainder of the other

(Continued)

fragments, and it was held with temporary fixation with two 0.045 K-wires. Again, two 0.045 K-wires were placed at volar to dorsal, again, to better stabilize the coronal fragment. After placing this, we did distract the joint and looked intraarticularly and ensured that we had a narrow anatomic reduction with greater than 1 mm gapping of the fracture fragments.

The Stryker volar plate was then used and placed in the appropriate position on this distal fragment. Again, the fracture of the shaft still separated it from these articular fragments. The plate was placed onto the distal fragments. After appropriate position was confirmed and after we confirmed that we had good articular reduction, both visually and using C-arm fluoroscopy, we placed the plate and distal row of screw holes. All 2.3 screws were drilled, measured, and put into place, ensuring that we continued to have good reduction as well as adequate fixation of these fragments. We also placed the proximal hole via 2 distal rows. The proximal styloid screw was also placed, so a total of 5 screws were placed into these distal fragments. We ensured that we had good fixation, that they moved as a unit.

After this, we then reduced these fragments into the shaft and as well brought the plate down to the shaft, restoring some volar tilt. One screw was placed in the oblong hole. It was drilled, appropriately measured, and the appropriate-sized screw was put into position. We again checked this under fluoroscopy and ensured that we had a good reduction of the distal fragments to the proximal shaft and metadiaphysis. After we ensured that this was the case, 3 additional screws were placed into the proximal shaft and the metadiaphysis. We again ensured under C-arm fluoroscopy that it was in the appropriate position and that we had an appropriate reduction.

We then checked to ensure that there were no screws in the joint. It was difficult to tell using the main C-arm, so we got plain films in the room. When these came back, we did note that the most distal ulnar screw was intraarticular. The distal ulnar screw was backed out, redirected, and replaced. Again under C-arm it appeared that all these screws were out of the joint. We again got plain films, and they confirmed that the screws were extraarticular.

The patient also had good wrist motion. We again visualized the joint prior to closing to ensure that no screws were inside the joint.

Cancellous allograft as well as some metaphyseal bone that had been removed to assist with reduction were then placed and tamped into the comminuted areas.

The wound was then well irrigated. The deep tissues were gently reapproximated with 2-0 PDS. The skin was then closed with 3-0 nylon in a running horizontal mattress fashion. The tourniquet was deflated prior to doing any of the closure, and we ensured that the patient had meticulous hemostasis. A sugar-tong splint was then applied.

The patient tolerated the procedure well and was transferred back to the patient bed, then back to the PACU in stable condition. There were no complications.

POSTOPERATIVE PLAN
The patient will remain in a sugar-tong splint. We will then plan on putting her into a cast for approximately 4 to 6 weeks; however, this will be determined based on radiographic evidence of healing. This is secondary to her significantly comminuted fracture. She will be kept overnight for monitoring to make sure there are no adverse events, and we will plan on discharging her in the morning barring any complications.

_____

Raquel Rodriguez, MD
Orthopedic Surgery

RR:pai
D:10/27/----
T:10/28/----

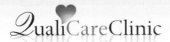

Ear, Nose, and Throat Surgical Report

Patient Name: Anthony L. Duckett   **ID#:** S-47

Date of Operation: 17 April ----   **Age:** 49   **Sex:** Male

PREOPERATIVE DIAGNOSES
1. Snoring.
2. Obstructive sleep apnea.

POSTOPERATIVE DIAGNOSES
1. Snoring.
2. Obstructive sleep apnea.

SURGEON: Leela Pivari, MD

ASSISTANT: Jimmy Dale Jett, RN, Circulating Nurse

ANESTHESIA: Local by Dr. Delaney.

OPERATION PERFORMED: Palatal radiofrequency ablation (RFA).

SPECIMEN REMOVED: None.

INDICATIONS: Mr. Duckett has had one previous treatment while he underwent repair of his nasal septum and inferior turbinates on 14 Feb ----. He actually had worsening of his snoring after that, and patient is here for his second RFA therapy.

PROCEDURE IN DETAIL: The patient was seated in the examination chair, and he had a chance to ask questions. Once these had been answered to his satisfaction, he signed the informed consent, and the procedure was begun.

The patient was anesthetized initially with a Hurricaine lollipop supplemented with 2 separate injections of 5 mL of 1% lidocaine with 1:100,000 epinephrine. Once the patient had been adequately anesthetized, the radiofrequency probe was bent to an angle of 45 degrees and inserted into the midline of the palate. At a temperature of 85 degrees, 650 joules was administered to the midline of the palate. Supplemental anesthesia was required for the lateral treatments, and then 325 joules at 85 degrees Celsius was administered in the lateral palatal areas.

DISPOSITION: The patient was instructed to neither eat nor drink for 1 hour until oral anesthesia has completely resolved. He was then discharged to home with Vicodin and a Medrol Dosepak. He was given instructions for his postop care and phone numbers at which to reach us if he has any problems. He was discharged from the ENT clinic in stable condition. We will see him in the office in followup in 1 week.

_____
Leela Pivari, MD
ENT Clinic

LP:pai
D:4/17/----
T:4/18/----

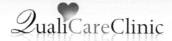

General Surgery Report

Patient Name: Lori Anne Richey   **ID#:** S-49

Date of Operation: 22 Aug ----   **Age:** 18   **Sex:** Female

PREOPERATIVE DIAGNOSIS
Papillary thyroid cancer.

POSTOPERATIVE DIAGNOSIS
Papillary thyroid cancer.

SURGEON: James A. McClure Jr, MD

ASSISTANT: Bernard Kester, MD

ANESTHESIA: General endotracheal anesthesia given by Dr. Carl Erickson Avalon.

OPERATION PERFORMED: Total thyroidectomy.

MATERIAL FORWARDED TO LABORATORY FOR EXAMINATION: Right and left lobes of thyroid were passed off as specimen.

INDICATIONS: Lori is an 18-year-old girl who presented to her PCM and was found to have a neck mass. Workup proved to be papillary thyroid cancer. The mass was found on CT to be approximately 3 x 6 cm in her right thyroid gland. Preoperative imaging revealed no lymphadenopathy within the neck.

FINDINGS
1. Bilateral inferior parathyroid glands identified and preserved in situ.
2. Likely left superior parathyroid gland preserved in situ, although not specifically identified.
3. Right superior parathyroid gland, likely sacrificed due to proximity and involvement with the tumor.
4. Bilateral recurrent laryngeal nerves fully preserved and able to be stimulated with less than 0.5 on the nerve integrity monitor (NIM) stimulator at the end of the case.

PROCEDURE IN DETAIL: Patient was brought to the operating room and placed on the operating room table in supine position. General endotracheal anesthesia was induced using a nerve integrity monitor tube as the endotracheal tube. The head of the bed was turned. The incision was marked on the neck with a skin marker in a skin crease in a low transverse position approximately 3 cm above the clavicles. This incision was of a length of about 7 cm. Methylene blue and needle were used to mark several dots along the edges of the incision for reapproximation at the end of the case.

Lidocaine with epinephrine, 1% and 1:100,000, was injected into the incision, and the patient was prepped and draped in the usual sterile fashion. Incision down through the skin, subcutaneous tissue, and platysma was undertaken with a No. 15-blade scalpel followed by elevation of superior and inferior subplatysmal flaps, also with scalpel. Hemostasis was with bipolar cautery. The superior subplatysmal flap was raised as high as the thyroid notch and the inferior as low as the cuticular heads. The strap muscles were divided along the midline raphe in a vertical orientation using cautery. The skin edges were then retracted with dural hooks and rubber bands. The strap muscles were elevated from the face of the thyroid gland using cautery and blunt dissection bilaterally out to the lateral border of the gland.

Next, attention was turned to the right, and the right middle thyroid vein was ligated. Dissection then was undertaken along the right superior pole, taking meticulous care to ligate blood vessels as they were encountered. Most of the superior pole vessels were ligated, but it was found at this point in the case that there was a large portion of the nodule that extended up into the superior pole, very high, beyond where the superior pole would normally lie. This also extended posteriorly as far back as the posterior edge of the thyroid cartilage. Some of the inferior attachments at the inferior pole were then divided to allow more mobility.

(Continued)

Next, dissection was undertaken on the superior-lateral portion of the gland to allow visualization of the area where the recurrent laryngeal nerve would be entering the cricothyroid joint. Once this region was closed, the inferior parathyroid gland on the right side was identified and preserved at all times. The recurrent laryngeal nerve was identified near its entrance into the cricothyroid joint by gently spreading through tissues without cutting any tissues until the nerve had been positively identified, both visually and confirmation obtained using the NIM stimulator. The nerve was then traced a small bit inferiorly to ensure that there were no branches prior to the point at which we had identified the nerve. The nerve was then traced superiorly to the cricothyroid joint, and the overlying tissues were divided carefully, using a combination of cautery and suture ligation of vessels when needed. Once the nerve had been taken down as far as the cricothyroid joint, dissection was undertaken through Berry ligament and the remaining attachments of the inferior portion of the gland to the trachea until the gland was free. The isthmus of the gland was then divided, and the right lobe was passed off as specimen.

Attention was then turned to the left side of the gland, which was approached in a similar fashion, beginning first with ligation of the middle thyroid vein followed by division of the superior pole vessels. The inferior parathyroid gland was identified and preserved in situ. There was a fatty deposit near where we expected to find the superior parathyroid gland. Dissection of this fatty deposit was not undertaken for a desire to preserve any blood supply to that gland, if it was contained within that deposit of fatty-appearing tissue. Once the gland had been freed from its superior pole attachments, attention was turned to the cricothyroid joint region. Gentle spreading motions were utilized to identify the recurrent laryngeal nerve. No tissues were cut until the nerve had been identified. In similar fashion to the right side, the nerve was traced slightly inferiorly to confirm that there were no branches prior to our identification point, followed by tracing the nerve superiorly to the cricothyroid joint. Overlying tissues were divided. The nerve was quite closely adherent to a nodule of the thyroid gland, directly approaching the tracheoesophageal groove on the left side. Careful dissection was used to separate the gland from the nerve. Berry ligament was then dissected through, and the gland was removed from its remaining attachments to the trachea medially and inferiorly and passed off as specimen. The wound was copiously irrigated. Hemostasis was confirmed followed by a Valsalva maneuver to confirm that the increased pressure would cause no problem with hemostasis.

During the case it was noted that there was a burn through the skin superior to our incision by approximately 2 cm to 3 cm. When this was identified, it appeared that it had been caused by conduction of electrocautery current to the Army-Navy retractor that had been used to retract the skin in that region, possibly during separation of the strap muscles. The burned skin edges were excised. The wound was closed meticulously with 4-0 subdermal Vicryl followed by a running 5-0 Monocryl subcuticular suture. The total length of this incision when closed was approximately 2.5 cm.

The main incision was then closed over a No. 1-0, fully perforated, flat Blake drain. The wound was closed in layers using 3-0 Vicryl in the strap muscles, 3-0 Vicryl in the platysma, 4-0 Vicryl in the subdermal tissues, and a running 5-0 subcuticular Monocryl to close the skin. Steri-Strip was placed over the wound as a dressing.

Patient was then awakened and brought to the PACU breathing spontaneously and in stable condition with no further complications.

_____

James A. McClure Jr, MD
General Surgery

JAM:pai
D:8/22/----
T:8/23/----

c: Patrick Keathley, MD, Endocrinology

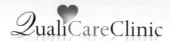

QualiCareClinic

Orthopedic Surgical Report

Patient Name: Jose Tijerina   **ID#:** S-50

Date of Operation: 9 Feb ----   **Age:** 19   **Sex:** Male

PREOPERATIVE DIAGNOSIS
Left index finger metacarpal nonunion.

POSTOPERATIVE DIAGNOSIS
Left index finger metacarpal nonunion.

SURGEON: Raquel Rodriguez, MD

ASSISTANT: Jack Zullig, MD

ANESTHESIA: General endotracheal.

OPERATIONS PERFORMED
1. Left index finger metacarpal nonunion takedown and intercalary bone graft (iliac crest bone graft).
2. Open reduction, internal fixation.

SPECIMEN REMOVED: None.

INDICATIONS: Jose is a 19-year-old male who sustained an injury to his left hand several weeks ago. The patient was initially treated with open reduction, internal fixation of the long finger metacarpal; however, pinning of the index finger metacarpal demonstrated no evidence of significant healing. Treatment options then were reviewed with the patient and his family. The patient subsequently elected surgical intervention.

PROCEDURE IN DETAIL: The patient was identified, brought to the operating room, and placed supine on the operating room table. Preoperative antibiotics were given. General endotracheal anesthesia was obtained. Left upper extremity was then prepped and draped in the usual sterile fashion after the tourniquet had been applied. The contralateral right iliac crest was also prepped and draped in the usual sterile fashion.

Attention was first placed to the left hand. The extremity was exsanguinated, and the tourniquet was inflated to 250 mmHg. Utilizing the previous dorsal longitudinal incision, which was extended both distally and proximally, careful dissection was made through the skin and subcutaneous tissue with hemostasis obtained with bipolar cautery. The extensor tendons were identified and released. Significant scar tissue noted between the underlying fascia of the intrinsics as well as the index metacarpal. This was released. Utilizing sharp dissection, the index metacarpal was then exposed through a longitudinal incision dorsally. Nonunion noted in the distal one-third of the metacarpal. This was removed with sharp dissection.

Attention was then carried to release a portion of the capsule dorsally as well as on the radial aspect. Increased motion was noted at the metacarpophalangeal joint. The wound was copiously irrigated with normal saline solution.

Attention was then focused to the right iliac crest. Careful dissection made through skin and subcutaneous tissue with hemostasis obtained with bipolar cautery. Careful attention was noted to stay posterior to the anterior superior iliac spine. The fascia was identified and released to expose the iliac crest. A 2 x 1.5 cm portion of the iliac crest was removed. The wound was copiously irrigated with normal saline solution. Gelfoam was placed for hemostasis. The wound site was anesthetized with 1% lidocaine and 0.5% Marcaine, approximately 10 mL. Fascial layer was closed in interrupted fashion using 2-0 Vicryl suture. Subcutaneous layer was closed with 2-0 Vicryl suture. The skin closed with a running subcuticular 3-0 Monocryl suture. Dry sterile dressings were placed as well as Steri-Strips.

(Continued)

ID#: S-50   PAGE 2

Attention was then placed to the left hand. The iliac crest was then fashioned and secured in the nonunion site. The index metacarpal was then rigidly fixed with a 2.3 mm T-plate. Intraoperative imaging confirmed proper placement of all hardware as well as adequate bony contact. Additional cancellous bone graft was then placed in the nonunion site. Full range of motion of the wrist demonstrated no evidence of significant angular or rotational deformities. The portion of sagittal band was repaired radially with 4-0 PDS suture in interrupted fashion. The fascia overlying the index metacarpal was also repaired with 4-0 PDS suture in interrupted fashion. In order to prevent adhesions, a bioabsorbable cold polyester sheet was used (VivoSorb). This was secured to the soft tissues with 4-0 PDS suture in interrupted fashion. Again, range of motion of the wrist demonstrated good flexion/extension of the index digit without evidence of significant rotational or angular deformities.

Once this had been accomplished, the wound was copiously irrigated with normal saline. The skin was closed with 4-0 nylon suture in an interrupted fashion. Dry sterile dressings were placed. The patient was placed in a dorsal block splint in intrinsic-plus position. The tourniquet was released up to 111 minutes. The patient was awakened from general anesthesia and taken to the recovery room in stable condition.

_____
Raquel Rodriguez, MD
Orthopedic Surgery

RR:pai
D:2/9/----
T:2/9/----

c: Marie Aaron, DO, Family Practice

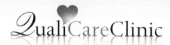

Ophthalmologic Surgery

Patient Name: Rosalinda Celio   **ID#:** S-52

Date of Operation: 12/21/----   **Age:** 75   **Sex:** F

PREOPERATIVE DIAGNOSIS
Mature cataract, left eye.

POSTOPERATIVE DIAGNOSIS
Mature cataract, left eye.

OPERATION PERFORMED: Placement of intraocular lens implant, left eye.

SPECIMEN REMOVED: Cataract, left eye.

SURGEON: Yasmin Naimi, MD

ASSISTANT: Jimmy Dale Jett, RN, Circulating Nurse

ANESTHETIC: Monitored anesthesia care by Dr. Delaney.

PROSTHETIC DEVICES: Lens used is Model SA 608T, power 20.0 diopter, length 13 mm, optic 6 mm, and serial #997052.029.

PROCEDURE IN DETAIL: Patient was brought into OR 3 and placed under monitored anesthesia control while under intravenous sedation. A retrobulbar block was administered. Following this, intermittent digital compression was placed over the surgical eye. Operating eye is the left eye. Limbal peritomy was created. Hemostasis was achieved with a razor-tipped cautery. Crescent knife was used to create a scleral incision posterior to the surgical limbus and then used to create a tunnel wound into the clear cornea. A limbal paracentesis was then created with the 75 blade, and Viscoat was injected into the anterior chamber through this wound.

A phacoblade was then used to enter the anterior chamber through the corneoscleral tunnel wound. A cystitome was used to initiate capsulotomy. Utrata forceps was used to complete a continuous curvilinear capsulorrhexis. Balanced salt solution on a blunt cannula was used to hydrodissect the lens. The lens nucleus then phacoemulsified and was aspirated from the eye. Residual lens cortex was removed from the lens capsular bag with the automated I&A handpiece. Healon was injected into the lens capsular bag.

The phacowound was then enlarged with the phacoblade. The intraocular lens was then folded and inserted into the lens capsular bag. Residual Viscoat elastic material was then removed from the eye with the automated I&A handpiece. Paracentesis wound was hydrated and found to be tight. The subconjunctival wound was closed with a single 8-0 Vicryl suture. The wound integrity was checked and found to be watertight.

Postoperatively, subconjunctival injections of 0.5 mL of Decadron and Ancef were placed in the inferior fornix. Maxitrol ointment and pilocarpine gel were applied to the eye along with a pressure patch and Fox shield. Patient was then transferred to the ward in stable condition.

_____

Yasmin Naimi, MD
Ophthalmology

YN:cks
D:12/21/----
T:12/23/----

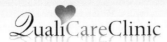

General Surgery

Patient Name: DeMarcus Collins

Date of Operation: 07/10/----   Age: 47

ID#: S-54

Sex: M

PREOPERATIVE DIAGNOSIS
Motor vehicle collision with resultant closed-head injury.

POSTOPERATIVE DIAGNOSIS
Motor vehicle collision with resultant closed-head injury.

OPERATIONS PERFORMED
1. Percutaneous tracheostomy, #8-Shiley.
2. Percutaneous endoscopic gastrostomy, 20-French.

SPECIMEN REMOVED: None.

SURGEON: James A. McClure Jr, MD

INDICATIONS: This is a 47-year-old man who was involved in a motor vehicle collision approximately 1 week ago, sustaining a significant closed-head injury. He remains ventilator dependent and requires intraoral nutrition. He is now taken for tracheostomy and feeding tube placement.

DESCRIPTION OF OPERATION: The patient was brought to the operating room where the ophthalmology team stabilized a left orbital fracture. Following this procedure we proceeded with the tracheostomy and percutaneous endoscopic gastrostomy (PEG) placement.

We started with the tracheostomy. His cervical spine had not been formally cleared, so we used in-line stabilization. He had a transversely positioned shoulder roll placed, exposing his cervical landmarks. We made a small transverse incision about 2 cm below the cricoid cartilage. We then used bronchoscopic guidance through the endotracheal tube to assist with tracheostomy tube placement.

We entered the trachea with an access needle and passed a guide wire through the needle. We then serially dilated the tracheostomy tube tract, and then we placed a #8-Shiley tracheostomy tube into the trachea under direct visualization without difficulty. We had confirmation of placement with end-tidal CO_2. We then anchored the tracheostomy in place with Prolene sutures and a tracheostomy tube holder.

We then performed a bronchoscopy through the tracheostomy to evacuate moderate secretions identified earlier in the surgical procedure.

We then proceeded with the gastrostomy tube. We started by performing gastrostomy, which showed some small petechial hemorrhages within the stomach wall. None of them were bleeding at all. We then insufflated the stomach and placed the patient in steep reverse Trendelenburg. We were able to transilluminate easily and ballotted the stomach with a sharp indentation seen on the endoscopic image.

We prepped the left upper quadrant of the abdomen, made a small transverse incision, and passed the Angiocath into the gastric lumen. We then threaded a wire into the stomach, which we retrieved with the gastroscope. We then pulled the PEG tube down through the mouth and up through the abdominal wall. We re-endoscoped the patient and confirmed PEG tube position, which appeared to be appropriately placed with the tube at about 4 cm. We anchored the tube in place with interrupted sutures and desufflated the stomach.

(Continued)

ID#: S-54   PAGE 2

The patient tolerated the procedure well and was able to be taken to the recovery unit in good condition. He will continue to be followed by the neuro team.

_____
James A. McClure Jr, MD
General Surgery

JAM:cks
D:07/10/----
T:07/11/----

cc: Midori Okano, MD, Ophthalmology
       Anne Basswood, MD, Neurology

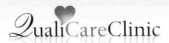

General Surgery

Patient Name: Joe Christopher Lanier   **ID#:** S-56

Date of Operation: 02/12/----   **Age:** 16   **Sex:** M

PREOPERATIVE DIAGNOSIS
Acute appendicitis.

POSTOPERATIVE DIAGNOSIS
Acute appendicitis.

OPERATION PERFORMED: Open appendectomy.

SPECIMEN REMOVED: Vermiform appendix, which was opened on the back table by me.

SURGEON: James A. McClure Jr, MD

ASSISTANT: Jimmy Dale Jett, RN

ANESTHETIC: General endotracheal by Dr. Delaney.

ESTIMATED BLOOD LOSS: 3 mL.

INDICATIONS: Joe is a 16-year-old young man who presented yesterday with abdominal pain and some nausea. This had been going on for several days. CT scan was obtained in the ED, which showed a retrocecal, dilated, and thickened appendix. On physical exam, his condition progressed overnight, and this morning he did have a positive Rovsing sign. He was tender to palpation at McBurney point. Due to the retrocecal location of his appendix, he had no anterior abdominal wall rebound tenderness. His white blood cell count was within normal limits, but he did have a significant bandemia of 20 bands. After discussion of his conditions, my findings, and reviewing the CT scan, I spoke with the patient's mother regarding the probable diagnosis of acute appendicitis. The patient's mother has verbalized her understanding of the procedure and all the risks, benefits, alternatives, and indications, as has the patient. Mother signed written, informed consent to have the patient taken to the operating room for appendectomy.

DESCRIPTION OF OPERATION: After being seen and identified in the holding area and ensuring that informed consent had been obtained, the patient was taken to the operating room and placed on the operating table in supine position. A satisfactory level of general endotracheal anesthetic was induced. His abdomen was prepped and draped in the usual sterile fashion using DuraPrep. An incision of approximately 3 cm was made over the area of McBurney point. The external oblique fascia was incised in line with the fibers, and a muscle-splitting technique was used. The posterior fascia was grasped, retracted anteriorly, and incised with Metzenbaum scissors. The abdomen was then entered. It was noted that there was a significant amount of omentum stuck down in the right lower quadrant.

The appendix was then visualized and grasped with a Babcock retractor and delivered up into the wound. The appendix was quite long, and the majority of it was retrocecal in origin. The cecum was mobilized off the lateral abdominal wall. The base of the cecum was delivered up into the wound. The vessels to the appendix were taken between clamps and silk ties without difficulty. The cecal base was then clearly visualized. It was freed of all surrounding adhesions. The appendix was crushed with a straight clamp, then ligated with a free tie and then a silk stick tie. The appendix was transected and passed off the field with a clamp. The mucosa of the appendiceal stump was then cauterized with a Bovie electrocautery.

(Continued)

ID#: S-56   PAGE 2

The abdomen was irrigated and suctioned, and the abdominal wall was then closed in layers. The posterior fascia was grasped with Kocher clamps and closed with a running 2-0 PDS suture. We irrigated between layers, and the anterior abdominal fascia was then closed with a running 2-0 PDS suture. Subcutaneous tissues were then irrigated. The skin was reapproximated with a series of interrupted inverted 3-0 Vicryl dermal sutures. The skin was closed with DermaBond. The patient was awakened, extubated in the operating room, and taken to the postanesthesia care unit in stable condition.

_____
James A. McClure Jr, MD
General Surgery

JAM:cks
D:02/12/----
T:02/12/----

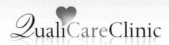

General Surgery

Patient Name: Rudolph Lochman   **ID#:** S-58

Date of Operation: 09/08/----   **Age:** 78   **Sex:** M

PREOPERATIVE DIAGNOSIS
Left inguinal hernia.

POSTOPERATIVE DIAGNOSIS
Direct left inguinal hernia.

OPERATION PERFORMED: Open left inguinal hernia repair with Prolene hernia system.

SPECIMEN REMOVED: Cord lipoma.

SURGEON: James A. McClure Jr, MD

ASSISTANT: Bernard Kester, MD

ANESTHETIC: General endotracheal by Dr. Delaney.

ESTIMATED BLOOD LOSS: 10 mL.

COMPLICATIONS: None.

INDICATIONS: This is an elderly gentleman with a long-standing history of left inguinal pain with bulge, worse with strenuous activity. He was referred to me for evaluation for a left inguinal hernia. After discussing all the options, he elected to have surgical repair of his left inguinal hernia.

DESCRIPTION OF OPERATION: After obtaining informed consent, the patient was brought back to operating room 1, placed in supine position, and general anesthesia was administered. Once patient was under anesthesia, he was prepped and draped in the usual sterile fashion. An approximately 7 cm incision was made in the left groin overlying the area of the inguinal ligament. The subcutaneous tissues were divided by the use of electrocautery down to Scarpa fascia. We went through Scarpa fascia all the way down to the level of the external oblique fascia. The external oblique fascia was cleaned free of subcutaneous tissues, and the external ring was identified. A small subcentimenter incision was then made in the external oblique fascia with an 11 blade. Once the external oblique fascia had been opened, Metzenbaum scissors were used to further divide the external oblique fascia.

Once the external oblique fascia was completely divided to the level of the external ring, the cord structures were readily identified and isolated using a Penrose drain. Once the spermatic cord and its structures had been isolated, the cord was skeletonized. We were able to identify a cord lipoma as well as a small indirect hernia. The hernia sac was dissected free of the cord structures and reduced into the opening of the internal ring. The cord lipoma was ligated and passed off the table as a specimen.

We then turned our attention to the direct floor. There was an obvious direct hernia defect. An incision was made in the transversalis fascia, and the preperitoneal space was bluntly dissected. Once the preperitoneal space had been bluntly dissected and the epigastric arteries identified, a large Prolene hernia system mesh was introduced into the preperitoneal space and the underlay deployed. Once the underlay was deployed and we were satisfied it was lying in a satisfactory position, we began to fix the overlay portion of the mesh. This fixed immediately to the pubic tubercle, inferiorly to the shelving border, superiorly to the conjoined tendon, and laterally to the internal oblique fascia. The wound was then irrigated thoroughly and inspected for hemostasis.

(Continued)

ID#: S-58   PAGE 2

We then closed the external oblique fascia using a running Vicryl suture. Once the external oblique fascia was closed, we irrigated the wound again, again ensuring hemostasis. At this point we used approximately 10 mL of local anesthetic and additionally performed an ilioinguinal nerve block. Scarpa fascia was closed using 3 interrupted 3-0 Vicryl sutures, and the subcutaneous layer was also closed using inverted interrupted Vicryl sutures. Dermabond was used to cover the rest of the wound. This concluded the operation.

The patient tolerated the operation well, and there were no complications.

_____
James A. McClure Jr, MD
General Surgery

JAM:cks
D:09/08/----
T:09/09/----

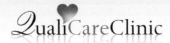

QualiCareClinic

Orthopedic Spine Surgery

Patient Name: Tanya K. Gordon **ID#:** S-59

Date of Operation: 12/14/---- **Age:** 14 **Sex:** F

PREOPERATIVE DIAGNOSIS
Adolescent idiopathic scoliosis, T4 to T11.

POSTOPERATIVE DIAGNOSIS
Adolescent idiopathic scoliosis, T4 to T11.

OPERATION PERFORMED: T4 to T11 posterior spinal fusion with instrumentation.

SPECIMEN REMOVED: None.

SURGEON: Gilbert M. Fields, MD

ASSISTANT: Howard H. Lee, MD

ANESTHETIC: GETA by Dr. Avalon.

DRAINS: Foley catheter.

SPONGE COUNT: Correct.

PROSTHETIC DEVICES: Implants—see operative report.
1. Seven titanium DePuy-Expedium spinal system polyaxial pedicle screws.
2. Two titanium DePuy-Expedium spinal rods.
3. Two titanium DePuy-Expedium horizontal rod interconnectors.
4. Five 6.2 sublaminar double-wires.

ESTIMATED BLOOD LOSS: 600 mL (100 mL returned to patient through Cell Saver).

INTRAOPERATIVE FLUIDS: 5500 mL crystalloid, 2 units donated packed red blood cells, and 1 unit fresh frozen plasma due to an intraoperative coagulopathy with an INR of 1.7. Also 1 liter 5% albumin and 500 mL Hespan.

INTRAOPERATIVE MEDICATIONS: Ancef 1000 mg intravenously x2, Amicar intravenous bolus, Amicar 10 mg/kg/hr intravenous drip intraoperatively.

URINE OUTPUT: Appropriate throughout the case.

COMPLICATIONS: None.

TOURNIQUET TIME: Not applicable.

INDICATIONS: Tanya Gordon is a healthy 14-year-old female with thoracolumbar scoliosis consistent with adolescent idiopathic type. She has a progressive 50-degree right-sided thoracolumbar curve extending from T4 to T11 with an associated right-sided thoracic hyperkyphosis. Her lumbar curve is a compensatory, nonstructural curve. She is not a candidate for bracing of this large, progressive curve and is indicated for posterior spinal fusion with instrumentation from levels T4 to T11.

(Continued)

ID#: S-59 PAGE 2

DESCRIPTION OF OPERATION: The patient's family was counseled regarding the risks, benefits, and outcomes of the proposed procedure, to include possible irreversible spinal cord or nerve root damage, bleeding, infection, wound breakdown or dehiscence, postoperative hematoma necessitating need for emergent return to operating room, hardware failure, pseudarthrosis, adjacent level osteoarthritis, thoracolumbar stiffness, and postoperative pain. The patient's family agreed to proceed with the stated T4 to T11 posterior spinal fusion with instrumentation.

Patient was taken to the operating room, and somatosensory and motor evoked potential neuromonitors were placed in standard fashion by the neuromonitoring representative. The patient was then turned onto a Jackson spine table in the prone position with the table at 0 degrees. The operative field was marked out from T3 to T12, and patient was prepped and draped in the usual sterile orthopedic fashion.

We then commenced with the procedure and made a direct midline posterior incision over the levels T4 to T11 on the back. Using sharp dissection with a 10-blade scalpel and electrocautery, we dissected down to the spinous processes of T3 to T12 and used direct fluoroscopic guidance to mark the appropriate T4 to T11 fusion levels. Then in standard fashion, the surrounding soft tissue over the posterior elements of these levels was cleared off the bone. We cleared off the transverse processes of all levels and identified the facet joints of all levels. We then performed facetectomies of the facet joints from the T10 to T11 level all the way up to the T4 to T5 level by performing ostectomies of the superior articular processes of T5 to T10. Similarly, we did the same on the right side of the spinal column. Meticulous hemostasis was performed throughout this portion of the procedure. All articular process osteotomies were collected and maintained for lateral bone grafting for the spinal fusion. All spinous process osteotomies performed were similarly collected for bone grafting later.

We then turned our attention to placement of posterior instrumentation. The hardware system selected was the DePuy-Expedium pedicle screw instrumentation and sublaminar wire spinal system. Three titanium DePuy polyaxial pedicle screws were placed at T4, T10, and T11 on the left side; four titanium DePuy polyaxial pedicle screws were placed on the right side at levels T11, T9, T7, and T4. The screw sizes ranged from 4.35 mm to 5 mm in diameter and from 30 mm to 40 mm in length. The screws on the left side were as follows: T4, 4.35 x 30 mm; T10, 4.35 x 35 mm; T11, 5 x 40 mm. The screws on the right side were as follows: T4, 4.35 x 30 mm; T7, 4.35 x 35 mm; T9, 4.35 x 35 mm; T11, 5 x 40 mm.

We then placed four 6.2 sublaminar double-wires at levels T6 to T9 on the left side without complication. Neuromonitoring during pedicle screw fixation and sublaminar wire placement showed no evidence of neurologic encroachment. Proper anatomic screw position and wire position at all levels was demonstrated using intraoperative fluoroscopy. Then in standard fashion, we determined the appropriate parallel rod lengths for the left and right sides of the patient's spine. The left rod was fashioned to be slightly hyperkyphotic while the right rod was fashioned to be slightly hypokyphotic to balance the patient's preoperative right hyperkyphosis.

We distracted the posterior spine on the left side and compressed the spine on the left side to correct the patient's preoperative right thoracolumbar scoliotic curvature. We were able to correct the deformity to approximately 6 degrees right T4 to T11 curvature, a significant improvement from her preoperative 50-degree curve.

After instrumentation, we thoroughly irrigated the surgical field with warm sterile normal saline, ensuring adequate hemostasis of the wound. After irrigation, we turned our attention to bone grafting of our posterior spinal fusion. Corticectomy was performed at all levels using a MicroAire-Legend hand-held bur. Throughout the case we prepared an autologous platelet-rich plasma sample using the patient's own blood and the DePuy Symphony II system. We mixed this preparation with our autologous bone graft obtained from the ostectomies. We mixed that solution with freeze-dried allograft bone chips on the back table. We then placed bone graft from T4 to T5 down to T10 to T11. We did not bone graft at T3-T4 or at T11-T12. The bone grafting was performed bilaterally from T4 to T11. We then interconnected the two parallel spinal rods with two DePuy-Expedium rod interconnectors proximally and distally.

(Continued)

The wound was then irrigated thoroughly one final time, and a deep Hemovac drain was placed. Hemostasis was confirmed. The wound was closed in standard fashion over the drain by reapproximating the posterior spinal musculature over the T3 to T12 spinous processes using buried interrupted 0 Vicryl suture and a running interlocking 0 Vicryl suture. The subcutaneous tissue was closed with buried interrupted 2-0 Vicryl suture in standard fashion, and the skin was closed with a running subcuticular absorbable 4-0 Monocryl suture. The skin was cleaned, and sterile occlusive dressing was placed. The patient's drapes were removed, and radiograph of the thoracolumbar spine was taken. The patient was extubated in the operating room without complication.

Wake-up test was negative for nerve injury. She tolerated this procedure without complication and was taken directly to the pediatric intensive care unit in excellent condition. The pediatric intensivist specialty group will monitor and treat her while she is in the PICU. Urine output was appropriate throughout the case, her Foley catheter was left in place, and she was ordered to remain on Ancef 1000 mg q.8 h. until removal of Foley and drain. She will remain on bed rest at least until postoperative day 1. Her drain and Foley will likely be removed on either postop day 2 or day 3.

_____

Gilbert M. Fields, MD
Orthopedic Surgery

GMF:cks
D:12/14/----
T:12/15/----

cc: Patricia Kofos, MD, Pediatric Intensivist

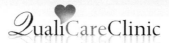

Ear, Nose, and Throat Surgery

Patient Name: Ana Marta Gutierrez   **ID#:** S-60

Date of Operation: 01/25/----   **Age:** 67   **Sex:** F

PREOPERATIVE DIAGNOSES
1. Presbylaryngis.
2. Glottic insufficiency.

POSTOPERATIVE DIAGNOSES
1. Presbylaryngis.
2. Glottic insufficiency.

OPERATIONS PERFORMED
1. Fiberoptic laryngoscopy.
2. Injection laryngoplasty (Cymetra).

SPECIMEN REMOVED: None.

SURGEON: Leela Pivari, MD

ASSISTANT: Anna Marie Iaccarino, RN

ANESTHETIC: Topical.

INDICATIONS: Ms. Gutierrez is a 67-year-old Hispanic female who has dysphonia and hypofunctional voice. After going through several weeks of voice therapy, she has not improved greatly. On repeat stroboscopy, it was demonstrated that she had continued hypofunction with what appeared to be glottic insufficiency.

DESCRIPTION OF OPERATION: The patient was seated in the examination chair where the procedure was explained to her in detail. She had the opportunity to ask questions, and these were answered to her satisfaction. She signed the informed consent, and the procedure began.

The patient was anesthetized in her nasal passages using a mixture of Afrin and lidocaine. A transnasal digital laryngoscope was placed through the left naris and passed to the level of the pharynx. Her sensation was tested using both the flexible laryngoscope and the transoral catheter without a needle on it. She tolerated the anesthesia well.

Cymetra was mixed and placed on the injection syringe. The syringe was transferred via her oral cavity through her larynx, and approximately 0.3 mL was injected on each side of her larynx. Injections were spread both in the middle of the muscular membranous vocal fold and just lateral to the vocal process. This allowed excellent medialization of both vocal folds with only mild subglottic filling on the right.

The patient tolerated the procedure well and had a slightly strained voice at the end. Several injections were done, and in between each injection, the voice was tested for quality. It improved in quality to a point, and then more Cymetra was added to make it a slightly worse quality and over-filled.

The Cymetra that was injected was from lot #B300A, expiration date April ----, PIN 134339, Life Cell Corporation 903829473829 REV C.

_____

Leela Pivari, MD
Otorhinolaryngology

LP:cks
D:01/25/----
T:01/25/----

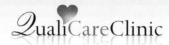

Obstetrics/Gynecology Surgery

Patient Name: Mary Louise Bright   **ID#:** S-61

Date of Operation: 05/23/----   **Age:** 25   **Sex:** F

PREOPERATIVE DIAGNOSES

1. Intrauterine pregnancy at 39-0/7 weeks with breech/breech, dichorionic-diamniotic twin gestation. Patient desires primary low transverse cesarean section.
2. Patient also desires permanent sterilization via bilateral tubal ligation.

POSTOPERATIVE DIAGNOSES

1. Intrauterine pregnancy at 39-0/7 weeks with breech/breech, dichorionic-diamniotic twin gestation. Patient desires primary low transverse cesarean section.
2. Patient also desires permanent sterilization via bilateral tubal ligations.

OPERATIONS PERFORMED

1. Primary low transverse cesarean section.
2. Bilateral tubal ligations via Parkland method.

SPECIMENS REMOVED: Placenta, portions of bilateral fallopian tubes, blood gases.

SURGEON: Tillman Risha, MD

ASSISTANT: Rosemary Bumbak, MD

ANESTHESIA: Spinal by Dr. Delaney.

DRAINS: Foley.

ESTIMATED BLOOD LOSS: 700 mL.

INTRAVENOUS FLUIDS: 4600 mL of lactated Ringer's.

URINE OUTPUT: 300 mL.

INDICATIONS: Patient is a 25-year-old G3, P2-0-0-2, at 39-0/7 weeks with dichorionic-diamniotic twin gestation with breech/breech presentation with concordant growth who desires permanent sterilization. She understood the high regret rate for permanent sterilization in patients younger than 30 years old, and she desires no future fertility even if something tragic happens to her current children.

FINDINGS

1. Live-born female infant A delivered at 0908 in complete breech presentation, with Apgars of 8 and 9, weighing 3153 g (6 pounds 15.2 ounces).
2. Live-born female infant B delivered at 0909 in complete breech presentation, with Apgars of 8 and 9, weighing 3224 g (7 pounds 1.7 ounces).
3. Cord gases for twin A: 7.23/56/8.3/24.7 with base excess of -1.3.
4. Cord gases for twin B: 7.27/57/6.2/23 with a base excess of -3.5.
5. Patient had normal uterus, bilateral tubes, and ovaries.
6. Parkland bilateral tubal ligations were performed without difficulty in a standard fashion with approximately 2 cm portions of bilateral fallopian tubes resected. Patient tolerated procedure well and was transferred to PACU. Infants stable to LDR.

(Continued)

DESCRIPTION OF OPERATION: Informed consent was obtained and placed on the chart. Patient was taken to the operating room where she underwent spinal anesthesia. A Foley catheter was then placed, and she was prepped and draped in the usual sterile fashion and placed in supine position with a leftward tilt. A Pfannenstiel skin incision was then made in the lower abdomen 2 cm above the pubic symphysis. Incision was carried down sharply with a scalpel. The fascia was nicked in 2 places with the scalpel. The fascial incision was then extended laterally using Mayo scissors. Two Kocher clamps were then used to elevate the superior fascia, which was then tented up and separated from the rectus muscle bellies. In a similar fashion, the posterior rectus muscle bellies were separated from the rectus muscle bellies. The peritoneum was then entered bluntly. Bladder blade was inserted. Vesicouterine peritoneum was identified and entered sharply, and the bladder flap was created digitally.

A low transverse incision was then made in the lower uterine segment, and infant A was delivered in complete breech presentation without difficulty. Cord clamped, infant was bulb suctioned, then handed over to waiting pediatricians. In a similar fashion, infant B was delivered in a complete breech presentation. Cord was clamped, and infant was handed over to waiting pediatrician. Placenta was then delivered spontaneously. Uterus was exteriorized from the abdomen and cleared of all clots and debris. The uterine incision was then closed using 0 Vicryl in a running locked fashion, and a second suture with 0 Vicryl was used to imbricate the uterus.

Parkland tubal ligation was then performed in a standard fashion. An approximately 2 cm portion of each fallopian tube was resected and handed over as specimen for pathologic evaluation. After all pedicles were inspected and found to be hemostatic, the uterus was returned to the abdomen. Pericolic gutters were irrigated. Uterine incision was reinspected and found to be hemostatic. Fascia was then closed using 0 Vicryl in a running unlocked fashion, and subcutaneous tissues were irrigated copiously. Bovie cautery was used to achieve sufficient hemostasis. The skin was then closed in a subcuticular fashion using 3-0 Monocryl.

Patient tolerated the procedure well and was taken to PACU. Infants stable to LDR.

_____

Tillman Risha, MD
Obstetrics/Gynecology

TR:cks
D:05/23/----
T:05/25/----

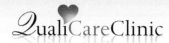

Ophthalmologic Surgery

Patient Name: Brandon R. Cavanaugh   **ID#:** S-62

Date of Operation: 08/31/----   **Age:** 20   **Sex:** M

PREOPERATIVE DIAGNOSIS
Severe globe trauma, status post globe repair and blind eye, right.

POSTOPERATIVE DIAGNOSIS
Severe globe trauma, status post globe repair and blind eye, right.

OPERATION PERFORMED: Enucleation, right eye.

SPECIMEN REMOVED: Right globe.

SURGEON: Yasmin Naimi, MD

ASSISTANT: Jimmy Dale Jett, RN, Circulating Nurse

ANESTHETIC: General endotracheal with MAC by Dr. Delaney.

DESCRIPTION OF OPERATION: After being properly identified in the preop holding area, the patient was brought back to room #3 and placed under monitored anesthesia control. General endotracheal was initiated and endotracheal tube was placed without difficulty. A retrobulbar block was administered immediately followed by intermittent digital compressions over the eye. Patient's eye was then prepped with 5% povidone-iodine solution and draped in the usual sterile fashion for eye surgery. A lid speculum was placed, and a 360-degree peritomy was performed. The lateral rectus muscle was hooked with a Jameson muscle hook along its insertion. A second Jameson muscle hook was then placed under the lateral rectus muscle in the opposite direction. All fascial attachments to the muscle were then severed anteriorly. The muscle was then cauterized approximately 4 mm posterior to its insertion. A double-armed 6-0 Vicryl suture was then woven through the muscle and locked in place in both directions. The muscle was then disinserted from the globe using Westcott scissors.

Attention was then turned to the medial rectus muscle, which was hooked, cauterized, tagged, and disinserted in the same fashion. Attention was then turned to the inferior rectus muscle, which was hooked, cauterized, tagged, and disinserted in a similar fashion. Locating the superior rectus muscle proved difficult, and what muscle attachments could be found were disinserted from the globe with Westcott scissors. Iris tenotomy scissors were then used to free the globe of its fascial attachments as much as possible. A 5-0 Vicryl suture was whip-locked through the stump of the lateral rectus muscle; it was then also whip-locked through the stump of the medial rectus muscle. This suture was then used to put traction anteriorly and temporally on the globe. Enucleation scissors were then used to strum the optic nerve posterior to the globe and then used to sever the optic nerve as it entered into the globe. The remaining fascial attachments of the globe to the orbit were then bluntly and sharply dissected, and the globe was removed from the orbit.

Hemostasis was obtained with gauze packing and direct pressure first and then with bipolar cautery. A 22 mm PMMA diving sphere was placed in the remaining pocket and found to be the correct size. The superior rectus muscle was located in the superior Tenon area and whip-locked with a 6-0 Vicryl double-armed suture. Then a 1 x 1 cm piece of a larger reconstituted piece of AlloDerm was created. A 22 mm Medpor implant was then placed in a 60 mL syringe along with a solution of injectable normal saline and gentamicin. Negative pressure created in this syringe assisted in removal of the air from the Medpor implant and infusion of the gentamicin solution. The implant was then placed in the inserter and inserted into the right orbit. The aforementioned AlloDerm segment was then placed on the surface of the Medpor implant. The inferior oblique muscle was then identified and tagged with a 5-0 Vicryl suture. The rectus muscles were then sutured to the AlloDerm tissue segment at adjacent sides, and the inferior oblique muscle was sewn to the inferotemporal corner of the AlloDerm graft.

(Continued)

ID#: S-62   PAGE 2

Tenon capsule was then closed over the surface of the AlloDerm patch using simple interrupted 5-0 Vicryl sutures. Closure was inspected and found to have no gaps. The conjunctiva was then closed over the surface of Tenon capsule using running and simple interrupted 5-0 plain gut suture. Bacitracin ointment was then placed on the back of a small, rigid PMMA lid conformer and placed over the surface of the covered implant. The lids were then brought over the conformer. A pressure patch with several layers of tape was then placed over the right orbit.

The patient was then awakened from anesthesia and extubated without difficulty. Patient was taken to the PACU in stable condition.

_____

Yasmin Naimi, MD
Ophthalmology

YN:cks
D:08/31/----
T:08/31/----

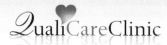

QualiCareClinic

Genitourinary Surgery

Patient Name: Tuong Van Nguyen   **ID#:** S-63

Date of Operation: 04/20/----   **Age:** 51   **Sex:** M

PREOPERATIVE DIAGNOSIS
Bilateral ureteral obstruction from recurrent retroperitoneal fibrosis.

POSTOPERATIVE DIAGNOSIS
Recurrent retroperitoneal fibrosis with bilateral ureteral obstructions.

OPERATIONS PERFORMED
1. Bilateral ureteral lyses.
2. Left ureteral resection.
3. Left ileal ureter interposition.
4. Right omental flap.

SPECIMENS REMOVED: (1) Left ureter and (2) right retroperitoneal biopsy.

SURGEON: Charles Mendesz, MD

FIRST ASSISTANT: Ken Miller, MD

SECOND ASSISTANT: Jimmy Dale Jett, RN

ANESTHETIC: General with epidural regional block by Dr. Avalon.

DRAINS: 10 mm flat Jackson-Pratt, left lower quadrant; 20-French Foley catheter in bladder; nasogastric tube.

SPONGE COUNT: Verified x3.

PROSTHETIC DEVICES: None.

INDICATIONS: This is a 51-year-old Vietnamese male with a history of retroperitoneal fibrosis who underwent a laparoscopic bilateral ureterolysis 2 years ago, after which he did well until early this year when on surveillance it was noted that his creatinine had increased from 1.1 to 1.8. Cystoscopy, retrograde pyelograms, and stent placements were performed in February of this year. His creatinine level returned to normal. Followup CT scanning demonstrated recurrent retroperitoneal fibrosis, which had extended down into his midureters previously. The obstruction was at the level of the proximal ureters. Patient was informed of his options for treatment to include medical treatment alone, surgical treatment alone, and combination therapy. Indwelling ureteral stents were also offered. He has had significant side effects from the ureteral stents, and he decided to be stent-free. After an extended consultation with the patient, it was decided that his best chance for long-term success is to undergo repeat ureterolysis in an open fashion, then have medical therapy postoperatively. In this regard, postop consultation with Rheumatology has already been arranged. Patient was informed of the indications, risks, benefits, and alternatives of the ureterolysis and possible need for ileal ureter interposition. He desired to proceed with the operation and was consented and scheduled as such.

DESCRIPTION OF OPERATION: Patient was taken to the operating room where an epidural catheter was placed by the anesthesia team. He was then placed in the supine position. General anesthetic was administered. He was prepped and draped in the usual sterile fashion. A 20-French Foley catheter was placed into his bladder on the field and clamped to the drapes. A midline laparotomy incision was made from the xiphoid process to near the pubic symphysis. Bovie electrocautery was continued down to the fascia. He had a lot of venous collaterals that required coagulation. Of note, on his preoperative imaging, he has an occluded vena cava from the retroperitoneal fibrosis.

(Continued)

SECTION 3 SURGICAL REPORTS 289

ID#: S-63   PAGE 2

We incised to his anterior abdominal wall fascia, sharply incised his peritoneum, and entered his abdomen. Cautery was used to incise the transversalis fascia and peritoneum. Initially we noticed not a great deal of intraabdominal adhesions noted from his previous laparoscopic procedure. The urachal remnant was isolated from his anterior abdominal wall, cut, and incised to allow better mobilization of the bladder. The Bookwalter retractor set was assembled over the wound and used for retraction as needed throughout the case.

We turned our attention first to identifying his right ureter. The right colon was reflected medially off the kidney. There were a great deal of adhesions in reflecting the colon off his retroperitoneum. Again, a lot of venous collaterals were noted, but hemostasis was adequate. Sharp and blunt dissection was used. We eventually found the right ureter as it crossed the pelvic brim. It was adhesiolysed from a dense, rock-hard, fibrotic mass surrounding the ureter. This was particularly evident at the pelvic brim and crossing down into the true pelvis.

Several centimeters into the true pelvis, the ureter became normal again and was easily mobilized in its most distal extent toward the bladder. Once the ureter was completely mobilized up toward the renal pelvis, an inspection of the ureter demonstrated what appeared to be an otherwise viable ureter. There was about a 1 cm segment that was perhaps slightly ischemic, but it was felt that it would probably be viable, especially given our plans for an omental wrap. We sharply excised a small portion of the fibrotic mass near the portion of the ureter that was most encased and sent this for permanent pathologic examination as a right retroperitoneal biopsy.

We then turned our attention to the left side. Of note, on his previous surgery, the left ureter was apparently placed outside the retroperitoneum by tacking the left colonic mesentery underneath the ureter. In the process of reflecting the left colon, again we found dense adhesions. We did, in fact, find the left ureter to be tented up over the left colonic mesentery in an intraabdominal fashion. We completely mobilized the ureter from the mesentery and reflected the mesentery back medially in its normal anatomic location. We mobilized the left ureter with great difficulty down to the pelvic brim. At this point, however, it was completely adherent to the surrounding retroperitoneal mass. Furthermore, the part of the ureter that was draped over the colon appeared severely ischemic and nonviable. For this reason it was decided to incise the ureter at the level of the pelvic brim. This was done sharply, such that the previous indwelling ureteral stent could be removed intact. This was, in fact, done. With the ureter incised, we then mobilized it proximally until the ureter appeared pink and viable. It appeared viable no more than 2 to 3 cm away from the renal pelvis. When we found what appeared to be viable ureter, we excised the nonviable portion of the ureter and sent it for permanent pathology examination. In doing so, we had a gap of approximately 15 to 20 cm that needed to be bridged. We decided that ileal ureter interposition would be required on this side. We mobilized the bladder on both the left and right sides slightly; however, neither bladder pedicle required ligating. This allowed the bladder to be lifted just to the level of the pelvic brim, slightly beyond the level of the previously incised ureter on the left side.

We turned our attention to the bowel. Some adhesiolysis was required around the terminal ileum and ileocecal valve in order to properly identify the ileocecal valve. Approximately 20 cm proximal to this we marked the distal end of our bowel segment and went about another 15 to 20 cm proximal and marked the most proximal end of our bowel segment. We ensured that the mesenteric vascular pedicle of this segment would be adequate to maintain viability of the excised ileal segment. This proved to be the case. We marked the peritoneum overlying the mesentery with Bovie electrocautery, then incised and ligated the small mesenteric vessels with interrupted silk sutures. This was done on both the proximal and distal extents. The GIA stapler was passed through the incised mesentery, completing the bowel resection proximally and distally.

We then returned bowel continuity by approximating the butt ends of the more distal ileum, excising the tips and passing the GIA 75 stapler into the bowel lumen, then firing the stapler, ensuring that the bowel was anastomosed in a side-to-side fashion with the one antimesenteric border approximating the other antimesenteric border. The GIA stapler was removed. The butt ends of the bowel anastomosis were closed with the TA 55 stapler, which was also fired without difficulty. The crotch of the anastomosis was secured with 3-0 silk sutures, and Lemberts on the butt end of the anastomosis were used to bury the staple line.

(Continued)

We then turned our attention to the isolated portion of ileum, which would be used for the ileoureter. We attempted to mobilize the left colonic mesentery enough to pass the ileum through a hole in the mesentery so that it would be able to lie in a retroperitoneal fashion; however, due to his retroperitoneal fibrosis, his left colonic mesentery had been sucked into the fibrotic mass somewhat, and it was very short. It did not allow adequate mobility for the ileal segment to pass. We decided to drape the ileal segment over the top of the left colon. In doing so, it appeared to have more than adequate length to reach both the bladder and the incised ureter up near the left ureteropelvic junction. It also did not seem to impinge upon the left colon, such that we felt that it would function normally and be at low risk for obstruction.

With the ileal segment isolated and placed in a proper position, we first turned our attention to the proximal anastomosis. We made an approximately 1 cm incision in the proximal butt end of the ileal segment and in an end-to-side fashion anastomosed the ileum to the left proximal-most ureter. Prior to doing so the ureter was spatulated widely. After spatulation, we passed Van Buren sounds through the ureter into the left renal pelvis to calibrate the remaining lumen, and this calibrated up to 20-French easily. He was also given an ampule of intravenous indigo carmine, and there was seen to be blue efflux from the proximal end of the ureter. Interrupted 5-0 Vicryl sutures were used to make the anastomosis between the ileum and proximal ureter. Approximately 8 to 10 anastomotic sutures were placed circumferentially in a clockwise fashion through full-thickness ureter and full-thickness bowel from mucosa to serosa. Once approximately 180 degrees of the anastomosis was completed, we opened the distal end of the ileal segment, passed a right angle through the distal end up through and into the anastomosis, grasped a 0.035-inch floppy-tipped guide wire, retracted it back through the distal end of the ileum, and then placed the proximal end into the right renal pelvis. Over this a 6-French x 30 cm double-J ureteral stent was passed through the ileum across the anastomosis and into the left renal pelvis. The wire was subsequently removed, allowing good stent placement across the proximal anastomosis with the distal end exiting the butt end of the ileal segment. The anastomosis was completed with the 5-0 Vicryl sutures proximally. It appeared to be watertight.

We then turned our attention to the distal end. The dome of the bladder was identified. The peritoneum overlying the dome was incised. The perivesicular fat was divided. Detrusor was identified, and 2-0 Vicryl stay sutures were placed on either side of the expected location of the anastomosis. The bladder was incised with Bovie electrocautery to a lumen that approximated the luminal size of the small bowel. Approximately 180 degrees of the anastomosis were again made with full-thickness bites, including the bladder mucosa and detrusor in both the serosa and mucosa of the small bowel. This was done with 3-0 Vicryl interrupted sutures. Once approximately 180 degrees of it had been completed, the distal tail of the double-J stent was placed inside the bladder, and the anastomosis was completed with interrupted sutures in 360 degrees. A second layer of closure was completed by closing the serosa and peritoneum overlying the bladder to the serosa of the small bowel with interrupted 3-0 Vicryl sutures. Again, this portion of the anastomosis appeared to be watertight. We copiously irrigated his abdomen at this point. Hemostasis appeared to be adequate. We closed the small bowel mesentery from the previous bowel resection with interrupted silk sutures, then secured the bowel anastomosis to the root of the ileal ureter mesentery and closed any surrounding mesenteric defects with interrupted silk sutures. This included the defect that occurred where the ileal ureter passed over the top of the left colon.

We then turned our attention to wrapping the right ureter with an omental wrap. We split the patient's omentum in the midline up to the transverse colon and mobilized a portion of this omentum off the transverse colon to allow a tongue that would reach deeply into his pelvis, passing behind the right colon. In doing so we were allowed to have piece of omentum that wrapped circumferentially around the lysed portion of the ureter circumferentially. The omentum extended down to normal distal ureter. With the omentum wrapped 350 degrees around the ureter at the level of the fibrotic mass, we secured it there with interrupted Vicryl sutures. We quickly ran his small bowel and identified no injuries. Earlier in the case, in mobilizing his right colon, there was a partial deserosalization of the cecum. This was repaired with interrupted silk Lembert sutures. Inspection of this at the conclusion of the case demonstrated an intact repair. A #10 mm flat Jackson-Pratt drain was brought into the abdomen through

(Continued)

ID#: S-63   PAGE 4

the left lower quadrant and was placed along the left colonic gutter near the left ileal ureter. The abdomen was subsequently closed with #1 looped PDS up to the level near the xiphoid process. Interrupted #1 Vicryl suture closed the most proximal extent of this incision near the xiphoid and allowed us to bury the knot from the PDS suture. Once all these sutures were tied and cut, his wound was copiously irrigated. Hemostasis in the superficial tissues was assured, and the skin was approximated with stainless steel staples. Sterile dressing was applied. His Jackson-Pratt drain was hooked up and secured.

Patient tolerated the procedure well, was extubated in the operating room, then taken to SICU in stable condition. He received 1250 mL of colloid and 9000 mL crystalloid. Estimated blood loss 900 mL. Urine output 1200 mL. Gastric output was 50 mL.

It should be noted that the nasogastric tube that had been placed at the start of the case was left indwelling at the conclusion of the case. It was verified in good position prior to closure.

_____

Charles Mendesz, MD
Urology

CM:cks
D:04/21/----
T:04/22/----

cc: Luke Mosbacker, MD, Rheumatology
     Ken Miller, MD, Gastroenterology

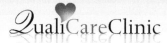

Vascular Surgery

Patient Name: Jerry Watson

Date of Operation: 01/18/----   **Age:** 54

ID#: S-64

Sex: M

PREOPERATIVE DIAGNOSIS
Acquired defect of mandible and intraoral mucosa.

POSTOPERATIVE DIAGNOSES
1. Acquired defect of mandible and intraoral mucosa.
2. Acquired defect of left lower extremity.

OPERATIONS PERFORMED
1. Vessel preparation in the neck.
2. Left free fibula microvascular reconstruction of mandible.
3. Split-thickness skin graft to left neck.

SPECIMEN REMOVED: None.

SURGEON: Ly An Tabor, MD

FIRST ASSISTANT: Leah Pittfield, MD

SECOND ASSISTANT: Danila R. Fry, MD

ANESTHETIC: General endotracheal via transoral approach by Dr. Delaney.

TOTAL TOURNIQUET TIME DURING FLAP HARVEST: 93 minutes.

TOTAL ISCHEMIA TIME: 4 hours 9 minutes.

INDICATIONS: Jerry Watson is a 54-year-old gentleman who was evaluated a year ago and found to have a squamous cell carcinoma of his right mandibular gingiva. He was staged as a T4N0M0 squamous cell carcinoma of the right mandibular gingiva. He was referred to Hillcrest Medical Center for definitive care. The risks, benefits, indications, and alternatives to reconstruction of the surgical defect with a free fibular flap were thoroughly described to the patient and his wife preoperatively by me. I reiterated some of these risks with Mr. Watson on the morning of the surgery as well. I explained that the risks would include but not be limited to infection, bleeding, scarring, fistula formation, delayed healing, failure of the flap with loss of the flap, requiring additional surgery, or partial failure of the flap. The risk of additional procedures was also discussed. Time was allowed for questions, and all questions were answered to his apparent satisfaction. Informed consent was obtained.

FINDINGS: The resultant mandibular defect extended from the inferior portion of the ascending ramus, just past the angle of the mandible, to the contralateral parasymphysis. The total mandibular defect measured 15 cm. Three closing-wedge osteoectomies were performed with some additional trimming of the inferior edge of the fibula, which turned into the posterior aspect of the neomandible in an angulated fashion to achieve a good bone approximation posteriorly. The neomandible was secured to the 2-0 Synthes reconstruction bar with locking screws. The arterial anastomosis was performed in an end-to-end fashion to the facial artery. The venous anastomosis was performed from the dominant venae comitantes into the internal jugular vein in an end-to-side fashion.

DESCRIPTION OF OPERATION: Patient was identified in the holding area and was then transferred to the operating room. He was placed supine on the operating table, then intubated transorally by the anesthesiology service. The account of the resection of the tumor, direct laryngoscopy, tracheotomy, and neck dissection will be dictated by Dr. Pittfield. The microvascular team assisted in prepping and draping the patient and positioning the left leg in anticipation of dissection of the left leg.

(Continued)

After the resecting team was well into their portion of the procedure, we began the dissection of the flap. The fibular head and lateral malleolus were marked. The posterior edge of the fibula was also marked. A line was placed 7 cm below the head of the fibula in order to protect the common peroneal nerve. Similarly, 8 cm of inferior fibula was left in the ankle for stability. The left leg had previously been prepped and draped in the usual sterile fashion.

A sterile tourniquet was placed and inflated to 300 mmHg pressure. The procedure was initiated by making an anterior incision on the skin panel, which had been centered on the lower half of the leg with its midpoint being the posterior border of the fibula. The flap was oriented vertically. The anterior incision was made through the skin, subcutaneous tissue, and the deep fascia. Subfascial dissection was then performed posteriorly until the anterior intermuscular septum was identified. Once the anterior intermuscular septum was identified, we transitioned to a more medial course of dissection following the septum toward the fibula. The peroneal muscles were then retracted anteriorly. Once we reached the fibula, the peroneal muscles were dissected off the lateral aspect of the fibula and retracted further anteriorly. A small cuff of muscle was preserved. We then encountered the next intermuscular septum between the peroneus muscles and the extensor muscles. This was divided. The extensor muscles were also subsequently dissected off the anterior aspect of the fibula. Care was taken to preserve a small cuff of muscle measuring roughly 1 to 2 mm on the fibula bone. Care was taken to not delve deeply into the extensor muscles. The extensor muscles were retracted further medially and then the inner osseous membrane was identified. It was carefully incised with a #15 blade and the posterior tibialis muscles identified. This was done along the entire course of the exposed fibula, which measured about 30 cm. At this point we transitioned to posterior dissection.

Posterior skin incision was then made and carried down to the deep fascia. The fascia over the soleus muscle was divided and anteriorly directed dissection was performed over the soleus until it got within about 1 cm of its lateral edge. The perforating vessels, which had been previously identified from the anterior aspect, were located again on the posterior aspect. Their sanctity was confirmed. Once we reached this point, we returned to an anterior approach. The fibula was exposed over about a 20 cm length from approximately 9 cm above the ankle to about 8 cm below the superior limit of the fibula. With this amount of fibular exposure, this was deemed adequate for reconstruction of the mandibular defect. We then used a Satinsky clamp to dissect around the medial edge of the fibula with care taken to stay right on the bone. Once the Satinsky was placed, both at the inferior and then at the superior limits of the bone, an oscillating saw was used to perform osteotomies. Now that the bone was free, it was retracted laterally. This allowed identification of the common peroneal vessels. The pedicle was dissected superiorly toward the upper limit of our visualization, essentially to the take-off of the common peroneal vessels from the posterior tibialis vessels. The pedicle was isolated and swept laterally with the flap. The posterior tibialis muscles were divided and then, moving from medial to lateral around the pedicle, a small cuff of flexor hallucis longus and soleus was taken with the flap. This allowed freedom of the flap from the lateral leg, at which point it was attached only by its vascular pedicle.

Under loupe magnification, intensive dissection of the proximal aspect of the pedicle was then performed. The artery and two venae comitantes were identified and isolated. In the course of pedicle elevation, several large venous communicating branches were noted that were communicating with the posterior compartment. These were doubly clamped, divided, and ligated with 2-0 silk. At about one-third the distance down the fibula, there was a communicating artery toward the posterior compartment, which was also doubly clamped, divided, and ligated with 2-0 silk. Prior to ligating this, it was confirmed that the anterior tibial vessels were visualized and patent in the extremely anterior and medial aspects of our field.

At this point we were apprised that the mandibular defect measured 15 cm in length. This was confirmed on the specimen and on the preplated mandible. The resecting team had preformed a 2-0 Synthes locking reconstruction plate to the mandible. We used this as our template for ultimate mandibular shaping. At this point it was felt that we had more than enough bone, and the flap was set for transfer. We then moved up to the neck and carefully dissected out the facial artery well into the periphery. This was to serve as our recipient artery. The internal jugular vein was skeletonized and isolated with vessel loops. Once the greater vessels were prepared, the flap was then transferred. The common peroneal artery was clamped, divided, and ligated with a 2-0 silk suture ligature

(Continued)

ID#: S-64   PAGE 3

and a medium clip. Next the venae comitantes were clamped and tied off with suture ligatures and clips as well. The flap was now free, and it was transferred to the neck.

We began by first orienting the flap with the skin paddle intraorally and the latter surface of the fibula adjacent to the bar for reconstruction. The pedicle was then draped down into the neck in preparation for the microvascular anastomosis. In order to trim down the excess bone, the periosteum was stripped from the superior edge of the fibula down toward the upper reaches of the bone that we would need. In doing so, the pedicle was carefully identified and protected. Closing wedge osteoectomies were then performed in 3 sites to allow contouring of the fibula to the plate for re-creation of the medial mandible. Once this was accomplished, the neomandible was secured in place with 8 mm and 10 mm screws to the locking reconstruction bar. There were good bony contact areas throughout. In a few areas where the bony contact was less than ideal, some of the bone chips from bone shaping were inserted.

With the flap securely in place, attention was then turned to the microvascular anastomosis. The pedicle vessels were dissected under the operating microscope to adequate length. There seemed to be a dominant vein, dominant venae comitantes, and this was chosen for our end-to-side anastomosis into the internal jugular vein. Due to flap geometry concerns, the vein anastomosis was performed first. This was performed in an end-to-side fashion with interrupted 9-0 nylon sutures to the internal jugular vein after adequate cleaving under the microscope of both the pedicle vessel and the internal jugular vein.

Next the arterial anastomosis was performed under the operating microscope with interrupted 9-0 nylon suture. There was a small amount of mismatch, essentially a 1.5:1 mismatch between the facial artery, which was a smaller artery, and the common peroneal artery. Once the anastomoses were completed, the clamps were removed, and the vessel loops were removed from around the internal jugular vein. (The venous outflow tract was unblocked first.) Excellent flow to the flap was evidenced by a palpable pedicle pulse up underneath the mandible and by improvement in the skin color of the intraoral paddle and bleeding from the skin edges. After the flap was allowed to perfuse for several minutes, the pedicle was inspected. The vagus anastomoses were patent. There was good flow through each, as was also determined by Doppler.

The flap was then inset beginning posteriorly. In the region of the left anterior tonsillar pillar, the mucosa was reapproximated to itself primarily. Then the flap was reapproximated to the mucosa in the region of the retromolar trigone, moving anteriorly along the floor of the mouth. Interrupted vertical mattress sutures of 3-0 Vicryl were used for closure. Excess flap was located laterally, which was deepithelialized. The lip, which had been split as part of the resection, was then brought into its normal anatomic position, and this facilitated accurate mapping of what areas of the flap needed to be deepithelialized. Some of the anterior aspects of the deepithelialized flap were draped over the neomandible and reconstruction bar. The suprahyoid muscles were resuspended to the mandible with 2-0 Prolene suture. This was accomplished by figure-of-8 stitches around the reconstruction bar itself. The flap inset continued until the lip was closed. The resultant neck wound was then closed in layers by the resecting team. A 3-layer closure was accomplished on the lip.

An excellent Doppler signal was found in the flap, in the anterior aspect, and this was marked with a 2-0 silk suture placed very superficially. At this point, with only closure of the neck remaining, care of the patient was returned to Dr. Pittfield.

_____

Ly An Tabor, MD
Vascular Surgery

LAT:cks
D:01/18/----
T:01/18/----

cc: Leah Pittfield, MD, Otorhinolaryngology
      Danila R. Fry, MD, Plastic Surgery

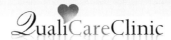

Oromaxillofacial Surgery

Patient Name: Trent R. Lockwood   **ID#:** S-65

Date of Operation: 01/04/----   **Age:** 30   **Sex:** M

PREOPERATIVE DIAGNOSIS
Left zygomaticomaxillary complex fracture.

POSTOPERATIVE DIAGNOSIS
Left zygomaticomaxillary complex fracture.

OPERATION PERFORMED: Open reduction, internal fixation of left zygomaticomaxillary complex fracture.

SPECIMEN REMOVED: None.

SURGEON: Leela Pivari, MD

ASSISTANT: Jimmy Dale Jett, RN, Circulating Nurse

ANESTHETIC: General endotracheal by Dr. Delaney.

ESTIMATED BLOOD LOSS: Minimal.

INDICATIONS: Patient sustained an assault to the face with a fist 2 days ago. He was found to have a left zygomaticomaxillary complex fracture based on both physical exam and computer tomography scan of the face. He wishes to proceed with the above operative procedure to correct these fractures.

DESCRIPTION OF OPERATION: The patient was brought into the operating room and placed on the operating table in supine position. He was intubated, and the bed was turned 90 degrees. He was prepped and draped in the usual sterile fashion. Then 1% lidocaine with 1:100,000 epinephrine was injected into the conjunctiva of the left lower lid. In addition, injection was placed into the left lateral upper brow and intraorally into his gingivobuccal crease.

Left lateral canthotomy and cantholysis was completed. First, the canthus was clamped with a mosquito, and tenotomy scissors were used to sharply cut the canthus. Dissection was then made down to the canthal tendon, which was cut as well, thereby freeing the lower lid. A corneal protector was placed at this point. The conjunctiva was incised with a #15 blade, and dissection was carried down through the muscle into the orbital septum. At this point, the corneal protector was removed and a portion of the conjunctiva was draped over the cornea, thereby protecting it.

Dissection was carried down to the inferior orbital rim. The orbital septum had already been penetrated by the traumatic injury. The separation of the inferior orbital rim had effectively incised the periorbita at this point; therefore, dissection was carried down to the orbital rim, and the periosteum was elevated from the fracture site both medially and laterally. Once dissection down the face of the maxilla was carried out, attention was then brought to the gingivobuccal sulcus. Bovie was used to make an incision in the left gingivobuccal sulcus on the maxillary aspect. Dissection was carried down to the maxillary bone. Dissection with a Freer was carried out and brought superiorly, thereby connecting the previous dissection from above with the dissection below. In doing so, the infraorbital matter was carefully preserved. Its bundle was seen coursing in vivo.

Finally, the zygomaticofrontal suture was exposed using a 2 cm incision immediately superior to the left eyebrow at its lateral aspect. Dissection was carried down to the bone, and a Freer elevator was used to remove the periosteum from the bone. The bony fragment was apparent at the zygomaticofrontal suture. At the zygomaticomaxillary buttress there was a hairline nondisplaced fracture. A Sayre elevator was then introduced into the intraoral incision and placed medial to the zygomatic arch. Using careful but firm pressure, the zygomatic arch was popped laterally into position. This effectively reduced the zygomaticofrontal and inferior orbital rim fractures. A Synthes craniofacial set was then used to plate the inferior orbital rim and zygomaticofrontal

(Continued)

fractures. A gently curved, 6-hole, 1.3 plate was used on the inferior orbital rim. Two holes spanned the fracture, 2 screws were placed on either side of the fracture, and 4 mm screws were placed. A gently curved, 5-hole, 1.5 plate was placed on the left zygomaticofrontal fracture. One hole spanned the fracture and 2 holes spanned the lateral and medial aspects of the fracture. Then 4 mm screws were placed into the holes.

Next the gingivobuccal sulcus incision was closed with a running 4-0 chromic. We attempted to close the area of the periosteum of the orbital floor and the anterior face of the maxilla; however, the trauma had mangled much of this periosteum. Therefore, unfortunately, not a stitch could be placed in an effective and safe fashion. The left lateral canthal tendon was resuspended using a 5-0 PDS. It was sutured to the medial and superior aspect on the inside of the lateral orbital rim in the region of the Whitnall tubercle. An overcorrection was carried out to allow for postoperative relaxation. Then 5-0 fast-absorbing gut was used to approximate the canthotomy incision. A simple interrupted 5-0 fast-absorbing gut was used to close the zygomaticofrontal incision. This skin suture was placed after interrupted 4-0 Vicryl sutures had been used to approximate the deep portion of the incision.

Once all the incisions had been closed, the patient was turned over to the anesthesia team. He was extubated and brought back to the PACU, from where he will be discharged home when he meets criteria. Patient will return in 1 week for wound evaluation.

Leela Pivari, MD
Oromaxillofacial Surgery

LP:cks
D:01/04/----
T:01/06/----

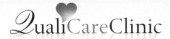

QualiCareClinic

<u>**General Surgery**</u>

Patient Name: Michael R. Turnbow   **ID#:** S-66

Date of Operation: 06/12/----   **Age:** 17   **Sex:** M

PREOPERATIVE DIAGNOSIS
Bilateral gynecomastia.

POSTOPERATIVE DIAGNOSIS
Bilateral gynecomastia.

OPERATION PERFORMED: Bilateral subcutaneous mastectomies.

SPECIMENS REMOVED: (1) Right breast. (2) Left breast.

SURGEON: James A McClure Jr, MD

ASSISTANT: Bernard Kester, MD

ANESTHETIC: General via endotracheal intubation and Marcaine infiltration by Dr. Avalon.

SPONGE COUNT: Verified correct x3.

COMPLICATIONS: None.

INDICATIONS: Gynecomastia, persistent for greater than 1-1/2 years, affecting social development and behavior.

DESCRIPTION OF OPERATION: After discussion of risks, benefits, and alternatives, and after answering all questions, the patient was taken to the operating room, sleep induced, intubated, and fully anesthetized by Dr. Avalon. He was positioned squarely and symmetrically on the board with both arms out without hyperextension of the arms and with a pillow under the knees. Sterile prep and drape with Betadine scrub and paint, sterile towels and drapes, was performed of the bilateral chest, shoulders, arms, and upper abdomen, and the patient was draped out.

An incision was made in a semicircle under each breast with a 5 mm extension to the right and left of the nipple. The incision was at the edge of the areola. Leaving an adequate depth of tissue behind the nipple to avoid nipple necrosis, the breast was divided under the nipple. Then the breast and fat pads surrounding the breast were excised using electrocautery dissection on the right and left sides. Care was taken to avoid making the flap too thin. Good hemostasis was achieved. The pectoralis fascia was left intact, and the axillary fat pad was left undisturbed.

Both wounds were irrigated with warm sterile saline solution. Good hemostasis was achieved. With the patient symmetric and midline marked, the breast tissue was examined with the skin flaps reapproximated. A small amount of trimming of the duct bundle behind the nipple was made to allow for a symmetric and healthy appearance. Following this a 3-0 Vicryl was used to tack down the backside of each nipple to the pectoralis fascia at an appropriate point for upright posture.

(Continued)

ID#: S-66   PAGE 2

Deep dermis was reapproximated using inverted 3-0 Vicryl, and the subcutaneous tissue was run with 4-0 Vicryl. Steri-Strips and a compressive dressing with foam tape and wads of fluff were placed. Patient tolerated this procedure well without complications. All sponge and instrument counts were correct. Wound was closed in 2 layers. The patient was transported to the recovery room in satisfactory condition.

_____

James A. McClure Jr, MD
General Surgery

JAM:cks
D:06/12/----
T:06/12/----

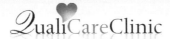

QualiCareClinic

<u>Gastroenterology Surgery</u>

Patient Name: Charisse Moore   **ID#:** S-67

Date of Operation: 06/22/----   **Age:** 21   **Sex:** F

PREPROCEDURE DIAGNOSES: Acute left lower quadrant abdominal pain and peritonitis.

POSTPROCEDURE DIAGNOSES: Colonic edema, gastritis, gastric polyp.

PROCEDURES PERFORMED
1. Esophagogastroduodenoscopy.
2. Colonoscopy.

SPECIMENS REMOVED
1. Distal esophagus.
2. Antrum.
3. Gastric polyp.
4. Second portion of duodenum.
5. Surveillance biopsies, colon.

PROCEDURES PERFORMED BY: Michael Panagides, MD

ANESTHETIC: Propofol.

INDICATIONS: This is a 21-year-old female with a history of Wilms tumor, status post right nephrectomy, and total abdominal radiation therapy as a young child. She has a history of several years of abdominal pain. She presented acutely with onset of left lower quadrant abdominal pain 4 days prior to this procedure. She had had a history of fever prior to admission. She was found on CT scan to have diffuse bowel wall thickening as well as ascites. Her ascitic fluid was drained by Interventional Radiology 1 day prior to this procedure, and it appears to be infected with neutrophil counts greater than 5000. She has been on antibiotics for 4 days. The concern was, given her abdominal radiation, whether she had an area of ischemia, small area of volvulus, or colitis that was contributing to the onset of peritonitis. Patient does have a history of chronic recurring ascites, likely from destruction of lymph tissue from previous radiation therapy. She has been occult-blood positive while in the hospital. Stools cultured no growth at the time of endoscopy. Fecal leukocytes were zero at the time of endoscopy. She underwent the procedure given concern for significantly inflamed colon and risk of perforation.

FINDINGS
1. Esophagus: The esophagus was normal in appearance. There was no evidence of esophagitis, extrinsic mass, compression, varices, erosions, or other abnormalities. Photo documentation was obtained. Biopsies were obtained from the distal esophagus.
2. Stomach: The stomach had a hypertrophic mucosal appearance, which was evidenced by scattered erythema. The gastric mucosa was easily friable with biopsy as well as with passage of the scope. No discrete ulcerations or varices were noted. A small gastric polyp approximately 0.5 cm in diameter was noted along the greater curvature of the stomach. This was isolated in appearance. Pylorus appeared normal. Photo documentation of all the above was obtained. Biopsies were obtained in the antrum as well as of the gastric polyp. They were sent to pathology for evaluation.
3. Duodenum: The duodenum was normal in appearance. No evidence of duodenitis, ulcers, nodules, polyps, masses, or vascular malformation was seen. Photo documentation of the duodenum was obtained. Biopsies were obtained from the second portion of the duodenum.

(Continued)

ID#: S-67   PAGE 2

4. Colon: The visualized colonic segments were all abnormal in appearance. The mucosal surface of the colon appeared edematous with loss of vascular markings as well as crypt hyperplasia. No true structures were identified; however, segments of the colon appeared to be less distensible than others. There were no polyps, ulcers, or masses identified on examination. No areas of ischemia were noted. The colonic mucosa did appear to be slightly friable throughout. Photo documentation of colonic segments was obtained. Surveillance biopsies were obtained throughout the entirety of the colon.

DESCRIPTION OF PROCEDURE: H&P was performed prior to the procedure. Before the patient was taken from the floor, the procedure indications, potential complications, and alternatives available were explained to the patient and her mother, who was present. Patient has been on Dilaudid for pain control. Because of this, Mother co-signed the consent forms, even though the patient is older than 18 years. Opportunities for questions were provided, and informed consent was obtained prior to the procedure.

In the procedural room, Betadine diluted with saline was administered via 3-way Foley intrarectally. The patient had a total of 1000 mL administered prior to the procedure in order to clear out remaining stool. Patient had been n.p.o. for 6 days prior to the procedure. Scant clots of greenish stool were noted to come out of the 3-way Foley after administration of only 250 mL of diluted Betadine; thus, the full 1000 mL was administered. Stools became clear after administration of an additional 750 mL of diluted Betadine. After this preparation enema and after sedation in the OR, an upper endoscope was passed through the incisural orifice into the oral cavity. Under direct visualization, the esophagus was intubated. The endoscope was passed down the esophagus through the stomach and into the duodenum. Careful inspection was made as the endoscope was advanced and withdrawn.

After the upper endoscope was removed, a colonoscope was inserted into the rectum, and under direct visualization it was advanced to the cecum. The terminal ileum was unable to be intubated. Careful inspection was made as the colonoscope was inserted as well as withdrawn. The quality of the preparation was good, allowing visualization of all mucosal surfaces. The patient tolerated the procedure well, and there were no complications.

RECOMMENDATIONS

1. Follow up with pathology for results of biopsies.
2. Continue Dilaudid for pain control.
3. Continue Timentin for antibiotic of choice for infected peritoneal fluid.
4. Follow up with lab for culture results, when available.
5. Encourage p.o. intake.
6. Continue total parenteral nutrition for now.
7. Patient has a PICC line in place for administration of antibiotics and TPN. Continue to monitor for clinical signs of sepsis, fever, or other bacterial infections in the line.
8. Patient to have flat and abdominal upright films after colonoscopy to allow free air, although there was no suggestion of perforation on either colonoscopic or clinical exam after the procedure.

_____

Michael Panagides, MD
Gastroenterology

MP:cks
D:06/22/----
T:06/23/----

c: Trevor Jordan, MD, Nephrology
    Sherman Loyd, MD, Internal Medicine

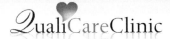

General Surgery

Patient Name: Robert Kent Wentworth   **ID#:** S-68

Date of Operation: 10/14/----   **Age:** 20   **Sex:** M

PREOPERATIVE DIAGNOSIS
Bilateral inguinal hernias.

POSTOPERATIVE DIAGNOSIS
Bilateral inguinal hernias.

OPERATION PERFORMED: Bilateral laparoscopic inguinal hernia repair.

SPECIMEN REMOVED: None.

SURGEON: James A. McClure Jr, MD

ASSISTANT: Jimmy Dale Jett, RN

ANESTHESIA: General endotracheal by Dr. Delaney.

COMPLICATIONS: None.

INDICATIONS: This is a 20-year-old black male who presented with a symptomatic left inguinal hernia with a latent right inguinal hernia. Patient desired repair.

FINDINGS: Left indirect inguinal hernia and right direct inguinal hernia.

DESCRIPTION OF OPERATION: Patient lay in the supine position in the operating suite after being given general endotracheal anesthetic. The patient's abdomen was prepped and draped in the usual sterile fashion. An infraumbilical incision was made and carried down to the posterior fascial layer. The anterior fascia and rectus muscles were elevated using the surgeon's finger and an S retractor down to the pubic symphysis. Once this space was dissected bluntly, a balloon dilator was inserted into this space and blown up with 20 compressions to completely delineate the preperitoneal space of Retzius. Once that was accomplished, the dilator was removed. An 0 Vicryl suture was placed on the anterior fascia, and a laparoscopic port was placed and insufflated.

The space was then insufflated, and the lateral margins were dissected bluntly after the placement of 2.5 mm trocars bilaterally. Dissection was then carried toward the spermatic cord and the indirect inguinal hernia on the left, which was carefully dissected from the spermatic cord. No other abnormalities were noted. The Hunter graspers were then used bluntly to dissect the right spermatic cord and other structures. There was noted to be a direct inguinal hernia present medial to the inferior epigastric vessels. A small rent was made in the peritoneum, which was decompressed through the abdomen with a Veress needle in the right upper quadrant.

Following this procedure, the mesh was rolled, after having been fashioned. It was placed into the abdomen and tacked to Cooper ligament with a spiral tacker. Several anterior tackers were placed above the direct inguinal potential space bilaterally. Two tacks were placed laterally for fixing the mesh in place. Good coverage of all hernias was noted, and the femoral space was accordingly covered once the mesh had been placed bilaterally. The site was then desufflated gradually with the camera still in place. Trocars were removed. No bleeding was noted from the trocars. The abdomen was desufflated with the Veress needle.

(Continued)

ID#: S-68   PAGE 2

The anterior fascia was reapproximated with the preplaced Vicryl suture, and the skin was closed using interrupted Vicryl suture followed by Dermabond. The patient tolerated the procedure well and was transferred to the recovery room in good, stable condition.

_____
James A. McClure Jr, MD
General Surgery

JAM:cks
D:10/14/----
T:10/15/----

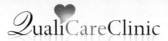

Vascular Surgery

Patient Name: Leena O. Martin   **ID#:** S-70

Date of Operation: 05/25/----   **Age:** 58   **Sex:** F

PREOPERATIVE DIAGNOSIS
Right common femoral artery hematoma and pseudoaneurysm.

POSTOPERATIVE DIAGNOSIS
Right common femoral artery hematoma and pseudoaneurysm.

OPERATION PERFORMED: Right femoral artery pseudoaneurysm thrombin injection under ultrasound guidance.

SPECIMEN REMOVED: None.

SURGEON: Ly An Tabor, MD

ASSISTANT: Anna Marie Iaccarino, RN

ANESTHETIC: Lidocaine.

INDICATIONS: This is a 58-year-old female who has a significant history of respiratory failure. She was admitted for exacerbation of this and had a femoral A-line placed. This was removed yesterday evening, and then she developed a large hematoma. She had a CT scan that suggested active extravasation, and ultrasound today showed a small pseudoaneurysm with a large hematoma. Her distal blood flow was within normal limits. It was felt that injection of this was the best temporizing measure, although she did have some early changes of the skin from the pressure underneath the blood and hematoma that may require operative intervention. Patient fully understands the risks, benefits, and alternatives of the thrombin injection and desires to proceed.

DESCRIPTION OF OPERATION: The patient was in the intensive care unit on the ventilator. The right groin was prepped using Betadine and draped in the usual sterile fashion. Using sterile Doppler ultrasound probe, 1% lidocaine was used to anesthetize over the area of the pseudoaneurysm, which had a to-and-fro Doppler signal. We then used the micropuncture kit to access this area, confirming the area with the aspirations. There was no flash of blood with this. Thrombin was injected into this area, getting cessation of the color flow on the Doppler. Roughly 0.5 mL was used. The patient then had the distal wave forms checked on the blood flow at her ankle, and this was noted to be the same. She complained of no toe pain and no foot pain.

After that had been completed, the patient had a pressure dressing placed on the right groin. The patient tolerated the procedure well. She remains in the intensive care unit on a ventilator and with full cardiovascular monitoring.

_____

Ly An Tabor, MD
Vascular Surgery

LAT:cks
D:05/25/----
T:05/26/----

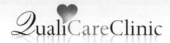

Ear, Nose, and Throat Surgery

Patient Name: Leslie S. Hunter   **ID#:** S-71

Date of Operation: 04/20/----   **Age:** 60   **Sex:** F

PREOPERATIVE DIAGNOSIS
Laryngotracheal papillomatosis.

POSTOPERATIVE DIAGNOSIS
Laryngotracheal papillomatosis with involvement of her nasal passages, soft palate, larynx, and trachea, with some lesions in segmental bronchi.

OPERATIONS PERFORMED
1. Microdirect laryngoscopy.
2. Flexible bronchoscopy.
3. Microdebridement of laryngeal and tracheal papillomatosis.
4. Ablation of papillomata via KTP-pulsed laser application using both rigid and flexible tracheoscopy and bronchoscopy techniques.

SPECIMENS REMOVED: All microdebridement specimens were collected and sent to Pathology for review.

SURGEON: Leela Pivari, MD

ASSISTANT: Joshua Stephen Gatlin, MD

ANESTHETIC: General by Dr. Delaney.

INSTRUMENT AND SPONGE COUNT: Verified correct at the end of case.

INDICATIONS: This is procedure #108 for Ms. Hunter regarding her papillomatosis.

DESCRIPTION OF OPERATION: The patient was taken to the operating room and placed in the supine position on the operating room table. After successful induction of the appropriate level of anesthesia, the patient's mouth preformed tooth guard was inserted. The table was turned 90 degrees, and a shoulder roll was placed. Attempted visualization of the larynx using a Lindholm laryngoscope failed, and a large Dedo laryngoscope afforded good view of the anterior commissure. The laryngoscope was let down every time the patient needed to be ventilated, and the procedure was performed using an apneic intermittent intubation ventilation technique.

Bronchoscopy was performed using the flexible bronchoscope. Papillomatous lesions were noted in the trachea at the carina, in the lingular segmental bronchi on the left, and in the medial segmental bronchus of the middle lobe of the right lung. Pulmonology was present in the operating room for this procedure and directed its accomplishment. There was some concern about one of the subsegmental bronchi on the right.

After bronchoscopy was complete, a laryngeal Skimmer blade was used to debride as many papillomata as could be debrided in the trachea using a Hopkins rod telescope and the microdebrider. A significant portion of papillomata were treated in this fashion. Blood was suctioned out of the trachea, and the KTP laser was used on the setting of 15 watts and 35 watts at a 15-millisecond pulse width using 2 and then 4 pulses per second. The initial lasing was done using Hopkins rod telescope and rigid fiber carriers. The patient and all operating room staff were protected with the use of amber glasses.

The patient was then rinsed with sterile water and suctioned free of blood and fluid from her lungs. The laryngoscope was removed from her mouth, and she was returned to the care of the anesthesia team, who awakened her in the operating room. All microdebridement specimens were collected and sent to Pathology for review. The patient was given Decadron and antibiotics in the operating room and was started on Levaquin postoperatively.

(Continued)

ID#: S-71 PAGE 2

Instrument and sponge counts were correct. The teeth were in good condition at the end of the case. The tongue suspension had been released about every 5 minutes during the case. There were no oropharyngeal or laryngeal lacerations.

_____

Leela Pivari, MD
Otorhinolaryngology

LP:cks
D:04/20/----
T:04/21/----

c: Joshua Stephen Gatlin, MD, Pulmonology

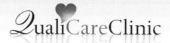

Orthopedic Surgery

Patient Name: Stephen M. Joyner   **ID#:** S-72

Date of Operation: 10/13/----   **Age:** 32   **Sex:** M

PREOPERATIVE DIAGNOSIS
Left knee patella, trochlea, and medial femoral condyle chondral defects with medial meniscal deficiency.

POSTOPERATIVE DIAGNOSIS
Left knee patella, trochlea, and medial femoral condyle chondral defects with medial meniscal deficiency.

OPERATIONS PERFORMED
1. Left knee diagnostic arthroscopy.
2. Left knee autologous chondrocyte implantation of the medial femoral condyle, trochlea, and patella.
3. Left medial meniscal transplant.
4. Left Fulkerson tibial tubercle osteotomy.

SPECIMEN REMOVED: None.

SURGEON: Gilbert M. Fields, MD

ASSISTANT: Jesse D. Smith, MD

ANESTHETIC: General endotracheal by Dr. Delaney.

PROSTHETIC DEVICES: Implants, autologous chondrocytes x3 vials. Medial meniscal allograft. Two 4.5 mm screws, one 17 mm Smith & Nephew button.

INTRAOPERATIVE MEDICATION: 0.5% Marcaine without epinephrine, a total of 20 mL injected following skin closure and Ancef 1 g IV given prior to skin incision as well as q.4 h. subsequently.

FLUIDS: 4200 mL crystalloid.

ESTIMATED BLOOD LOSS: 350 mL.

URINE OUTPUT: 1300 mL.

COMPLICATIONS: None.

INDICATIONS: Capt. Joyner is a 32-year-old active duty Air Force male who has had continued left knee pain as a result of anterior cruciate ligament (ACL) reconstruction and subsequent revision with failed medial meniscal repair as well as a chondral defect over his trochlea, patella, and medial femoral condyle. Although he has no shell deficiency at this point, he continues to have knee pain and medial meniscal deficiency. He has undergone harvest for ACL and is to undergo left knee medial meniscal allograft placement. Risks, benefits, indications for surgery were discussed with patient, and he wishes to proceed with surgery.

FINDINGS: Grade IV chondral changes in the trochlea measuring 1.5 x 1 cm. Medial femoral condyle measuring 2 x 1.5 cm, and the lateral patellar facet measuring approximately 1 x 1 cm.

DESCRIPTION OF OPERATION: Patient was met in the preoperative holding area. Informed consent was confirmed and operative extremity was initialed. He was brought to the operating room where he was placed supine on the table. Anesthesia then placed a lumbar plexus injection. He was subsequently returned to the supine position and general endotracheal was begun. Patient was prepped and draped in the usual sterile fashion. Nonsterile tourniquet had been placed on the left leg. Sterile Alvarado leg holder was placed on the left leg.

Diagnostic arthroscopy was then performed. Superolateral outflow portal was established. Inferolateral camera portal was established as well. Diagnostic arthroscopy revealed fissuring as well as surrounding chondral defect

(Continued)

ID#: S-72   PAGE 2

over the trochlea approximately 1.5 x 1 cm in size. There was also an approximately 1 x 1 cm chondral defect in the far lateral aspect of the lateral patellar facet. Lateral gutter revealed no loose bodies or other pathology. Camera was then placed in the medial compartment. Medial portal was established under direct visualization, and a probe was inserted. Medial femoral condyle lesion was seen relatively far in the posterior aspect of the condyle.

Surrounding softening of the cartilage was noted as well. There was significant deficiency of the medial meniscus primarily posteriorly and laterally. Examination into the notch revealed an intact ACL graft and an intact PCL. Lateral compartment showed no chondral damage. The lateral meniscus was intact. The shaver was placed in through the medial portal, and the remainder of the medial meniscus was debrided. This was done back to a healthy rim of vascular tissue for placement of the meniscal allograft. This was done circumferentially.

At the same time, the medial meniscal allograft was prepared. This was soaked in normal saline until it was adequately thawed. Using a combination of saws and rongeurs, bone plug for the posterior root and bone plug for the anterior root were formed. FiberWire suture was placed through the bone plug both anteriorly and posteriorly to assist with passage of the graft.

The tunnels were then prepared for passage of the meniscus. This was done initially arthroscopically so that the posterior horn and root and insertion site could be visualized behind the ACL. Once this had been debrided adequately, a guide was placed. Next a midline incision was made in the anterior aspect of the knee extending down to the proximal tibia. An arthrotomy was made in the medial aspect of the knee joint. Under direct visualization with assistance from the camera, the tunnel for the posterior meniscal root was made. This was done using guide pin guidance followed by overdrilling and dilation. Next the anterior tunnel was drilled. This was done at the insertion site of the anterior horn of the medial meniscus. This tunnel intersected the posterior tunnel. Once the tunnels had been debrided and found to be in adequate position, the prepared meniscal allograft was ready to be passed.

Prior to passage, a Fulkerson tibial tubercle osteotomy was made. This was done primarily as an elevation procedure rather than a medialization osteotomy. This was done using an oscillating saw followed by osteotome. Once the tibial tubercle had been freed from the tibia, the chondral lesions in the medial femoral condyle, trochlea, and lateral patellar facet were identified. These were debrided using a ring curette and a sharp blade. These were taken back to healthy chondral border. Following this preparation, the sockets were measured using a glove paper. The glove paper was then taken to the medial face of the tibia. These were used as templates for the periosteal patches for the ACL procedure. The periosteal patches were harvested and kept moist on the back table while the meniscus was being passed. The bone plugs were then used to pass the posterior horn of the meniscal allograft through the posterior tunnel. Next the anterior bone plug was passed through the anterior tunnel. The button was used to have the sutures tied over on the medial tibial face where the tunnel had exited. Once we had good fixation over the button, attention was then directed toward placement of the ACL patches.

The moist periosteal patches were sutured into place using 6-0 Vicryl sutures. Nearly all the periphery was sutured followed by water testing to be sure there was a seal. Once these periosteal patches had a good seal, 1 vial for each lesion was then mixed with the chondrocytes and injected into the periosteal patch. The remainder of the periosteal patch was sutured to the surrounding cartilage. Fibrin glue was then placed around the periphery to add the additional seal. This was done in the same manner for the trochlea and the medial femoral condyle. When the patella periosteal patch was being sewn, 2 small holes were noted. Because of this, we harvested an additional piece of periosteum to serve as the patch. Also, 2 Mini Mitek suturing kits were used at the far border because this lesion was uncontained. After all 3 of the chondral defects were patched with periosteum and filled with autologous chondrocytes, attention was directed toward completion of the fixation for the medial meniscus.

Inside-out technique was used with 2-0 PDS sutures. This was done around the periphery, and each suture was tied over the posterior and medial capsule. Anteriorly we were able to secure the meniscus under direct visualization. The sutures were then checked to ensure that the meniscus was adequately secured in proper location. After this had been completed, attention was then directed toward fixation of the tibial tubercle.

(Continued)

The tibial tubercle was elevated approximately 1 cm and was then fixed using two 4.5 large fragment screws using a lag technique. Once we were pleased with the fixation of the tubercle, the wound was copiously irrigated. The arthrotomy was closed using 0 Vicryl. The skin was closed using 2-0 Vicryl, 3-0 Monocryl, Steri-Strips, and Xeroform. Dressings included flats, Webril, EBIce, and an Ace wrap. He was placed in a hinged knee brace.

Patient was then extubated without difficulty and transferred to PACU for recovery.

POSTOPERATIVE PLAN
He will be nonweightbearing and will begin CPM during this admission. He will follow up with us in 2 weeks for suture removal.

_____

Gilbert M. Fields, MD
Orthopedic Surgery

GMF:cks
D:10/14/----
T:10/15/----

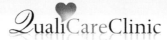

Plastic Surgery

Patient Name: Linda A. Hargrove　　　　　　　　　　　　　　　　　　　**ID#:** S-73

Date of Operation: 02/09/----　　　　　　　　**Age:** 18　　　　　　　　**Sex:** F

PREOPERATIVE DIAGNOSIS
Symptomatic macromastia.

POSTOPERATIVE DIAGNOSIS
Symptomatic macromastia.

OPERATION PERFORMED: Bilateral vertical reduction mammoplasties.

SPECIMENS REMOVED: Right breast: 242 g breast tissue. Left breast: 228 g breast tissue.

SURGEON: Danila R. Fry, MD

ASSISTANT: Anna Marie Iaccarino, RN

ANESTHETIC: General endotracheal by Dr. Delaney.

DRAINS: None.

SPONGE COUNT: Verified correct at end of case.

PROSTHETIC DEVICES: None.

ESTIMATED BLOOD LOSS: Minimal.

INTRAVENOUS FLUIDS: 1500 mL crystalloid.

COMPLICATIONS: None.

INDICATIONS: Patient is an 18-year-old female with a 3-year history of progressively worsening upper back and neck pain due to the large size of her breasts. She presented to the plastic surgery clinic requesting breast reduction. She was marked in the plastic surgery clinic 1 day prior to her surgery with a standard mosque-type pattern. The areolar inset was marked at 14 cm. The most cephalad portion of the vertical incision was marked 3 cm above the inframammary fold. The nipple was placed at the inframammary fold bilaterally.

DESCRIPTION OF OPERATION: On the day of surgery, patient was taken back to the operating room where she was placed on the operating table in supine position. Cardiac monitors were attached. The general endotracheal anesthesia was induced. The patient was administered 1 g Ancef for antibiotic prophylaxis prior to starting the case. The surgical markings were reinforced with methylene blue dye, and the breasts were infiltrated with local anesthetic solution consisting of 0.25% lidocaine with a 1:400,000 dilution of epinephrine. Then 30 mL of local anesthetic was injected into each breast. The breasts were prepped and draped in the usual sterile fashion.

The new areola was demarcated with a 40 mm cookie cutter. A 6 cm medial pedicle was marked out. The medial pedicle was then deepithelialized. The pedicle was developed perpendicular to the chest wall, down to the chest wall. The remaining skin incisions were made, and a small wedge of breast tissue was resected from the superior aspect with the majority of resection taking place in the inferolateral aspect of each breast. A total of 242 g was resected from the right breast and 228 g from the left. The areolar inset was closed at the 6-o'clock position with a 3-0 Monocryl suture, and the medial and lateral pillars were approximated with 3-0 PDS sutures. The most cephalad stitch was placed at the base of the medial pedicle and brought straight across to approximate the medial and lateral pillars at 2 cm from the skin surface. Once the breast parenchyma had been closed, the dermal margins were approximated with interrupted 2-0 Monocryl sutures.

(Continued)

The patient was placed in a semi-upright position and assessed for asymmetry. Once this was deemed satisfactory, she was placed back in the supine position, and a running subcuticular 3-0 Monocryl suture was used for final skin closure. Mastisol and Steri-Strips were applied, and the incisions were dressed with sterile gauze 4 x 8 dressings. A surgical bra was placed on the patient. She was awakened from her general anesthetic and transferred to the recovery room in good condition. No known complications at the time of this dictation.

_____

Danila R. Fry, MD
Plastic Surgery

DRF:cks
D:02/09/----
T:02/10/----

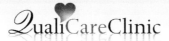

<u>Obstetrics/Gynecology Surgery</u>

Patient Name: Kimberly A. Grantham   **ID#:** S-74

Date of Operation: 04/20/----   **Age:** 34   **Sex:** F

PREOPERATIVE DIAGNOSES
1. Nonreassuring fetal heart tracing.
2. Intrauterine pregnancy at 39 weeks 0 days.

POSTOPERATIVE DIAGNOSES
1. Nonreassuring fetal heart tracing.
2. Intrauterine pregnancy at 39 weeks 0 days.

OPERATION PERFORMED: Primary low transverse cesarean section.

SPECIMENS REMOVED: Placenta and cord gases were sent.

SURGEON: Tillman Risha, MD

ASSISTANT: Rosemary Bumbak, MD

ANESTHETIC: Epidural by Dr. Avalon.

DRAINS: Foley.

SPONGE COUNT: Verified correct x2.

ESTIMATED BLOOD LOSS: 800 mL.

INTRAVENOUS FLUIDS: 2500 mL.

URINE OUTPUT: 250 mL.

COMPLICATIONS: None.

INDICATIONS: This is a 34-year-old G1, P0, at 39 weeks 9 days who progressed to complete, complete, and +2 after presenting with premature rupture of membranes. Pushed for 2 hours with development of nonreassuring fetal heart rate tracing and late decelerations.

FINDINGS: Normal gravid uterus with normal tubes and ovaries bilaterally. Live-born female infant with Apgars of 6/9. Tight nuchal cord present x2 and small, narrow pelvis noted.

DESCRIPTION OF OPERATION: Patient was taken to the operating room where epidural anesthesia was found to be adequate. She was then prepped and draped in the usual sterile fashion and placed in dorsal supine position with a leftward tilt. A Pfannenstiel skin incision was then made with a scalpel and carried through to the underlying layer of fascia with the scalpel. The fascia was then incised in the midline, and the incision was extended laterally with the Mayo scissors. The superior aspect of the fascial incision was grasped with Kocher clamps, elevated, and underlying rectus muscles were dissected bluntly.

Attention was then turned to the inferior aspect of this incision, which in a similar fashion was grasped, tented up with Kocher clamps, and the rectus muscles dissected off bluntly. The rectus muscles were then separated in the midline and the peritoneum identified and entered bluntly. The peritoneal incision was then extended superiorly and inferiorly with good visualization of the bladder. Bladder blade was then inserted and the vesicouterine peritoneum identified, grasped with pick-ups, and entered sharply with Metzenbaum scissors. Incision was then extended laterally and a bladder flap created digitally. The bladder blade was then reinserted into the lower uterine segment and incised in a transverse fashion with a scalpel. The uterine incision was then extended laterally. The bladder blade was removed, and the infant's head was delivered from +2 station and brought up to the uterine

(Continued)

hysterotomy and delivered. The nose and mouth were then bulb suctioned. The cord was clamped and cut. The infant was handed over to waiting pediatricians. Cord gases were sent.

The placenta was then removed manually. The uterus was exteriorized and cleared of all clots and debris. The uterine incision was repaired with 0 Monocryl in a running, locked fashion. A second imbricating stitch of the same suture was then used to obtain excellent hemostasis. The posterior cul-de-sac was then cleared of all clots and debris, and the uterus was returned to the abdomen. The gutters were then cleared of all clots and debris. The peritoneum was closed with 2-0 chromic. The fascia was approximated with 0 Vicryl in a running fashion. The subcutaneous layer was closed with 2-0 chromic, and the skin was closed with 3-0 Monocryl.

The patient tolerated the procedure well. Sponge, lap, and needle counts were correct x2. One gram of Ancef had been administered 30 minutes prior to the procedure. The patient was taken to the recovery room in stable condition.

_____
Tillman Risha, MD
Obstetrics/Gynecology

TR:cks
D:04/20/----
T:04/20/----

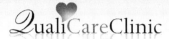

QualiCareClinic

<u>**General Surgery**</u>

Patient Name: Laura I. Benson   **ID#:** S-75

Date of Operation: 07/11/----   **Age:** 62   **Sex:** F

PREOPERATIVE DIAGNOSES
Cirrhosis and colon cancer with abdominal wound dehiscence.

POSTOPERATIVE DIAGNOSES
Cirrhosis and colon cancer with abdominal wound dehiscence.

OPERATION PERFORMED: Exploratory laparotomy with abdominal washout and replacement of temporary abdominal closure.

SPECIMEN REMOVED: None.

SURGEON: James A. McClure Jr, MD

ASSISTANT: Bernard Kester, MD

ANESTHESIA: General endotracheal by Dr. Delaney.

INDICATIONS: This is a 62-year-old woman with hepatitis C and Child's B cirrhosis who presented with a colonic adenocarcinoma in her right colon requiring right colectomy. Postoperatively she developed abdominal wound dehiscence with evisceration that, with her morbid obesity and loss of abdominal domain, had to be managed with temporary abdominal closure. She is now taken back to the operating room for washout of her peritoneal cavity.

In addition, she has developed progressive renal insufficiency, now requiring hemofiltration. She was found on physical examination to have a purulent central venous line site. With the anesthesiology service, we replaced all her lines as well as placing a dialysis catheter while under general endotracheal.

FINDINGS: There was no gross purulence. There was some fibrinous exudate along the abdominal wound edges. Her transverse colon is still massively dilated, although the small bowel and descending colon appear to be decompressed.

DESCRIPTION OF OPERATION: The patient was brought from the intensive care unit to the operating room and placed supine on the operating room table. She was on mechanical ventilation. General endotracheal was initiated. The anesthesiology team put in a right subclavian central venous catheter. We removed her right internal jugular central venous catheter. The anesthesiology team then proceeded to place a left subclavian central venous dialysis catheter. Once her lines were in place, we proceeded with the abdominal washout.

We removed her temporary abdominal closure, prepped her abdomen with Betadine, and draped sterilely. We explored her peritoneal cavity, and we found no new pockets of purulent fluid. We irrigated with about 3 L of warm saline. We ended up having to place a little bit of Surgicel along the liver edge near the falciform ligament,

(Continued)

which controlled a small amount of bleeding. We then replaced the temporary abdominal closure, starting with an x-ray cassette cover and then fashioning a towel closure covered over with an Ioban.

The patient tolerated the procedure well and was able to be taken back to the intensive care unit in critical but stable condition.

_____
James A. McClure Jr, MD
General Surgery

JAM:cks
D:07/11/----
T:07/12/----

c: Eric J. Lopez, MD, Oncology
     Leon Medina, MD, Internal Medicine

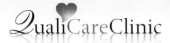

Genitourinary Surgery

Patient Name: Annette L. Capt   **ID#:** S-76

Date of Operation: 02/02/----   **Age:** 50   **Sex:** F

PREOPERATIVE DIAGNOSIS
Right distal ureteral stone.

POSTOPERATIVE DIAGNOSIS
Right distal ureteral stone.

OPERATION PERFORMED: Right semirigid ureteroscopy with basket stone extraction.

SPECIMEN REMOVED: Right ureteral stone.

SURGEON: Charles Mendesz, MD

ASSISTANT: Jimmy Dale Jett, RN

ANESTHETIC: General endotracheal by Dr. Delaney.

SPONGE COUNT: Verified correct at end of case.

FLUIDS: 500 mL normal saline.

ESTIMATED BLOOD LOSS: Zero.

URINE OUTPUT: Not recorded.

INDICATIONS: This is a 50-year-old female with a 6 mm right distal ureteral stone. Patient was originally treated for a urinary tract infection last month by the ED doctors. She returned with fevers of 101, persistent bilateral flank pain, and suprapubic pain. She was noted to have a distal right ureteral stone on CT and was admitted for intravenous antibiotics. She received a stent the next day. This is the patient's first episode of stone; however, because of the complications associated with her stone, she will receive a metabolic workup after her stone extraction.

DESCRIPTION OF OPERATION: Patient was met in the holding area where site verification and patient identification were obtained. She was then taken to the operating room where general endotracheal anesthesia was induced. She was placed in the low dorsal lithotomy position with care taken to pad her lower extremity bony prominences and pressure points. KUB done showed the stent in place across the proximal and distal edge as well as a stone in the same position as it had been for the preop KUB.

The indwelling double-J stent was then pulled through the urethra. A sensory guide wire was placed up to the kidney and noted to be there by fluoroscopic guidance. The stent was removed. The wire was secured. A semirigid scope was then placed and guided into the right ureter. The stone was easily seen. It was not impacted. There was no evidence of inflammation or injury to the ureter. Basket was placed, and the stone was easily removed with no trauma to the ureter. The wire was removed afterward.

The bladder was drained, and the procedure was completed. The stone was passed off the field as a specimen. Patient tolerated the procedure without complication, was extubated in the operating room, and was taken to PACU for recovery.

(Continued)

ID#: S-76   PAGE 2

DISPOSITION: As stated earlier, the patient will undergo a metabolic workup within 4 weeks along with a renal ultrasound to rule out ureteral stricture. The likelihood of a stricture is extremely low, based on the appearance of the ureter and the lack of trauma or inflammation surrounding the stone.

_____
Charles Mendesz, MD
Urology

CM:cks
D:02/02/----
T:02/03/----

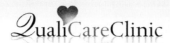

General Surgery

Patient Name: Bobby Schlecter   **ID#:** S-77

Date of Operation: 12/08/----   **Age:** 19   **Sex:** M

PREOPERATIVE DIAGNOSIS
Bilateral gynecomastia, grade IIA.

POSTOPERATIVE DIAGNOSIS
Bilateral gynecomastia, grade IIA.

OPERATION PERFORMED: Bilateral gynecomastectomies.

SPECIMENS REMOVED: Left breast, 4 g subareolar disk. Right breast, 8 g subareolar disk.

SURGEON: James A. McClure Jr, MD

ASSISTANT: Bernard Kester, MD

ANESTHETIC: General endotracheal with local by Dr. Delaney. Local anesthetic: 20 mL of 1:1 mixture of 0.5% Marcaine with 1% lidocaine and 1:100,000 epinephrine.

TUMESCENT FLUID: Left breast: 220 mL of 0.05% lidocaine with 1:100,000 epinephrine. Right breast: 235 mL of same tumescent.

SPONGE COUNT: Verified as correct at end of case.

INTRAVENOUS FLUIDS: 1300 mL.

ESTIMATED BLOOD LOSS: 20 mL.

INDICATIONS: This 19-year-old male presented with a several-year history of gynecomastia. Workup was unremarkable. Patient with extensive workout history but no history of illicit drug use. Unable to rid himself of the subareolar abnormalities. Preoperative consent obtained.

DESCRIPTION OF OPERATION: Patient was appropriately identified and brought back to the operating room. After induction of general endotracheal intubation, he was prepped and draped in the usual sterile fashion. One gram Ancef administered preoperatively. Bilateral lower extremity SCDs placed. While patient was still in the upright position, the inframammary folds in midline position were demarcated.

Beginning with the patient's left breast, a 15-blade scalpel was then used to place a 5 mm incision along the lateral axillary fold. Similar incision was made in the contralateral right breast. Then 235 mL was administered into the right breast while 220 mL tumescent was dispensed within the left breast. Pretunneling was then performed with No. 3 flat cannula. This was performed significantly bilaterally until ease of tunneling was without difficulty. We then made small inferior areolar incisions along the left and right breast tissue with electrocautery down to the subareolar depth of approximately 1 cm. Pretunneling was then performed through the infra-areolar incisions bilaterally, paying particular attention to cross-tunneling all regions as well as disrupting the inframammary folds.

At this point we began with the patient's right breast, completing our subareolar incision, resecting a small, 8 g disk in the subareolar region. A similar 4 g disk was resected from the contralateral left breast. The same No. 3 cannula was then used to perform feathering liposuction bilaterally through both the lateral and infra-areolar incisions until we felt we had excellent, smooth contour. Our dissection used a combination of sharp and electrocautery dissection.

Wound was inspected for hemostasis. We felt we had excellent contour in bilateral chest walls. A flat No.7 Blake drain was then placed bilaterally through the lateral incision sites and secured with nylon suture. Then 3-0 monofilament was used to close the dermis as well as a running intracuticular suture. Reston compression

(Continued)

ID#: S-77   PAGE 2

was then placed bilaterally, exposing the nipple-areola complex. Then 10 mL of 1:1 solution with Marcaine and lidocaine was infiltrated in bilateral drains for local anesthesia. Compression garment placed.

Patient tolerated this procedure well and was transferred to recovery room in stable condition. Sponge, needle, and instrument counts were correct at the end of the case.

DISPOSITION: Patient will be discharged home per routine recovery room protocol. Follow up in 3 days.

_____
James A. McClure Jr, MD
General Surgery

JAM:cks
D:12/09/----
T:12/10/----

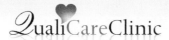

Ear, Nose, and Throat Surgery

Patient Name: Audrey Bohannon   **ID#:** S-78

Date of Operation: 07/12/----   **Age:** 1 year   **Sex:** F

PREOPERATIVE DIAGNOSIS
Recurrent acute otitis media.

POSTOPERATIVE DIAGNOSIS
Recurrent acute otitis media.

OPERATION PERFORMED: Bilateral myringotomies and pressure equalization (PE) tube placement.

SPECIMEN REMOVED: Polyp sent to histology.

SURGEON: Leela Pivari, MD

ASSISTANT: Anna Marie Iaccarino, RN, Scrub Nurse

ANESTHETIC: General mask anesthesia by Dr. Avalon.

INTRAVENOUS FLUIDS: None.

ESTIMATED BLOOD LOSS: Minimal.

COMPLICATIONS: None.

INDICATIONS: Patient is a 1-year-old female with complaint of recurrent acute otitis media, greater than 6 episodes in the last year. Preoperative audiogram showed sound fields with mild hearing loss and type B tympanic membranes bilaterally.

FINDINGS: Bilateral thick, mucoid, purulent middle ear effusions.

DESCRIPTION OF OPERATION: Patient was brought to the operating room, and after adequate general mask anesthesia was obtained, attention was first turned to the left ear. This was examined under binocular microscopy and cleaned of any cerumen. Anterior inferior radial incision was made with the myringotomy knife, and purulent middle ear effusion was suctioned from the middle ear space as well as a polyp from the middle ear space. A Pope pressure equalization tube was placed within the myringotomy, and the ear canal was filled with Floxin drops and plugged with a cotton ball.

Attention was turned to the right ear where the same exact operation was performed with the same exact findings. There were no complications. Patient tolerated the procedure well and was taken to the recovery room in satisfactory condition.

_____
Leela Pivari, MD
Otorhinolaryngology

LP:cks
D:07/12/----
T:07/12/----

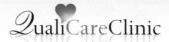

QualiCareClinic

Orthopedic Surgery

Patient Name: Gladys R. Franklin   **ID#:** S-79

Date of Operation: 01/13/----   **Age:** 59   **Sex:** F

PREOPERATIVE DIAGNOSIS
Infected left total knee arthroplasty.

POSTOPERATIVE DIAGNOSIS
Infected left total knee arthroplasty.

OPERATIONS PERFORMED
1. Explantation, left knee hardware components.
2. Irrigation and debridement.
3. Insertion of antibiotic spacer.

SPECIMEN REMOVED: Left knee hardware components.

SURGEON: Gilbert M. Fields, MD

ASSISTANT: David Castillo, MD

ANESTHETIC: General endotracheal by Dr. Avalon.

INTRAVENOUS FLUIDS: 1400 mL crystalloid.

ESTIMATED BLOOD LOSS: Less than 100 mL.

TOURNIQUET TIME: Approximately 80 minutes.

COMPLICATIONS: None.

INDICATIONS: The patient is a 59-year-old female with a history of previous infected left total knee arthroplasty treated with a 2-stage revision. The infecting organism was methicillin-resistant *Staphylococcus aureus* (MRSA). The cultures from both her current admission and her previous irrigation and debridement procedures were positive for MRSA. We discussed with the patient her options, including component retention and antibiotic suppression versus 2-stage revision. The patient was interested in proceeding with 2-stage revision surgery. She is being brought to the operating room for removal of her components and insertion of antibiotic spacer.

DESCRIPTION OF OPERATION: Patient was seen by Anesthesia in the preoperative holding area. She was brought to the operating room and placed in supine position on the operating table. After the appropriate monitoring devices were placed, general endotracheal anesthesia was induced by Anesthesia without difficulty. A nonsterile tourniquet was applied to patient's left upper thigh. The left lower extremity was prepped and draped in the usual sterile fashion.

The patient's left leg was maintained in an elevated position. Tourniquet was then inflated to 300 mmHg. The patient's staples were removed, and the knee was entered by opening her previous sutures. The sutures were removed. The patella was gently everted after securing the tibial tubercle with two-headed pins. The polyethylene insert was removed. The femoral component was separated from the underlying bone/cement interface with reciprocating saw. After the femoral component had been loosened, it was removed without difficulty. The femoral condyles remained intact, and no substantial bone was removed with the implant. The patient's tibia was subluxed forward, and the tibia was released from the underlying bones/cement interface using reciprocating saw. Multiple osteotomes were then used to gently wedge the tibial base plate away from the underlying tibia. The tibial component was then removed without difficulty. Excess cement was also removed. The bone surfaces were then gently curetted. The patient's patellar component was removed without difficulty using an oscillating saw and osteotomes. The knee was thoroughly lavaged with 12 liters of pulsatile lavage.

(Continued)

ID#: S-79   PAGE 2

Three batches of Palacos cement were mixed on a back table with 6 grams of vancomycin. The cement came premixed with gentamicin as well. The spacer was formed and, part of final hardening, was inserted into the joint space with the joint in full extension. The spacer was contoured to fit the space. An additional piece of cement was compressed into a flat disk, and this was positioned underneath the extensor mechanism to separate it from the underlying femur. The patient's wound was closed over a quarter-inch Hemovac drain using 0 Vicryl suture in the peripatellar retinaculum, a 2-0 Vicryl suture in the subcutaneous tissue, and the skin was closed with staples. The wounds were cleaned and dried. Sterile dressings were applied. The patient's leg was wrapped from toe to groin with 6-inch Ace wrap.

The tourniquet was deflated at the conclusion of the procedure. The patient's knee was placed in an immobilizer. She was transferred to postop recovery in stable condition. She tolerated the procedure well without complication. All sponge and instrument counts were reported as correct.

PLAN
The patient is to return to the operating room in 3 weeks to place another total knee prothesis.

_____
Gilbert M. Fields, MD
Orthopedic Surgery

GMF:cks
D:01/13/----
T:01/14/----

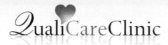

QualiCareClinic

General Surgery

Patient Name: Verna Hibberd   **ID#:** S-80

Date of Operation: 02/09/----   **Age:** 47   **Sex:** F

PREOPERATIVE DIAGNOSIS
Right breast radial scar.

POSTOPERATIVE DIAGNOSIS
Right breast radial scar.

OPERATION PERFORMED: Right medial localization lumpectomy.

SPECIMEN REMOVED: Excisional biopsy of right breast tissue.

SURGEON: James A. McClure Jr, MD

ASSISTANT: Jason Wagner, PA

ANESTHETIC: Local with MAC by Dr. Delaney.

SPONGE COUNT: Correct at end of case.

ESTIMATED BLOOD LOSS: 10 mL.

COMPLICATIONS: None.

CONDITION: Good.

FINDINGS: Right breast radial scar identified by needle localization. Successfully retrieved by excisional biopsy.

DESCRIPTION OF OPERATION: The morning of surgery the patient was taken to the mammography suite where she underwent needle placement into the region of the radial scar that had been previously identified. She was identified in the holding area. She had undergone wire placement prior to coming to the operating room. She was brought back to operating room #5 and placed in supine position. Local monitored anesthesia care was achieved. The right breast and wire were prepped and draped in the usual sterile fashion. Intravenous antibiotics were given.

A 6 cm skin incision was made, and the skin and dermis were incised. Flaps were created with the Bovie cautery. A core of tissue was circumferentially dissected around the wire. The entire wire was surrounded by tissue and removed at the base. The mass was labeled with a short stitch superior, a long stitch lateral, and the wire exiting as superficial. This was sent to Radiology, and the microcalcifications were noted by the radiologist.

The wound bed was copiously irrigated. Hemostasis was achieved with the Bovie. The wound was closed using a running subcuticular stitch, and Dermabond was applied. All counts were correct.

The patient was extubated in the operating room and taken back to recovery. There were no complications.

_____
James A. McClure Jr, MD
General Surgery

JAM:cks
D:02/09/----
T:02/10/----

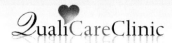

Genitourinary Surgery

Patient Name: Jonathan T. Weeks   **ID#:** S-81

Date of Operation: 11/17/----   **Age:** 2 years   **Sex:** M

PREOPERATIVE DIAGNOSIS
Distal hypospadias.

POSTOPERATIVE DIAGNOSIS
Distal hypospadias.

OPERATION PERFORMED: Distal hypospadias repair.

SPECIMEN REMOVED: None.

SURGEON: Charles Mendesz, MD

ASSISTANT: Elizabeth Cole, MD

ANESTHETIC: General endotracheal and caudal block by Dr. Avalon.

DRAINS: 6-French Silastic catheter to a diaper drain.

COMPLICATIONS: None.

INDICATIONS: Jonathan is a 2-year-old white male who was born with a distal hypospadias. He now presents for an elective repair.

DESCRIPTION OF OPERATION: Once the proper patient was identified and informed consent obtained, he was brought to the operating room where anesthesia was attained via general endotracheal anesthesia and caudal block. He was then laid supine upon the operating table where he was prepped and draped in the usual sterile fashion. Visual inspection of the phallus revealed an obviously tethered penis with coronal hypospadias.

A circumferential subcoronal incision was marked, and the skin of the shaft was mobilized as a sleeve, taking care not to injure the delicate urethral wall. Corpora were cleared of all tissue that was causing tethering, releasing the urethral meatus, advancing it distally, as well as providing us with additional penile length.

Once the orthoplasty was complete, the margins of skin and glandular epithelium on either side of the glans groove were marked and incised, forming a "U" around the meatus. The urethral plate was then incised in its midportion from the level of the neomeatus to the meatus to assist in tubularization. A 6-French elastic catheter was then inserted, and the neomeatus was reapproximated with 7-0 Vicryl sutures. Urethroplasty was then performed using a running subcuticular 7-0 Vicryl suture. The glandular sponge was then reapproximated with 6-0 Vicryl suture with interrupted mattress sutures.

The skin was then closed using 4 quadrantal sutures that were reapproximated with a 5-0 Vicryl running mattress suture. At the conclusion of the case Tegaderm was applied over the phallus, securing the urethral catheter in place. Patient tolerated the procedure well. There were no complications. He was awakened and transferred from the operating table to the gurney in stable condition. He will be discharged from the recovery area when all discharge criteria have been met.

_____

Charles Mendesz, MD
Pediatric Urology

CM:cks
D:11/17/----
T:11/18/----

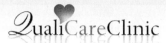

Obstetrics/Gynecology Surgery

Patient Name: Aimee J. Fitzgerald   **ID#:** S-82

Date of Operation: 06/10/----   **Age:** 30   **Sex:** F

PREOPERATIVE DIAGNOSIS
Spontaneous abortion with a missed abortion. Failed Cytotec x2.

POSTOPERATIVE DIAGNOSIS
Spontaneous abortion with a missed abortion. Failed Cytotec x2.

OPERATION PERFORMED: Suction dilatation and curettage.

SPECIMEN REMOVED: Products of conception sent for analysis.

SURGEON: Tillman Risha, MD

ASSISTANT: Jimmy Dale Jett, RN, Circulating Nurse

ANESTHETIC: General by Dr. Delaney.

INTRAVENOUS FLUIDS: 700 mL lactated Ringer's.

URINE OUTPUT: None.

ESTIMATED BLOOD LOSS: 50 mL.

COMPLICATIONS: None.

INDICATIONS: Ms. Fitzgerald is a 30-year-old G3, P0, with a last menstrual period of 03/23/---- who was seen initially at approximately 10 weeks' gestation for bleeding and cramping. Patient was noted to have a 6-week intrauterine fetal demise with no cardiac activity. Scan was repeated 4 days later, and results were confirmed. Patient attempted outpatient Cytotec management x2 without passing products of conception. At this time, it was decided to take patient to the operating room for a D&C.

FINDINGS: Moderate products of conception.

DESCRIPTION OF OPERATION: Patient was taken to the operating room where general anesthesia was found to be adequate. She was prepped and draped in the usual sterile fashion in the high lithotomy position. Surgical speculum was placed in the vagina, and the cervix was visualized. It was grasped with a tenaculum on the anterior lip, and it was dilated with a 13 Hanks dilator. The os was noted to be open at this point.

Because of the open os, 7-French suction catheter was passed without difficulty into the fundus. Suction was applied, and products of conception were removed with several passes. The suction curette was taken out, and a sharp curette was introduced with a good uterine cry noted. The suction catheter was replaced, with a small amount of products of conception and blood evacuated from the uterine cavity. The sharp curette was once again introduced, and an excellent uterine cry was noted in all quadrants of the uterus.

(Continued)

ID#: S-82   PAGE 2

The curette was removed and very little blood was noted coming from the os. The tenaculum was removed, and pressure was applied to the cervix with excellent hemostasis noted. The speculum was then removed, and the patient was taken to the PACU in stable condition.

The patient received 100 mg doxycycline intraoperatively. She will be discharged home this afternoon when all criteria for discharge are met.

_____
Tillman Risha, MD
Obstetrics/Gynecology

TR:cks
D:06/10/----
T:06/11/----

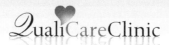

Nephrology Surgery

Patient Name: Doris Vanham   **ID#:** S-83
Date of Operation: 09/23/----   **Age:** 58   **Sex:** F

PREOPERATIVE DIAGNOSIS
Left pararenal mass.

POSTOPERATIVE DIAGNOSIS
Left pararenal mass.

OPERATION PERFORMED: Left radical nephrectomy, laparoscopic.

SPECIMEN REMOVED: Left kidney and mass. The adrenal gland was spared.

SURGEON: Charles Mendesz, MD

ASSISTANT: Trevor Jordan, MD

ANESTHETIC: General by Dr. Avalon.

SPONGE COUNT: Verified correct.

ESTIMATED BLOOD LOSS: 50 mL.

COMPLICATIONS: None.

INDICATIONS: This lady presented with a pulmonary embolism and on subsequent workup was found to have a large left pararenal mass adjacent the left kidney. The patient was counseled that this was not typical appearance for a renal cell carcinoma, in that it was not arising from within the renal parenchyma; however, it was adjacent to the kidney, and options were discussed. Malignancy could not be ruled out. She is here now for a left radical laparoscopic nephrectomy.

DESCRIPTION OF OPERATION: Patient was placed on the operating room table in the left-flank-up position. A Foley catheter and gastric tube were placed to decompress the urinary bladder and the stomach. The patient was prepped and draped in the usual sterile fashion. Veress needle was placed to produce pneumoperitoneum. Then 10 mm dilating trocars were placed in the left upper and lower quadrants as well as periumbilically. The Harmonic scalpel was used to reflect the left colon medially. The mass was easily seen on the anterior surface of the kidney. Care was taken to not enter the mass and to not enter Gerota fascia over the mass.

Next the plane between the tail of Gerota fascia and the aorta was developed. The psoas muscle was identified. The kidney was then hoisted up off the posterior wall, and dissection was carried superiorly in this plane up to the renal hilum. The renal vein and artery were identified. Stapling devices were used to take these. The artery was taken first. A 5 mm trocar was placed laterally to allow placement of a PEER retractor. This allowed retraction of this large renal mass to allow visibility for continued resection. The left adrenal was identified and was left in place. The plane between the kidney and adrenal was developed and continued. The upper pole was freed using the Harmonic scalpel. The spleen was not injured during the procedure. The posterior attachments of the kidney were freed with the Harmonic scalpel, and then Gerota tail was transected lastly using the stapling device.

Next the kidney was positioned on top of the spleen, and the ureter was grasped with a locking grasper. A 50 mm Endo Catch bag was placed through the left lower quadrant trocar site and opened in the renal fossa. The kidney was then slid off the spleen into the Endo Catch. The left lower quadrant incision was enlarged approximately 4 inches, and the kidney was extracted.

The incision was then closed in 2 layers with PDS. Laparoscope was then replaced into the umbilical trocar to check for hemostasis. Hemostasis was adequate. No distinct bleeders were seen. This was examined under low

(Continued)

ID#: S-83   PAGE 2

insufflation pressure. The trocars were then removed under direct vision, and the skin was approximated using a skin stapler at the extraction site and the trocar site. Sterile dressings were applied. Lap, sponge, and needle counts were correct. There were no complications. The patient was escorted to recovery in stable condition.

_____
Charles Mendesz, MD
Nephrology

CM:cks
D:09/23/----
T:09/25/----

cc: Lloyd Verlin, MD, Pulmonary

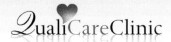

Plastic Surgery

Patient Name: Melinda R. Chadwick   **ID#:** S-84

Date of Operation: 01/05/----   **Age:** 50   **Sex:** F

PREOPERATIVE DIAGNOSIS
Disfiguring scar following abdominoplasty.

POSTOPERATIVE DIAGNOSIS
Disfiguring scar following abdominoplasty.

OPERATION PERFORMED: Abdominal scar revision.

SPECIMENS REMOVED: Abdominal skin and fat.

SURGEON: Danila R. Fry, MD

ASSISTANT: Jimmy Dale Jett, RN

ANESTHETIC: General endotracheal by Dr. Avalon.

DRAINS: 7 mm flat Blake drain x2.

SPONGE COUNT: Correct x2 at end of case.

PROSTHETIC DEVICES: None.

ESTIMATED BLOOD LOSS: Minimal.

INTRAVENOUS FLUIDS: 1400 mL crystalloid.

INDICATIONS: The patient is a 50-year-old female who has a history of gastric bypass with subsequent abdominoplasty. She was unhappy with the midportion of her scar in the lower half of her abdomen. She requested scar revision with reduction of the mons redundancy. The proposed operation along with its associated risks and benefits was discussed with the patient at length, and questions were answered to her satisfaction. She gave informed consent to proceed.

DESCRIPTION OF OPERATION: Patient was marked in the preoperative holding area to determine the amount of skin and fat that could be safely resected in the course of the scar revision. Once this had been accomplished, the patient was taken to the operating room where she was placed on the operating table in supine position. Cardiac monitors were attached, and general endotracheal was induced. Patient's abdomen was prepped and draped in the usual sterile fashion. The proposed incision sites were infiltrated with 0.5% Marcaine mixed 1:1 with 1% lidocaine with 1:100,000 epinephrine. A total of 20 mL was infiltrated into the proposed incision sites.

The inferior incision was incised sharply, and the subcutaneous tissues were divided with the electrocautery down to the anterior abdominal fascia. The overlying skin and fat were elevated from the underlying anterior abdominal fascia to an area just above the proposed superior incision. Once this was fully mobilized, the midline fascia was plicated with a series of interrupted 0 Ethibond buried figure-of-8 sutures. The wound was irrigated copiously with normal saline, and meticulous hemostasis was assured. The skin was then pulled down over the inferior incision to ensure that the previously marked incision site was appropriate. Once it was determined that it was, this was excised sharply and meticulous hemostasis was once again achieved.

The Scarpa fascia was closed with a series of interrupted 3-0 PDS sutures. The 7 mm flat Blake drains were then placed throughout the separate stab incisions in the mons and brought out on either side of the wound bed. They

(Continued)

ID#: S-84   PAGE 2

were secured in place with 3-0 nylon sutures. Dermal margins were closed with interrupted 3-0 Monocryl sutures followed by a running 3-0 Monocryl subcuticular suture. Steri-Strips were applied to the incision. It was dressed with sterile gauze 4 x 8 dressings. The abdominal binder was placed on the patient.

She was awakened from her general endotracheal anesthesia and transferred to the recovery room in good condition. No known complications at the time of this dictation.

_____

Danila R. Fry, MD
Plastic Surgery

DRF:cks
D:01/05/----
T:01/05/----

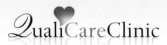

<u>**Ear, Nose, and Throat Surgery**</u>

Patient Name: Joaquin R. Mireles   **ID#:** S-85
Date of Operation: 03/10/----   **Age:** 35   **Sex:** M

PREOPERATIVE DIAGNOSIS
Chronic sinusitis and nasal airway obstruction.

POSTOPERATIVE DIAGNOSIS
Chronic sinusitis and nasal airway obstruction.

OPERATIONS PERFORMED
1. Functional endoscopic sinus surgery (FESS) with balloon sinuplasty with bilateral sphenoidotomies and bilateral frontal sinusotomies.
2. Revision rhinoplasty with left auricular cartilage harvest to include foot plate binding sutures and endonasal alar rim graft.

SPECIMEN REMOVED: None.

SURGEON: Leela Pivari, MD

ASSISTANT: Anna Marie Iaccarino, RN, Scrub Nurse

ANESTHETIC: General endotracheal by Dr. Delaney.

SPONGE COUNT: Verified correct x3 at the end of case.

COMPLICATIONS: None.

ESTIMATED BLOOD LOSS: Minimal.

INDICATIONS: This 35-year-old Hispanic male has a history of chronic sinusitis. He is status post functional endoscopic surgery in the past. He has failed maximal medical therapy. He also complains of nasal airway obstruction. He is status post open septorhinoplasty in the past. He is noted to have collapsed alar rims, and patient is taken to the operating room for surgical correction.

DESCRIPTION OF OPERATION: The patient was taken to the operating room and placed supine on the operating table. After general endotracheal anesthesia was induced, the head of the bed was turned 180 degrees from Anesthesia. The nose was packed with Afrin-soaked pledgets. Attention was first placed on the functional endoscopic sinus surgery.

Using the 0-degree scope, the middle turbinate and root were injected with 1% lidocaine with 1:100,000 epinephrine bilaterally. The sphenoid sinus was addressed first. Sphenoid os was identified, and the introducer was placed from the sinuplasty set. The guide wire was inserted using fluoroscopic guidance. The guide wire was seen inside the sphenoid sinus on the left side. Next the balloon was inserted. The balloon used was a 6 mm balloon. This was confirmed to be in place using fluoroscopic guidance, and the pressure was taken up to 8 atmospheres of pressure, thus dilating the sphenoid os. The exact same procedure was performed on the right side.

Attention was then placed on performing the frontal sinusotomy. The introducer was first placed in the left frontal recess using the guide wire. The guide wire was placed into the left frontal sinus. This was confirmed using fluoroscopic guidance. The 70-degree introducer was used. Next, the balloon was inserted into the frontal recess outflow tract using fluoroscopic guidance. Again, this was inflated up to 8 atmospheres of pressure. The exact same procedure was performed on the right frontal recess. Three separate balloon inflations were made along the frontal sinus outflow tract bilaterally.

With the FESS completed, attention was then placed on performing the revision septorhinoplasty. First the left conchal bowl auricular cartilage was harvested. A postauricular incision was made using a 15 blade. This was carried down to the level of the perichondrium. The conchal bowl cartilage was then harvested using a 15 blade

(Continued)

ID#: S-85

and a Freer elevator. This was resected and passed off the field for the alar rim cartilage graft. The postauricular incision was closed with a deep 5-0 PDS suture and running locking 5-0 chromic suture. A bolster dressing made of dental rolls was placed.

Next, a small pocket was made in the nasal portion of the alar rim area, and the harvested cartilage was placed in order to help reinforce the alar rim and keep it from collapsing. This was done bilaterally. The incision was closed using a 5-0 chromic suture. Next, a footplate binding suture was made x2 in the alar medial crural foot plates. This was performed using interrupted 5-0 clear nylon suture. The incisions that were created were closed using 5-0 chromic suture. Bacitracin was applied to the incisions. No complications in this case. Sponge, needle, and instrument counts were all correct at the end of the case.

The patient was handed over to Anesthesia, where he was extubated and transferred to the PACU in stable condition.

_____

Leela Pivari, MD
Otorhinolaryngology

LP:cks
D:03/10/----
D:03/11/----

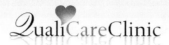

Genitourinary Surgery

Patient Name: Randall Oscar Doubletree   **ID#:** S-86

Date of Operation: 08/25/----   **Age:** 20   **Sex:** M

PREOPERATIVE DIAGNOSIS
Bulbar urethral stricture.

POSTOPERATIVE DIAGNOSIS
Bulbar urethral stricture.

OPERATIONS PERFORMED
1. Cystoscopy.
2. End-to-end anastomotic urethroplasty.

SPECIMEN REMOVED: Approximately 1.5 cm of urethra was excised, which was then passed off the table as specimen.

SURGEON: Charles Mendesz, MD

ASSISTANT: Jason Wagner, PA-C

ANESTHETIC: General endotracheal by Dr. Delaney.

INDICATIONS: The patient is a 20-year-old male who presented to the urology clinic with complaints of left flank pain and decreased force of his urinary stream. He has reported a history of difficult catheter placement as a child and has always had a decreased force of stream, nocturia, and incomplete voiding since then. A flow rate and postvoid residual were performed, revealing a poor maximum flow at 4.9 with an average of 2.3, a total volume of 300, and a postvoid residual of 324. A cystoscopy was performed that revealed a dense 6-French distal bulbar urethral stricture. Retrograde urethrogram was performed, which revealed a 1 cm distal bulbar stricture. The remainder of the distal urethra was normal in caliber. The patient was counseled regarding his options, to include direct visual internal urethrotomy versus end-to-end anastomotic urethroplasty. After discussion of the risks and benefits of each, the patient elected to undergo an end-to-end urethroplasty. The patient was kept on oral Levaquin preoperatively.

DESCRIPTION OF OPERATION: After obtaining informed consent and after correctly identifying the patient in the holding area, he was brought to the operating room and placed on the operating table. After induction of general anesthesia, he was put in high lithotomy position using the Yellofin-like holders. The patient's perineum was shaved, prepped, and draped in the usual sterile fashion, including the genitalia and the lower abdomen. A red rubber 16-French catheter was passed through the urethra and was felt to be at the level of the urethra at the anterior perineum.

A linear incision in the median raphe of the perineum was made. Dissection was then performed sharply down to the level of the bulbous spongiosum muscle. This was divided in the midline. As the spongiosum was identified, the spongiosum was dissected free of the corpora and its other attachments laterally and anteriorly at the level of the stricture. Once adequate urethral immobilization was achieved proximally and distally, a bulldog clamp was placed on the urethra approximately 1 cm distal to the level of the stricture. The urethra was then divided sharply. It was felt to be the distal end of the stricture.

At this point, it was noted that there was a small false passage that had been created by the red rubber catheter in the urethra. The stricture was actually distal to this level. The urethra was spatulated, and the stricture was identified. Approximately 1.5 cm of urethra was excised, which was then passed off the table as specimen.

Cystoscopy was then performed of the distal urethra, revealing no evidence of stricture, disease, or other abnormalities. Cystoscopy was also performed on the proximal urethra and bladder, revealing no proximal stricture or urinary bladder stones. The midline between the corporal bodies was then divided slightly with Bovie

(Continued)

electrocautery to reduce the tension on the urethral anastomosis. The proximal urethra was immobilized such that tensionless anastomosis could be created. The first suture was placed dorsally through both the urethral ends and the tunica of the corpora to secure an anchor at end position. This was performed as a 4-0 PDS. The next 2 dorsal sutures on either side were performed as 5-0 PDS and also were anchored to the tunica. From then on, interrupted 5-0 PDS sutures were used to create the anastomosis. Eventually this was done in 2 layers, first through the mucosa and then through the overlying spongiosum.

There was good hemostasis throughout. The wound was irrigated with antibiotic solution. The bulbous spongiosum muscle was then closed in the midline with a running 3-0 Monocryl. Colles fascia was then closed with a running 3-0 Monocryl. The skin was closed with a running 3-0 Monocryl as well. The patient had his wound cleaned. Bacitracin was applied.

He tolerated the procedure well, was extubated in the operating room, and was transferred to the recovery room in satisfactory condition. No complications were evident at the end of the case.

_____
Charles Mendesz, MD
Urology

CM:cks
D:08/25/----
T:08/25/----

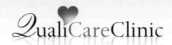

<u>Orthopedic Surgery</u>

Patient Name: Miguel Cantu   **ID#:** S-87
Date of Operation: 06/11/----   **Age:** 31   **Sex:** M

PREOPERATIVE DIAGNOSIS
Anteroposterior III pelvic ring disruption with concomitant right acetabular fracture from multiple trauma.

POSTOPERATIVE DIAGNOSIS
Anteroposterior III pelvic ring disruption with concomitant right acetabular fracture from multiple trauma.

OPERATIONS PERFORMED
1. Closed reduction, internal fixation with iliosacral screws of posterior pelvic ring.
2. Open reduction, internal fixation of anterior pelvic ring.

SPECIMEN REMOVED: None.

SURGEON: Raquel Rodriguez, MD

ASSISTANT: Howard H. Lee, MD

INDICATIONS: Preoperative History: The patient is a 31-year-old Hispanic male who was involved in a motorcycle accident against a minivan 4 days ago. Patient was severely injured with severe head injury, chest injuries, bilateral upper extremity injuries, and severe pelvic ring and right acetabular fractures. Dr. Howard Lee and his orthopedic team treated the patient initially with a pelvic binder and splinting. Patient also has T-11 compression fractures. He presented as a GCS 3. He had active bleeding from the right part of his neck. He was monitored in the ICU. He has severe pulmonary injuries as well. When it was finally deemed safe to bring the patient to the OR, it was still felt that he had to have limited procedures. Specifically, his right lung was a bad lung, and having him left-side down was considered much too dangerous.

DESCRIPTION OF OPERATION: The patient was positioned supine on a regulation table. He had facial injuries that were addressed by ENT, and he first underwent a tracheostomy by them.

The patient was then was prepped and draped in the usual sterile fashion. Preoperative antibiotics were used. We used standard technique with a small posterior approach after marking out the sacrum with a permanent marker and prepping and draping in sterile fashion. Under excellent image control, we carefully placed the guide wire for the 7.3 screw using the screwdriver guide. This was carefully placed into the S1 body. We confirmed it on inlet and outlet views. We then took the lateral view to check that the guide pin was in S1. We found this to be excellent, and we placed the screw after measuring. While doing this, we reduced the sacroiliac joint with a ball spike pusher. Monitoring was done throughout this portion of the procedure.

We then turned our attention to the S2 body. Again, in the same fashion, we carefully placed an S2 screw. We had confirmed this guide wire placement under lateral C-arm prior to this, and we confirmed it again on inlet and outlet views. Once both screws were placed and confirmed, we turned our attention anteriorly. We did a standard Pfannenstiel incision. We carefully elevated some of the rectus off the right anterior ramus and pubic region. The symphysis was completely disrupted. The left side rectus was completely torn off. We reduced this with a pointed reduction forceps, carefully protecting the urinary bladder throughout the procedure with a malleable retractor. We then placed our 4-hole Burgess plate on the reduced hemipelvis and carefully placed a screw of 60 mm anteriorly. We then reduced the pelvic ring completely and placed a screw on the left side, again 60 mm, a fully threaded 6.5 cancellous screw. When we were satisfied with this reduction, we placed the 2 lateral screws in slightly convergent fashion—a 50 on the right and a 60 on the left. All screws were 6.5 fully threaded cancellous screws. They had excellent purchase. We confirmed under C-arm that they were all well placed. Overall reduction of the pelvis was very good.

We elected at this time to not address his anterior column fractures. His acetabulum will be addressed at such time as the patient is stable and able to tolerate left-side-down positioning. He was monitored before and after, and we

(Continued)

ID#: S-87   PAGE 2

confirmed afterward that there were no EMG changes with stimulation of the screws and guide pins. We therefore thoroughly irrigated all the wounds. They were closed in standard fashion using 0 Vicryl for the deep, 2-0 for the more superficial, and staples for the skin. There were no complications during the procedure. The estimated blood loss was 250 mL. A good amount of that was old hematoma that came out at the Pfannenstiel incision.

POSTOPERATIVE PLAN
Give perioperative antibiotics. The ICU service is very capably managing him. He can be mobilized to a chair. We will keep traction on the right. He will be placed in a distal femoral traction pin, changing out from his tibial pin. This is for his acetabular fracture. He can have an upright chest as long as his spine is cleared by the trauma service.

_____
Raquel Rodriguez, MD
Orthopedic Surgery

RR:cks
D:06/11/----
T:06/12/----

cc: Leah Pittfield, MD, Otorhinolaryngology
     Lloyd Verlin, MD, Pulmonology
     Mack Stolga, MD, Trauma Surgery

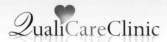

Obstetrics/Gynecology Surgery

Patient Name: Rebekah Renee Baxter   **ID#:** S-88

Date of Operation: 03/02/----   **Age:** 22   **Sex:** F

PREOPERATIVE DIAGNOSIS
Secondary infertility, status post bilateral tubal ligations.

POSTOPERATIVE DIAGNOSIS
Secondary infertility, status post bilateral tubal ligations.

OPERATIONS PERFORMED
1. Diagnostic laparoscopy.
2. Minilaparotomy.
3. Bilateral tubal anastomoses.

SPECIMEN REMOVED: None.

SURGEON: Tillman Risha, MD

ASSISTANT: Rosemary Bumbak, MD

ANESTHETIC: General endotracheal by Dr. Delaney.

DRAINS: Foley to gravity.

SPONGE COUNT: Verified correct x2 at the end of case.

INTRAVENOUS FLUIDS: 1400 mL of lactated Ringer's.

URINE OUTPUT: 175 mL clear urine at end of procedure.

ESTIMATED BLOOD LOSS: 50 mL.

COMPLICATIONS: None.

FINDINGS: Adequate tubal segments. Left proximal segment was 2 cm and distal was 3 cm. Right proximal segment was 2 cm and distal was 3 cm. Bilateral spill and fill, status post anastomoses. Condition was stable.

DESCRIPTION OF OPERATION: Patient was taken to the operating room where general endotracheal was found to be adequate. She was prepped and draped in the usual sterile fashion in the dorsal lithotomy position. A Foley was then placed into her bladder. A speculum was placed into the vagina. Cervix was visualized and grasped with a tenaculum, and a uterine manipulator was then placed. The tenaculum and the speculum were then removed.

Attention was then turned to the laparoscopy portion of the case. A 1 cm incision was made in the umbilicus, and the Hasson trocar was placed under direct visualization. It was confirmed to be in the abdomen, and the abdomen was insufflated. Thorough inspection of the abdominal cavity revealed a normal-appearing uterus with adequate segments for tubal reanastomosis. The decision was made to convert to a minilaparotomy to proceed. The camera was removed, and the trocar was subsequently removed.

An approximately 8 cm laparotomy incision was made in the skin through her old cesarean section scar and carried through to underlying layer of the fascia with the Bovie. The fascia was incised in the midline, and the incision was extended laterally with the Mayo scissors. The superior aspect of the fascial incision was grasped with Kocher clamps, tented up, and the underlying layer of the rectus muscle was dissected off bluntly. Attention was then turned to the inferior aspect of the incision, which was dissected off in a similar fashion. The rectus muscles were separated in the midline. Peritoneum was identified and entered bluntly. The uterus was then identified and exteriorized. The bilateral adnexa were then exteriorized. Approximately 2 cm of tube was noted proximally on

(Continued)

ID#: S-88   PAGE 2

each side, and about 3 cm of tube was noted distally on each side. The decision was made to proceed with bilateral tubal anastomoses.

Attention was turned to the left tube. The distal portion of the tube was grasped with an Allis clamp, elevated, and undermined with a combination of sharp and cautery dissection. Once this was performed, a 2.5 Pedicath was placed through the distal end of the tube and advanced toward where the original ligation was. The ligated portion of the tube was grasped with the pickups, and the lumen was then exteriorized with sharp dissection.

Attention was then turned to the proximal tube, which was undermined in a similar fashion with sharp and Bovie cautery. The tip of the tube was then grasped, and the lumen was exteriorized with sharp dissection. The mesosalpinx at the base of the bilateral tubes was then grasped and reapproximated with a 6-0 Vicryl interrupted stitch. The tube was then reapproximated with four 7-0 Vicryl sutures in the 3-, 6-, 9-, and 12-o'clock positions. Indigo carmine was then flushed through the tube from the uterus with spill noted at the distal portion of the tube. The serosa was then closed with a 6-0 Vicryl in a running fashion. Again the indigo carmine was flushed through the tube and noted to have spill at the fimbria.

Attention was then turned to the right side, which was reapproximated. Indigo carmine was then flushed through the uterine cavity once again, and spill was seen at the right fimbria. The tubes were then cleared of all indigo carmine, and indigo carmine was once again flushed through the uterus. Good fill was noted in both tubes, and good spill was noted from both fimbriae. The uterus was then returned to the abdomen. The peritoneum was closed with 2-0 Vicryl in a running fashion. The fascia was closed with 0 Vicryl in a running fashion. The subcutaneous tissue was then irrigated, and all bleeding was stopped with Bovie cautery until excellent hemostasis was noted. The skin was closed with 3-0 Monocryl in a running fashion. The umbilical port site was closed with Dermabond.

Patient tolerated the procedure well. Sponge, lap, and needle counts were correct x2. Patient was transferred to the PACU in stable condition.

_____
Tillman Risha, MD
Obstetrics/Gynecology

TR:cks
D:03/02/----
T:03/02/----

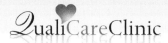

Plastic Surgery

Patient Name: Burgess T. Kline   **ID#:** S-89

Date of Operation: 01/05/----   **Age:** 60   **Sex:** M

PREOPERATIVE DIAGNOSIS
Brow ptosis and dermatochalasis.

POSTOPERATIVE DIAGNOSIS
Brow ptosis and dermatochalasis.

OPERATIONS PERFORMED
1. Bilateral upper lid blepharoplasty.
2. Bilateral direct brow lift.

SPECIMEN REMOVED: Skin of forehead.

SURGEON: Danila R. Fry, MD

ASSISTANT: Jason Wagner, PA

ANESTHETIC: Local monitored anesthesia care by Dr. Avalon.

ESTIMATED BLOOD LOSS: Minimal.

INDICATIONS: Patient has had problems with lateral gaze with the extensive lateral hooding that he has due to his dermatochalasis and brow ptosis. He presents for the above procedures.

DESCRIPTION OF OPERATION: The patient was brought into the operating room and placed on the operating table in supine position. He was prepped and draped in the usual sterile fashion. Then 2% lidocaine with 1:100,000 epinephrine was injected into bilateral upper brows and the bilateral upper lids. Incisions were planned. The upper blepharoplasty incision at the inferior extent was planned at the lid crease. An appropriate amount of skin was approximated so that the patient would have a slight lagophthalmos at the conclusion of the procedure.

The direct brow incisions were placed approximately 1 cm superior to the eyebrow in an elliptical fashion. The skin of the forehead was incised, and the portion of skin was removed. It was dissected down to the subcutaneous fat level. Some undermining was completed at the inferior extent of the incision. The wound was then closed in layers with 4-0 Monocryl in the deep layer and 5-0 nylon in the superficial layer. The upper blepharoplasty incision was made using a #15 blade. Incision was carried down to and including a portion of the orbicularis oculi muscle. Portions of the orbital septum were visible. The wound was then closed with a running 5-0 nylon to approximately the lateral limbus, at which point several vertical mattress sutures were placed and a couple of simple interrupted, again with a black nylon.

A similar procedure was performed on the contralateral side. At the conclusion of the procedure, the patient had a slight lagophthalmos of approximately 1 mm to 2 mm bilaterally. His brows were placed slightly above the supraorbital rim—therefore an appropriate position. The patient was then recovered from the procedure, and he will return in 1 week for suture removal.

_____
Danila R. Fry, MD
Plastic Surgery

DRF:cks
D:01/05/----
T:01/07/----

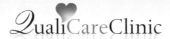

<u>**Genitourinary Surgery**</u>

Patient Name: Troy Gibbons   **ID#:** S-90

Date of Operation: 09/02/----   **Age:** 74   **Sex:** M

PREOPERATIVE DIAGNOSIS
Prostate cancer.

POSTOPERATIVE DIAGNOSIS
Prostate cancer.

OPERATION PERFORMED: Radical retropubic prostatectomy.

SPECIMEN REMOVED: Prostate.

SURGEON: Charles Mendesz, MD

ASSISTANTS: Jason Wagner, PA-C, and Jimmy Dale Jett, RN

ANESTHETIC: General endotracheal by Dr. Avalon.

FLUIDS: 4500 mL crystalloid fluid, 500 mL Hespan, and 1 unit packed red blood cells.

ESTIMATED BLOOD LOSS: 1200 mL.

COMPLICATIONS: None.

INDICATIONS: The patient is a 74-year-old male with significant urinary outlet obstructive symptoms, high postvoid residual, low flow, and an elevated PSA of 5.8. Patient underwent transrectal ultrasound and biopsy and was found to have adenocarcinoma of the prostate, Gleason's 3+3, on one biopsy core from the right base. After careful discussion of his options, including transurethral resection of the prostate for his outlet obstruction, radiation therapy, and brachytherapy, patient wanted to have radical retropubic prostatectomy. Patient therefore presented on this date for radical retropubic prostatectomy.

DESCRIPTION OF OPERATION: After the patient was correctly identified and informed consent obtained, he was taken to the operating room where he was given a general endotracheal tube anesthetic. An orogastric tube was placed. The patient was then prepped and draped in the usual sterile fashion. Foley catheter was placed in the bladder, 16-French in size. A low midline incision was made to approximately three-quarters of the way to the umbilicus. This was carried down through the fat and the abdominal fascia, and the rectus muscles were split in the midline. Space of Retzius was identified. Immediately we encountered dense adhesions from his prior left lower quadrant surgery. These dense adhesions were difficult to dissect. A small cystotomy was made in as much as the bladder had been tented up into the scarred area on the left side. The cystotomy site was closed using chromic suture in 2 layers.

The endopelvic fascia was finally identified on the left side. It was easily identified on the right side. It was cleaned of its fat, and the pelvic fascia was then sharply incised and followed posteriorly into the hypogastric vessels and anteriorly to the puboprostatic ligaments. Bunching sutures with 0 chromic suture material were placed, bringing the dorsal vein complex to the middle, occluding it, and also expressing Denonvilliers fascia, the prostate, and the lateral sides. After several bunching sutures were used, the dorsal vein complex was ligated using an 0 Vicryl suture. It was then divided. There was minimal bleeding, which was easily controlled with a second 9-0 Vicryl suture on a CTX needle. The urethra was then partially transected. While the urethra was transected, 4-0 Monocryl sutures were placed through the urethra. The catheter was then pulled up through the wound, the posterior aspect of the urethra dissected, and 2 additional sutures were placed in the posterior urethra.

The urethra was then completely transected, and using sharp dissection, the rectourethralis muscle was divided from Denonvilliers fascia, freeing the rectum from the prostate. Lateral pedicles were then carefully dissected out using right-angle clamps and right-angle clips. A nerve-sparing procedure was performed on both sides.

(Continued)

Once the nerve-sparing procedure had been performed and once the lateral pedicles had been carefully dissected and secured with clips, Denonvilliers fascia was incised, and seminal vesicles and ampulla of vas deferens were dissected in the usual fashion. There were marked scar tissue and adhesions in this area; nevertheless, the seminal vesicles and ampulla of vas were dissected.

This allowed us to see the posterior aspect of the bladder neck. Patient had a very large prostate with a moderate-sized median lobe, which was identified on palpation. Bladder neck was widely excised and left at the edge of the prostate. Next the mucosa of the bladder was carefully everted, and a tennis racquet closure was used. Ureteral orifices on the right and left sides were identified after the patient had been given indigo carmine. These were found to be away from the edge of the resection. Using a tennis racquet closure with 4-0 and 2-0 chromic sutures, the bladder neck was refashioned to approximately 30-French.

Next the anastomosis was performed over an 18-French Foley catheter with 10 mL left in the balloon. At the end of the case the Foley catheter irrigated easily. Before completing the anastomosis, the patient did have a small amount of bleeding from the fossa harboring the seminal vessel and ampulla dissection; 10 mL of FloSeal was inserted into this area to effect hemostasis.

The fascia was closed using double-stranded 0 PDS suture. A 7 mm Jackson-Pratt drain had been placed over the area of the anastomosis and secured to the skin on the right side using a 2-0 nylon suture. Subcuticular closure was performed using 4-0 Monocryl. The wound was sealed with Dermabond adhesive. The patient was then awakened, extubated, and transported to the recovery room awake and in stable condition. There were no complications. The patient tolerated the procedure well.

_____

Charles Mendesz, MD
Urology

CM:cks
D:09/02/----
T:09/03/----

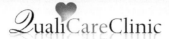

Ear, Nose, and Throat Surgery

Patient Name: Roberta L. Grissom   **ID#:** S-91

Date of Operation: 12/21/----   **Age:** 50   **Sex:** F

PREOPERATIVE DIAGNOSIS
Oral lesions and epiglottic mass.

POSTOPERATIVE DIAGNOSIS
Oral lesions and epiglottic mass.

OPERATIONS PERFORMED
1. Direct laryngoscopy with biopsy.
2. Excisional biopsy of chest lesions.

SPECIMENS REMOVED: Biopsies of the arytenoid, biopsies of the tongue, and biopsies of the skin on the anterior mid aspect of the chest.

SURGEON: Leela Pivari, MD

ASSISTANT: Jimmy Dale Jett, RN, Circulating Nurse

ANESTHETIC: General endotracheal by Dr. Delaney.

DRAINS: None.

SPONGE COUNT: Correct at the end of the case.

ESTIMATED BLOOD LOSS: Minimal.

INTRAOPERATIVE FLUIDS: See anesthesia record.

COMPLICATIONS: None.

INDICATIONS: The patient is a 50-year-old female with multiple medical problems who presented to the Hillcrest Medical Center ED with complaints of shortness of breath and worsening dysphagia over the past several days. On nasopharyngoscopy, the patient was noted to have what appeared to be an exophytic mass on the aryepiglottic fold extending up onto the epiglottis. The patient was admitted to the hospital on the evening of her evaluation with plans made to go to the operating room to obtain biopsy of the above-mentioned tissue.

DESCRIPTION OF OPERATION: The patient was brought to the operating room and placed supine on the operating table. At this point a final time-out and site verification were accomplished. The patient had awake fiberoptic intubation subsequently accomplished with some difficulty, given the patient's body habitus. The patient was successfully intubated, however, without significant desaturation or airway complication. Once the patient had been intubated, direct laryngoscopy was carried out utilizing a Dedo operating laryngoscope. The patient's oral cavity was inspected. A lesion was noted to be present on the base of the tongue, and a biopsy of this was subsequently taken. As the Dedo laryngoscope was further advanced, the soft palate, uvula, and posterior oropharynx were inspected, as were both tonsils. The base of tongue was systematically inspected, as were the valleculae, epiglottis, piriform sinuses bilaterally, aryepiglottic folds, posterior hypopharyngeal area, arytenoids, both true and false vocal cords, ventricles, and the subglottis.

Of note, the patient had an ill-defined, exophytic-appearing mass along the aryepiglottic fold. Several biopsies of this area were obtained. The patient was also noted to have several nodular-appearing growths on the anterior mid aspect of her thorax. These were also biopsied using a punch biopsy. At the end of the case, the rather small wounds were closed with several interrupted sutures of 4-0 nylon.

(Continued)

ID#: S-91   PAGE 2

At this time, the patient was turned back over to the anesthesia service. It was felt that the patient had a stable airway and was therefore extubated in the operating room and transferred back to the intensive care unit for continued close monitoring of her status and condition.

_____
Leela Pivari, MD
Otorhinolaryngology

LP:cks
D:12/21/----
T:12/23/----

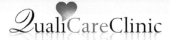

Orthopedic Surgery

Patient Name: Artie B. Copeland   **ID#:** S-92

Date of Operation: 02/17/----   **Age:** 59   **Sex:** M

PREOPERATIVE DIAGNOSIS
Chronic osteomyelitis of the left tibia.

POSTOPERATIVE DIAGNOSIS
Chronic osteomyelitis of the left tibia.

OPERATION PERFORMED: Irrigation and debridement of his left tibia with placement of antibiotic beads and wound V.A.C.

SPECIMEN REMOVED: The skin was sent for permanent section.

SURGEON: Raquel Rodriguez, MD

ASSISTANT: Jason Wagner, PA

ANESTHETIC: General endotracheal anesthesia by Dr. Delaney.

INTRAVENOUS FLUIDS: 2200 mL.

ESTIMATED BLOOD LOSS: 50 mL.

URINE OUTPUT: Not recorded.

TOURNIQUET TIME: 60 minutes at 300 mmHg.

BRIEF HISTORY: Artie is a 59-year-old male who sustained an open left tibial fracture 7 years ago. It was treated nonoperatively. He developed draining from his wound several months ago, and after initial conservative treatment, the decision was made to proceed with irrigation and debridement, curettage of the bone, to be followed by a gastrocnemius flap and split-thickness skin graft. The risks, benefits, alternatives, and indications were discussed with the patient, including the risks of pain, bleeding, infection, damage to adjacent structures, fracture, need for further surgery, loss of limb or life; and he agreed to proceed with the surgery.

DESCRIPTION OF OPERATION: The patient was identified in the holding area by the operating team. The correct extremity was marked. Consent was again reviewed with the patient, and he had no further questions. He was then turned over to Anesthesia and taken back to the operating room where he was placed supine on the operating table and underwent induction of general anesthesia and intubation without difficulty. He was given no antibiotics prior to the start of the procedure. The tourniquet was placed on the left lower extremity. Using the C-arm we identified the areas of bone that corresponded to his draining sinus tracts. The leg was exsanguinated by elevation, and the tourniquet was inflated. We then proceeded to ellipse the area of bad skin containing the sinus tracts in a large, oval fashion. This was carried down directly onto the face of the tibia and removed. The skin was sent to pathology for permanent section.

The areas of bone where the sinus tracts occurred were identified. These were opened using a curette and bur. The bone was curetted out thoroughly, and the edges of the bone were burred down. This was irrigated thoroughly with approximately 9 L of normal saline. Once we felt it was clean and all the infected, necrotic tissue had been debrided, we then placed a total of 14 antibiotic beads connected onto an Ethibond suture down into the 2 holes. The beads consisted of normal bone cement mixed with tobramycin. The 2 ends of the Ethibond suture were tied over to ensure the beads stayed in place.

The proximal and distal ends of the incision were closed as far as possible with 2-0 nylon. A wound V.A.C. was placed and sealed without difficulty. Patient was awakened by Anesthesia without difficulty and transferred to the PACU for recovery.

(Continued)

ID#: S-92   PAGE 2

PLAN

The plan will be for him to be weightbearing as tolerated. We will keep the patient on Lovenox for DVT prophylaxis, and we will plan on taking him back in approximately 3 to 5 days for repeat irrigation and debridement and replacement of the antibiotic beads and wound V.A.C. We will follow his cultures, consult Infectious Disease, and place the patient on appropriate antibiotics once his cultures have grown out bacteria. We will plan on covering the defect with the gastroc flap and skin grafting with the help of the hand team 1 week from this operative date if the cultures from his repeat I&D are negative.

_____

Raquel Rodriguez, MD
Orthopedic Surgery

RR:cks
D:02/17/----
T:02/17/----

c: Beth Brian, MD, Infectious Disease

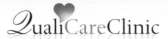

QualiCareClinic

Obstetrics/Gynecology Surgery

Patient Name: Cassandra Nolasco   **ID#:** S-93

Date of Operation: 06/09/----   **Age:** 35   **Sex:** F

PREOPERATIVE DIAGNOSIS
Undesired fertility. Desires permanent sterilization.

POSTOPERATIVE DIAGNOSIS
Undesired fertility. Desires permanent sterilization.

OPERATIONS PERFORMED
1. Diagnostic hysteroscopy.
2. Laparoscopic tubal ligation with bipolar cautery.

SPECIMENS REMOVED: Fallopian tubal segments.

SURGEON: Tillman Risha, MD

ASSISTANT: Anna Marie Iaccarino, RN, Scrub Nurse

ANESTHETIC: General endotracheal by Dr. Avalon. Also given was 9 mL of 1% lidocaine for a paracervical block and 8 mL 0.5% Marcaine for a local at abdominal incision sites.

DRAINS: Foley catheter removed at end of case.

INTRAVENOUS FLUIDS: 1200 mL of lactated Ringer's.

URINE OUTPUT: 600 mL clear at end of case.

ESTIMATED BLOOD LOSS: 10 mL.

COMPLICATIONS: None.

FINDINGS: Scarred endometrial cavity, status post ablation. Unable to see ostia. Normal tubes, ovaries, and uterus.

DESCRIPTION OF OPERATION: Patient was taken to the operating room where IV and local anesthesia were found to be adequate. She was prepped and draped in the usual sterile fashion in the low lithotomy position. A speculum was placed, and the os was grasped with a tenaculum. Local anesthesia was injected at both 4 and 7 o'clock to achieve an excellent paracervical block. The size 12 dilator was advanced without difficulty.

The 5 mm operative hysteroscope was placed into the internal os and advanced until what was thought to be a single ostium was observed. At this point, the Essure device was introduced through the operative port and deployed into what was thought to be the ostium. Approximately 13 coils were noted outside of the area in which it was deployed. The hysteroscope was removed, and the coil came back with the hysteroscope. The coil was grasped with the ring forceps and removed. The hysteroscope was reintroduced, and it was noted that this was actually the internal os that was very stenotic and not one of the ostia. Therefore, this stenotic internal os was gently dilated up, and the hysteroscope was again placed into the endometrial cavity at this time, which was noted to be extremely scarred from the previous NovaSure ablation that the patient had had performed several years ago. Neither ostium was able to be clearly identified secondary to the multiple synechiae present. The Essure procedure was aborted in favor of laparoscopic tubal ligation.

The patient at this time was put under general anesthesia. This anesthesia was found to be adequate. Patient was already prepped, so we moved on with the laparoscopic portion of the case. A small infraumbilical incision was made, and the 5 mm port was introduced into the abdominal cavity under direct visualization. An initial survey of the abdomen showed no injury where the port was placed. The abdomen was filled with gas, and a second port was placed suprapubically, 5 mm also, under direct visualization with the camera. After this a blunt probe was

(Continued)

ID#: S-93   PAGE 2

passed through the operative port, and a thorough abdominal survey showed no abnormalities. Normal uterus, ovaries, and tubes. Normal liver and normal appendix. The bipolar cautery was then introduced into the operative port, and the patient's right fallopian tube was grasped and burned in 3 different places.

Attention was then turned to her left tube, which was grasped in a similar fashion with the bipolar cautery and cauterized in 3 different places. Another survey of the abdomen showed no abnormalities and excellent cautery of bilateral tubes. The operative port was removed. Good hemostasis was noted at the area, and the gas was deflated from the abdomen. Camera port was removed.

Both 5 mm incisions were closed with 4-0 Monocryl and covered with an OpSite. Excellent hemostasis was noted. The patient was then taken to the recovery room in stable condition.

_____

Tillman Risha, MD
Obstetrics/Gynecology

TR:cks
D:06/10/----
T:06/11/----

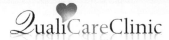

Nephrology Surgery

Patient Name: Amber K. Welch   **ID#:** S-94

Date of Operation: 09/16/----   **Age:** 36   **Sex:** F

PREOPERATIVE DIAGNOSIS
Right ureteropelvic junction obstruction with renal stones.

POSTOPERATIVE DIAGNOSIS
Right ureteropelvic junction obstruction with renal stones.

OPERATIONS PERFORMED
1. Right laparoscopic dismembered pyeloplasty.
2. Nephroscopic extraction of kidney stones.
3. Placement of ureteral stent.

SPECIMENS REMOVED: Kidney stones.

SURGEON: Charles Mendesz, MD

ASSISTANT: Trevor Jordan, MD

ANESTHETIC: General endotracheal tube by Dr. Delaney.

DESCRIPTION OF OPERATION: After the patient was correctly identified and informed consent was obtained, she was taken to the operating room where she was given a general endotracheal tube anesthetic. Foley catheter was placed in the urinary bladder, and patient was placed in a right modified lateral position. All pressure points were carefully checked and padded. Next she had a Veress needle inserted at the umbilicus, and its correct position was determined by drip test. Once the needle was found to be in the correct position, the abdomen was insufflated to 20 mmHg pressure. The abdomen was entered under directed vision using a Visiport device. There was no evidence of adhesions and no intra-abdominal pathology.

A 10 mm trocar was placed midway between the umbilicus and the xiphoid process and a 5 mm trocar placed in line with the umbilicus lateral to the rectus muscle. Using bipolar cautery, the colon was incised at the white line of Toldt and reflected medially. The ureter was identified along with a large gonadal vessel, which was somewhat adherent to the ureter. The gonadal vessel was divided to prevent shearing at the entry of the vena cava. The ureter was then completely mobilized, and there was no evidence of a lower pole crossing vessel. It appeared to be an intrinsic defect of the ureter with somewhat of a high insertion.

The ureter was then transected at the level of the ureteropelvic junction. The obstructing segment was removed. The ureter was spatulated for 1.5 cm. Then a reduction pyeloplasty was performed. Using the apex of the most dependent portion of the pelvis and the apex of the spatulated incision, the ureter was reapproximated back to the renal pelvis. There was no significant tension whatsoever to return the ureter back to the renal pelvis. A urologic wire was placed through a trocar and down the ureter into the bladder, over which a 28 cm 7-French, double-J stent was passed. Then the wire was removed. The upper portion of the stent was placed in the upper pole of the kidney.

A flexible cystoscope was then inserted through the open renal pelvis. After vigorous irrigation, the kidney stones, which had previously been identified, were flushed out. These were removed and sent for permanent evaluation. They appeared to be calcium oxalate stones. Using the flexible cystoscope, each calyx was inspected, and we were unable to find other stones. Using 4-0 PDS suture in a running fashion, the anterior portion of the anastomosis was performed. Then the posterior portion of the anastomosis was performed. This led to some of the renal pelvis that needed to be closed. This was closed using a running 4-0 PDS suture.

(Continued)

Next the patient had 5 mL of Hemaseel placed over the area of the repair. A 4 mm Jackson-Pratt drain was placed through a separate stab incision in the retroperitoneum and placed overlying the area of the anastomosis. The colon was then reflected back to its usual position and tacked using a hernia tacker. Patient was awakened, extubated, and transported to the recovery room awake and in stable condition. There were no complications. The patient tolerated the procedure well. There was minimal blood loss.

_____

Charles Mendesz, MD
Nephrology

CM:cks
D:09/16/----
T:09/17/----

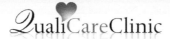

Orthopedic Surgery

Patient Name: Stefanie Woolsey   **ID#:** S-95

Date of Operation: 03/23/----   **Age:** 21   **Sex:** F

PREOPERATIVE DIAGNOSIS
Fracture-dislocation at T4-5 with incomplete spinal cord injury at the T5 level.

POSTOPERATIVE DIAGNOSIS
Fracture-dislocation at T4-5 with incomplete spinal cord injury at the T5 level.

OPERATIONS PERFORMED
1. T1 to T8 posterior spinal fusion with instrumentation.
2. Left iliac crest bone graft.
3. Decompression, left T4-T5 level with hemilaminoforaminotomy.
4. Application of Grafton putty (30 mL) allograft DBM.
5. T4-5 fracture-dislocation reduction.

SPECIMEN REMOVED: None.

SURGEON: Gilbert M. Fields, MD

ASSISTANT: Carol Dodds, MD

ANESTHETIC: General anesthesia by Dr. Delaney.

DRAINS: 7 mm JP drain.

PROSTHETIC DEVICES: Instrumentation: Stryker Xia 4.5 mm screws with 6.0 mm rod and Crosslinks.

COMPLICATIONS: None.

ESTIMATED BLOOD LOSS: 1 liter.

FLUIDS: Two units PRBCs given and 100 mL Cell Saver blood returned to the patient.

BRIEF HISTORY: Stefanie is a 21-year-old female who was involved in an MVA as the restrained passenger in a severe MVA with rollover. She had prolonged extrication. She presented to the Hillcrest Medical Center ED and was intubated. On exam when she was less sedated, and a further, more detailed exam when she was extubated, showed her to have a T5-level incomplete spinal cord injury. She has demonstrated no motor strength to the left lower extremity and has demonstrated 3/5 to 4/5 strength in the right lower extremity with abnormal sensation from T5 distally.

Due to the unstable nature of her fracture as well as the fact that she has a sternal fracture at the same level, it was elected to perform posterior spinal fusion for stabilization. The goal of this surgery is to stabilize her spine to allow her to be more mobile. We also feel that the overall spinal canal diameter is sufficient except for the superior facet of T5, which was displaced in the canal on the left side. Therefore, we decided to proceed with the above-described procedure.

I have discussed at length with the parents on multiple different occasions the significance and seriousness of the patient's injuries. We explained the potential for this to worsen, the potential for paralysis in the perioperative period. Appropriate consents have been obtained. Family has voiced understanding, and all questions have been answered at length.

DESCRIPTION OF OPERATION: Patient was brought to the operating room. She has been managed on spine precautions. She was transferred supine onto the Jackson table while awake. Again, she was able to demonstrate the same motor exam as noted above with movement of right lower extremity. We then proceeded with intubation. This went without difficulty. We then connected the patient to neuromonitoring, including transcranial motor

(Continued)

evoked potentials, as well as SSEP. At this time, they were able to obtain some baseline signal of SSEP but were unable to obtain motor signals for either lower extremity. We then decided to perform a wake-up test, even though at this time we had done no manipulation other than to put the patient to sleep. During the wake-up test the patient was cooperative in the sense that she would squeeze our fingers, give us a "thumbs-up," and blink her eyes upon command. But she demonstrated no motor function of either lower extremity. We then decided to proceed with the operation. Again, we encouraged Anesthesia to keep the patient's mean arterial pressure high so that we would not cause any vascular-related injuries to the cord. This had been discussed with them prior to the start of the case as well. At this time, we flipped the patient into the prone position using the Jackson table. Her SSEP remained constant during positioning. We then proceeded to prep and drape in the usual sterile fashion.

At that time a standard midline incision was carried out, centered over the T4 level. This was carried down through the subcutaneous tissues, and the fascia was identified. Subperiosteal dissection was carried out from T1 down to T8. The fracture site was easily defined by the large gap at the T4-5 level in the spinous processes as well as the malrotation of the upper thoracic relative to the lower thoracic regions. We proceeded with decompression of the superior facet on the left at T5. This was done through a hemilaminotomy at the T4-5 level. There was an enlarged, displaced superior fragment within the canal, which was removed. There was no evidence for dural leaks, but again, there was significant ecchymoses and contusion-type appearance to the tissue surrounding the dura.

We obtained bone graft through a separate fascial incision over the left posterior superior iliac spine. This was done as well through a separate skin incision. The incision was carried down to the fascia, and subperiosteal dissection was carried out over the posterior superior iliac spine. Four strips of the outer table were taken with an osteotome. The inner cancellous portion was removed and saved for future bone graft. The wound was copiously irrigated. Hemostasis was obtained with Surgiflo and bone wax as well as placement of a Gelfoam sponge soaked in thrombin along the crest. The wound was then closed watertight with No. 1 Vicryl in a running fashion followed by 2-0 Vicryl for the subcutaneous tissue and Monocryl for the skin.

Attention was then turned back to our main procedure. We proceeded with pedicle screw placement from T1 to T8 on the right and with T1 to T8 on the left with the exception of T4, which had a significant fracture not allowing placement of a screw, which we had determined preoperatively. All screws were placed without significant difficulty. We then stimulated the screws from T5 to T8 bilaterally with above 19 measurements in all screws. Again, instrumentation was Stryker Xia 4.5 mm screws. At this time we decorticated the facet joints bilaterally. The transverse processes were all decorticated. The dorsal surfaces were all decorticated. The iliac crest bone graft was packed within the facet joints, and our rods were contoured. We placed rods on both sides, providing gentle compression across the T3-4, T4-5, and T5-6 levels to help reduce some of the kyphotic deformity. We also compressed more on the left side than the right to, again, help reduce the fracture out of the translated position. Intraoperative x-rays confirmed excellent placement of our screws and good reduction after placement of our rods.

The wound was irrigated, and then 30 mL of Grafton putty cancellous mix was added to the dorsal and lateral fusion surfaces. Crosslinks were used for added stability. A 7 mm JP drain was placed, and the wound was closed watertight with No. 1 Vicryl for the fascia, 2-0 Vicryl for the subcutaneous tissues, and 3-0 nylon for the skin in an interrupted fashion.

Sterile dressings were applied. The patient was then awakened and returned to the supine position. Upon awakening, the patient was able to follow commands and demonstrate dorsiflexion and plantar flexion of the foot as well as flexion and extension of the toes on the right. Again, no motion was noted on the left. Neuromonitoring had reported a slight improvement of the SSEP signals during the case, moreso on the right than the left. Again, they were unable to obtain motor signals throughout the entire case.

The patient was then taken to the intensive care unit, intubated, but in a very stable condition. She required 2 units of PRBCs during the case and received 100 mL of Cell Saver.

DISPOSITION: We will plan at this time for intensive care unit observation for 24 hours. Then we will send patient to the floor where we will continue mobilization. She has been fitted for a cervicothoracic lumbosacral

(Continued)

ID#: S-95   PAGE 3

orthosis to be worn when she is up out of bed for at least the next 6 weeks to 3 months. This is just for additional support in light of the fact that she does have a sternal fracture as well. Again, we will begin mobilization to limit other postoperative complications. After her acute hospitalization, she will be transferred to Miami South Rehabilitation Center for intensive inpatient rehabilitation services.

_____

Gilbert M. Fields, MD
Orthopedic Surgery

GMF:cks
D:03/23/----
T:03/24/----

c: John G. Garcia, MD, Neurology
    Miami South Rehabilitation Center

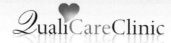

Ear, Nose, and Throat Surgery

Patient Name: Daniel T. Clark   **ID#:** S-96

Date of Operation: 07/31/----   **Age:** 2   **Sex:** M

PREOPERATIVE DIAGNOSES
Periodic fever, aphthous stomatitis, pharyngitis, and cervical adenitis.

POSTOPERATIVE DIAGNOSES
1. Periodic fever, aphthous stomatitis, pharyngitis, and cervical adenitis.
2. Patient had 2+ bilateral tonsils and approximately 50% obstructive adenoid tissue.

OPERATION PERFORMED: Bilateral tonsillectomies and adenoidectomies.

SPECIMENS REMOVED: Bilateral tonsils and adenoids.

SURGEON: Leela Pivari, MD

ASSISTANT: Jimmy Dale Jett, RN, Circulating Nurse

ANESTHETIC: General endotracheal by Dr. Delaney.

DRAINS: None.

SPONGE COUNT: Verified correct x2 at the end of case.

ESTIMATED BLOOD LOSS: Minimal.

INTRAOPERATIVE FLUIDS: See anesthesia record.

COMPLICATIONS: None.

DESCRIPTION OF OPERATION: Patient was brought to the operating room and placed supine on the operating table. A final time-out was accomplished, including surgical site verification. General endotracheal anesthesia was subsequently induced without difficulty. At this time, the operating room table was rotated 90 degrees from the anesthesia service. Shoulder roll was placed followed by the Crowe-Davis mouth gag, and the patient was subsequently suspended from the Mayo stand.

The oropharynx was inspected, palpated, and the patient was noted to have 2+ bilateral tonsils. There was a normal-appearing uvula and soft palate. No submucosal step-offs or lateral pulsations were identified. At this time, a red rubber catheter was placed through the left naris and used to secure the soft palate in standard fashion. Once this was accomplished, the Coblator on settings of 7 and 4 was used to remove the left tonsil from the tonsillar fossa in standard fashion. Once this had been accomplished, attention was turned to the right tonsil. In a similar fashion, the right tonsil was removed from the tonsillar fossa utilizing the Coblator.

At this time, attention was turned to the patient's adenoid pad, and a laryngeal mirror was used to inspect the nasopharynx. Patient was noted to have approximately 50% obstructive adenoid tissue. This tissue was subsequently ablated away using the Coblator on settings of 9 and 4. At this time the patient was taken off suspension, and the mouth gag was closed for approximately 1 minute. The patient was subsequently resuspended with no areas of brisk hemorrhage noted to be present.

Both tonsillar fossae were prophylactically cauterized using the Coblator with specific care being pointed out to both the superior and inferior poles. Once this had been accomplished, the patient was again taken off suspension. The red rubber catheter was removed. The Crowe-Davis mouth gag was removed followed by removal of the patient's shoulder roll.

(Continued)

The patient was then turned back over to anesthesia service to allow him to recover from general endotracheal. The patient was subsequently extubated in stable condition in the operating room, then transferred to PACU for continued observation with plans for admission to the hospital to ensure adequate pain control and, hopefully, to prevent any further episodes of fever, stomatitis, and cervical adenitis.

_____

Leela Pivari, MD
Otorhinolaryngology

LP:cks
D:07/31/----
T:08/01/----

c: Reed Phillips, MD, Pediatrics

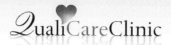

Obstetrics/Gynecology Surgery

Patient Name: Starr Kellogg   **ID#:** S-97

Date of Operation: 03/17/----   **Age:** 25   **Sex:** F

PREOPERATIVE DIAGNOSIS
Fetus at 19 weeks with posterior urethral valves.

POSTOPERATIVE DIAGNOSIS
Fetus at 19 weeks with posterior urethral valves.

OPERATION PERFORMED: Vesicoamniotic shunt.

SPECIMEN REMOVED: None.

SURGEON: Tillman Risha, MD

ASSISTANT: Rosemary Bumbak, MD

ANESTHETIC: Spinal by Dr. Avalon.

INDICATIONS: Fetus with posterior urethral valves.

FINDINGS: Fetus with significantly enlarged urinary bladder and what is known as a keyhole sign consistent with posterior urethral valves.

DESCRIPTION OF OPERATION: Patient was taken to the operating room and ultrasound was performed, which confirmed fetal heart rate motion and an enlarged urinary bladder consistent with posterior urethral valves. Patient then had a spinal anesthetic performed, and she was prepped and draped in the usual sterile fashion.

An ultrasound was then performed, and the ultrasound was draped. An attempt was made to paralyze the baby so that we could do the vesicoamniotic shunt. In order to do this we had to use a 7.5-inch, 22-gauge needle and go through the placenta into the baby's abdomen to give it an intramuscular injection. Attempts initially were made to give injections into the thigh, but these were unsuccessful. A total of 3 attempts were made, and the patient was paralyzed using vecuronium, and also the baby was given fentanyl. The dosing was appropriate for its size.

After this was performed, the needle was removed. A second location was used to insert a needle, again a 7.5-inch, 22-gauge spinal needle, away from the placenta in order to do an amnioinfusion of lactated Ringer solution. Some 300 mL of lactated Ringer's was injected into the amniotic fluid, enabling us to establish a normal amniotic fluid volume so that we would be able to do the vesicoamniotic shunt.

After this was done, another ultrasound was performed. The determination of the location into which to put the shunt was made. This location was on the lower fetal abdomen approximately halfway between the umbilicus and the fetal hip and as low into the pelvis as possible. The vesicoamniotic shunt was placed in the normal fashion by making a small skin puncture under ultrasound guidance, directing the trocar into the described, desired location. The trocar was then placed into the fetal abdomen without problems. This was done using Doppler color flow study to ensure that we did not damage the umbilical arteries.

Once the trocar was into the fetal abdomen, the shunt was placed by pushing the first coil that came out into the fetal bladder, removing the trocar, and extending the applicators so that the second coil would come out into the amniotic space. This was done successfully.

The trocar was then removed, and a fair amount of bleeding was noted to be coming from the placenta. In order to replace the vesicoamniotic shunt, we again had to go through the placenta with the trocar. The vesicoamniotic shunt that was used was a Harrison Fetal Bladder Stent Set.

(Continued)

ID#: S-97   PAGE 2

Again, this was done with a single attempt with good placement; however, bleeding from the placenta was noted. Fetal heart rate was normal after the procedure, and the patient was taken from the surgery suite down to the recovery room in stable condition.

_____
Tillman Risha, MD
Obstetrics/Gynecology

TR:cks
D:03/17/----
T:03/17/----

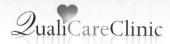

Genitourinary Surgery

Patient Name: Charles L. Looper   **ID#:** S-98

Date of Operation: 12/16/----   **Age:** 42   **Sex:** M

PREOPERATIVE DIAGNOSIS
Normal-volume azoospermia.

POSTOPERATIVE DIAGNOSIS
Normal-volume azoospermia.

OPERATIONS PERFORMED
1. Bilateral testis biopsies.
2. Bilateral scrotal explorations.
3. Bilateral vasograms.
4. Right-to-left crossover vasoepididymostomy.

SPECIMENS REMOVED
1. Right inguinal hernia sac.
2. Bilateral testis biopsies sent for frozen section.

SURGEON: Charles Mendesz, MD

ASSISTANTS: Jason Wagner, PA-C and Jimmy Dale Jett, RN

ANESTHETIC: General endotracheal by Dr. Delaney.

SPONGE COUNT: Correct at end of case.

INDICATIONS: Mr. Looper is a 42-year-old white male who is status post bilateral inguinal hernia repairs at 8 years of age who now has normal-volume azoospermia. After all options were discussed, the patient desired to have bilateral testis biopsies performed with scrotal exploration, vasogram, and possible inguinal vasovasostomy versus bilateral vasoepididymostomies. Patient understood the risks involved with this case and that we are unable to offer sperm cryopreservation at this facility. Preoperatively, the patient underwent chromosomal analysis, which revealed that he is a 46X, which revealed normal results of 46XY.

DESCRIPTION OF OPERATION: Once the proper patient was identified, informed, and consented, he was brought to the operating suite where the general anesthesia team obtained their general endotracheal anesthesia. Patient was then placed in dorsal lithotomy position. The lower abdomen and groin were then shaved, prepped, and draped in the usual sterile fashion. An incision was made over the left hemiscrotum, and the left vas deferens was carefully dissected. The left vas deferens was then transected using the Beaver blade, and a left vasogram was then attempted using 10 mL of Hypaque. A radiograph performed revealed that the Hypaque did not traverse beyond the pelvic inlet on the left side. Testis biopsy performed on the left testicle revealed the patient did have a few motile sperm present.

Attention was turned to the right testicle. The left vas deferens and epididymis were carefully dissected. The left epididymis was immediately noted to be cystic and atrophic in nature. The proximal vas deferens was carefully dissected transversely. Vasogram was performed, revealing that the vas deferens was patent with prompt filling of the seminal vesicles and emptying into the bladder. The right hemiscrotal exploration also revealed the patient to have a right inguinal hernia sac, which was excised and sent to pathology for prompt evaluation. This confirmed an inguinal hernia sac. Testis biopsy performed on the right testicle revealed no motile sperm.

At this time, it was therefore decided to perform a right-to-left crossover vasoepididymostomy with ligation of the left vas deferens. A small incision was performed in the median raphe in order to allow for the right epididymis to cross over into the left hemiscrotum. An end-to-side anastomosis was performed by opening the tunica vaginalis and selecting an area with dilated tubules just proximal to the site of obstruction. This was performed at the most

(Continued)

distal part of the epididymis, which was actually very proximal. A small, 3 mm circular patch of the epididymal capsule was excised just enough to expose an underlying tubule. The tubule was marked with a 10-0 nylon suture on the lateral wall. A touch preparation was performed, which revealed no sperm; therefore, this defect was cauterized and closed. The same procedure was done 1 cm more proximally. This time sperm were identified; therefore, the distal end of the vas was brought under the parietal tunica vaginalis and brought down to the site of the epididymis. Here it was fixed with three 8-0 Prolene sutures between the capsule and the adventitia of the vas. The mucosa of the vas was anastomosed through the opened epididymal tubule using 4 through-and-through 10-0 nylon sutures and 3 serosal stitches in between using 9-0 nylon.

The testis and the epididymis were returned to the scrotum, and the wounds were then closed using a 3-0 Vicryl stitch on the tunica vaginalis and chromic catgut on the dartos. A running subcuticular stitch was used to close both scrotal incisions, and Dermabond was applied. A red rubber catheter was then used to drain the bladder, which revealed only 400 mL of urine. Fluff dressings and scrotal support were applied. Patient was awakened and transferred to the recovery room in stable condition.

_____

Charles Mendesz, MD
Urology

CM:cks
D:12/16/----
T:12/16/----

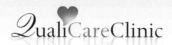

Orthopedic Surgery

Patient Name: Lee Weisenhantz   **ID#:** S-99

Date of Operation: 05/26/----   **Age:** 62   **Sex:** M

PREOPERATIVE DIAGNOSES
1. L2-3, L3-4 central canal stenosis with neurogenic claudication.
2. Status post L4 to S1 posterior instrumented fusion and decompression with pseudarthrosis at L5-S1 and pars defect at L3-4.

POSTOPERATIVE DIAGNOSES
1. L2-3, L3-4 central canal stenosis with neurogenic claudication.
2. Status post L4 to S1 posterior instrumented fusion and decompression with pseudarthrosis at L5-S1 and pars defect at L3-4.

OPERATION PERFORMED: L2-3, L3-4, L4-5, and L5-S1 anterior interbody fusion.

SPECIMEN REMOVED: None.

SURGEON: Gilbert M. Fields, MD

ASSISTANT: Howard H. Lee, MD

ANESTHETIC: General endotracheal by Dr. Avalon.

PROSTHETIC DEVICES: Allograft FRA spacers at L4-5 and L5-S1, femoral strut allograft at L2-3 and L3-4.

TOTAL FLUIDS: Crystalloid 6700 mL, Cell Saver 374 mL, albumin 500 mL, and potassium 20 mEq.

TOTAL URINE OUTPUT: 1550 mL.

ESTIMATED BLOOD LOSS: 1100 mL.

INDICATIONS: Patient is a 62-year-old gentleman, status post L4 to S1 posterolateral instrumented fusion and decompression 4 years ago. He was noted to have significant neurogenic claudication and adjacent level stenosis at L2-3 and L3-4. He was also noted to have an L3-4 spondylolysis and L5-S1 spondylolysis as well. He has a pseudarthrosis with a loose screw on the left at L4, which has penetrated the L3-4 disk space. The patient was therefore counseled in detail prior to the operative procedure regarding his options. After much deliberation and consideration, it was decided to perform an anterior interbody fusion of L2-3, L3-4, L4-5, and L5-S1 secondary to the patient's adjacent level stenosis and kyphosis at the L2-3 and L3-4 levels as well as his pseudarthrosis at L4-5 and L5-S1. The vascular surgeon assisted in the anterior exposure and approach and will be dictating this portion of the case.

DESCRIPTION OF OPERATION: After obtaining informed consent, identifying the patient, and confirming levels on which to be operated, the patient was placed in a supine position, intubated, and anesthetized. A bump was placed under the lumbosacral junction to offer extension of the lumbar spine, to ease exposure. Once this was done, the patient was prepped and draped in the usual sterile fashion, and he was given preoperative antibiotics in the form of Ancef 1 g and gentamicin 80 mg x1. Ancef was given at 4-hour intervals throughout the case. The vascular surgeon will dictate the initial portion of the exposure.

Once the iliac vessels were exposed and the segmentals were ligated by the vascular surgeon overlying the levels to be operated on, the L5-S1 junction was exposed at the bifurcation of the iliac vessels. The large diamond pins with a red rubber catheter were used to retract the vessels in combination with a renal retractor on each limb of the vessel. Careful retraction was placed with a malleable retractor over the sacral promontory. No Bovie cautery was used in this region of the dissection. Once this was performed, a long-handled 15 blade was used to perform a diskectomy in standard fashion at the L5-S1 level, after confirming our levels with a C-arm fluoroscopy. Once the knife was used to incise the disk at L5-S1, the large rongeur was used to remove the anterior annulus. This was

(Continued)

ID#: S-99   PAGE 2

followed by the periosteal elevator in a thorough removal of the cartilaginous end plates. A combination of curved and straight curettes were subsequently used to remove any remaining cartilaginous end plate down to bleeding bone, ensuring no penetration to the subchondral bone of the end plates. Once we were happy and had a satisfactory diskectomy, we used the trial sizers, increasing our sizers incrementally from a size 11 to a size 15. We noted size 15 to be the appropriate size; therefore, we used our trial 15 FRA spacer. Noting on fluoroscopy that this was adequate in size and position, we then replaced this with a femoral ring allograft. The femoral ring allograft was packed with BMP-soaked sponges, and a BMP-soaked sponge was also laid across the posterior aspect of the vertebral bodies.

Once this was performed, the diamond pins were removed, and the vessels were subsequently retracted to the right of the L4-5 disk space. A diskectomy was performed in a fashion similar to the L5-S1 level at this level and at the L3-4 and L2-3 levels. This was done in standard fashion using a combination of curettes and rongeurs to remove the entirety of the cartilaginous end plates down to bleeding bone, ensuring no damage or penetration through the subchondral bone. Once we were happy with the complete diskectomy at every level, the trial dilators were used followed by the sizers. At L4-5, a 13 mm lordotic FRA spacer was placed with BMP packed within the center and along the posterior aspect of the vertebral bodies as well. Similar procedures were performed at L3-4 and L2-3 using a 19 mm femoral ring allograft strut that was measured and fashioned using a sagittal saw to ensure adequate dimensions. It was also packed with BMP, and BMP was laid across the posterior aspect of the vertebral body at this level. A subsequent procedure, very similar, was performed at the L2-3 level using a size 15 mm strut, which was fabricated using the sagittal saw. Once this was done and the BMP was noted to be packed within the femoral ring and along the posterior aspect of each vertebral body, the patient's deep wound was evaluated.

It should be noted, the patient's sacral bump was also supplemented with flexion of the table to adequately extend the patient's back while performing our diskectomies and placing our femoral ring allografts. Once each of the allografts was in place, the table was flattened, and a Kocher test was used to try and pull each of the struts out of its place in the disk space. We were unsuccessful in removing the struts, noting that each of them was firmly seated and also subsided approximately 1 mm past the lip of the intervening vertebral bodies.

The wound was subsequently closed by Dr. Tabor of vascular surgery. Patient tolerated the procedure well and was subsequently taken to the intensive care unit where he will convalesce for the next 2 days. We will plan a second-stage procedure that will involve posterior instrumentation removal and exploration of the fusion mass, refusion in the posterolateral aspect of the patient's spine from L2 to S1. We will revise the patient's screws from L4 to S1 and place new screws at L2-3 and L3-4. We will also perform a decompression of L2-3 and L3-4. We will reevaluate our neural foramina at the L4-5 and L5-S1 segments, as a previous central decompression has already been performed.

Please note that the patient was evaluated by me prior to surgery, and a spinal was performed to ensure that repositioning of the patient's lumbar spine in lordosis would not adversely affect his stenosis and neurogenic claudication. Patient had no symptoms in his legs that would signify an indication for posterior decompression prior to the anterior surgery and reestablishing his lumbar lordosis. Please refer to Dr. Tabor's dictation regarding the vascular portion of this case.

_____

Gilbert M. Fields, MD
Orthopedic Surgery

GMF:cks
D:05/26/----
T:05/26/----

cc: Ly An Tabor, MD, Vascular Surgery
      Chris Salem, DO, Family Practice

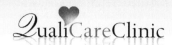

Genitourinary Surgery

Patient Name: Damaso Urribe   **ID#:** S-100

Date of Operation: 10/27/----   **Age:** 60   **Sex:** M

PREOPERATIVE DIAGNOSIS
Left proximal ureteral stricture.

POSTOPERATIVE DIAGNOSIS
Left proximal ureteral stricture with complete obstruction.

OPERATION PERFORMED: Cystoscopy under anesthesia with left retrograde pyelogram and left ureteral stent placement.

SPECIMEN REMOVED: 40 mL of grossly infected, catheterized, left ureteral specimen.

SURGEON: Charles Mendesz, MD

ASSISTANT: Jimmy Dale Jett, RN

ANESTHETIC: Laryngeal mask airway by Dr. Delaney.

SPONGE COUNT: Correct at conclusion of case.

INTRAVENOUS FLUIDS: 750 mL.

ESTIMATED BLOOD LOSS: Minimal.

INDICATIONS: Mr. Urribe is a 60-year-old gentleman who is status post left ureteroscopy for a 9 x 12 mm stone. He subsequently developed a left proximal ureteral stricture and is status post laser incision of this stricture with balloon dilation 4 weeks ago. The stent was removed 3 weeks after that procedure and followup IVP 4 days ago revealed that he had an approximately 2 cm to 3 cm visually obstructing, high-grade obstruction on the left. Patient was initially counseled to undergo a left open pyeloplasty; however, after all options had been discussed with the patient, he elected to undergo repeat attempt at a left endopyeloplasty.

FINDINGS: Completely obstructed left renal unit at the level of the left proximal ureter.

DESCRIPTION OF OPERATION: Once the proper patient was identified and informed consent obtained, he was brought to the operating room where the anesthesia team obtained laryngeal mask airway. He was then placed in the dorsal lithotomy position and prepped and draped in the usual sterile fashion. The urethra and bladder were then inspected with both 70-degree and 30-degree scopes and noted to have no abnormalities.

The left ureteral orifice was then cannulated with an open-ended ureteral catheter, and left retrograde pyelogram revealed a complete obstruction at the level of the left proximal ureter. A sensor guide wire was able to be advanced beyond the stricture, and the strictured segment was gently dilated with a #6-French open-ended ureteral catheter. Once the wire was removed, a hydronephrotic drip was noticed. A catheterized specimen was sent to microbiology for evaluation. The first 20 mL seemed to be straw-colored, but the subsequent 20 mL to 30 mL seemed to be grossly infected with frank pus. Microscopic evaluation confirmed that the catheterized specimen had too-numerous-to-count white blood cells and bacteria.

At this time, the decision was made to abort the planned endopyeloplasty. The decision was made to stent the patient. The open-ended ureteral catheter was removed over a wire, and a 7 x 24-French double-J ureteral stent was then advanced under both cystoscopic and fluoroscopic guidance with a nice coil noted in the left renal pelvis and in the urinary bladder.

(Continued)

ID#: S-100   PAGE 2

Patient tolerated the procedure well. There were no complications. He was awakened and transferred from the operating room table onto the gurney in stable condition.

_____

Charles Mendesz, MD
Urology

CM:cks
D:10/27/----
T:10/28/----

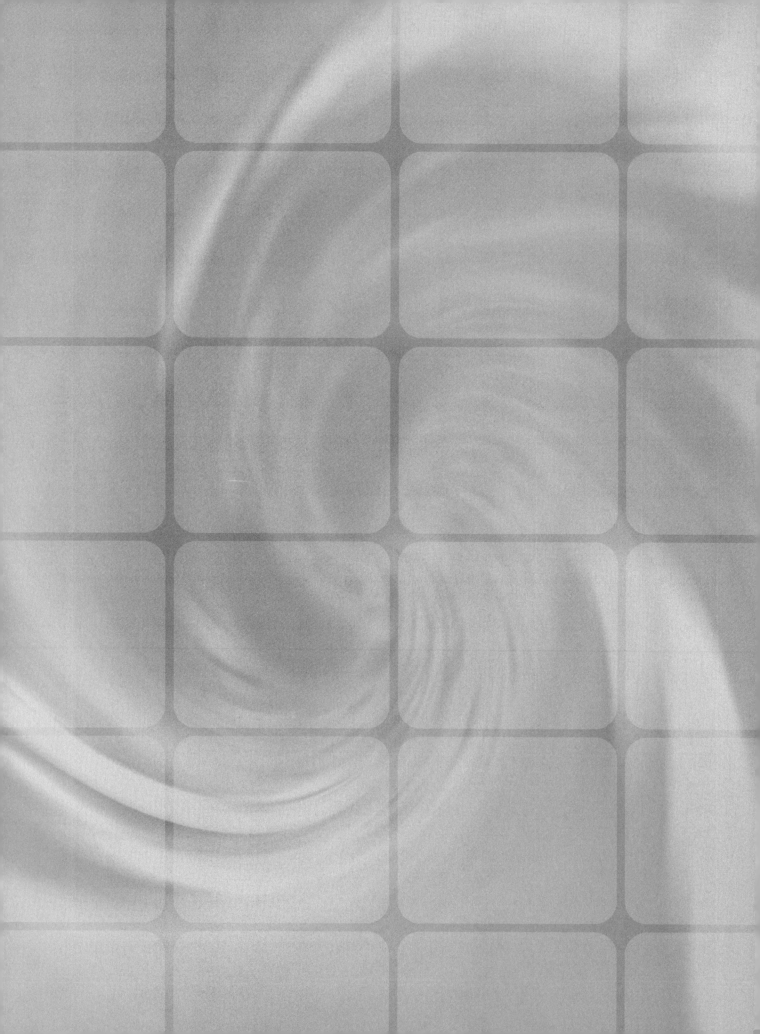

APPENDIX A

COMMON DICTATION ERRORS

...and how transcriptionists use medical language and editing skills to correct them, leaving their doctors' dictation medically intact yet grammatically correct and suitable for the legal and insurance fields, government agencies, research purposes, etc.,

OR

why verbatim transcription is a myth.

Key: Grammar/usage error = G
Sentence structure error = SS
Inappropriate words = IW
Dictionary or reference needed = DN
Medical Transcription Style = STY

	Type of error
D: There <u>is</u> interstitial changes... **T:** There <u>are</u> interstitial changes...	G
D: ...who appears to be in currently no acute distress... **T:** ...who currently appears to be in no acute distress...	SS
D: ...bilateral heel decubiti... **T:** ...bilateral heel decubitus ulcers...	DN, IW
D: ...right and left <u>groin</u> were... **T:** ...right and left <u>groins</u> were...	G
D: ...perioperative antibiotics were <u>administrated</u>... **T:** ...perioperative antibiotics were <u>administered</u>...	IW
D: ... with 1% lidocaine and <u>half</u> percent of Marcaine... **T:** ... with 1% lidocaine and <u>0.5%</u> of Marcaine...	STY
D: Patient handed over to anesthesia where <u>she</u> was extubated... **T:** Patient handed over to anesthesia where <u>he</u> was extubated...	DN, IW

(NOTE: Male patient from context of report.**)**

D: Thus the patient was converted to <u>open</u> for further exploration. **T:** Thus the patient was converted to <u>an open procedure</u> for further exploration.	SS
D: ... laryngoscope was passed through the left <u>nare</u> and passed to the level of the pharynx. **T:** ... laryngoscope was passed through the left <u>naris</u> and passed to the level of the pharynx.	DN
D: ... and approximately 0.3 <u>cc were</u> injected on each side... **T:** ... and approximately 0.3 <u>mL was</u> injected on each side...	G, STY
D: ...pulse is 20, respiratory rate is 61... **T:** ...pulse is 61, respiratory rate is 20...	DN
D: She had three <u>kiddos</u>. **T:** She had three <u>children</u>.	IW
D: Further dissection was <u>felt to be deemed</u> necessary. **T:** Further dissection was <u>felt to be</u> necessary. -OR- **T:** Further dissection was <u>deemed</u> necessary.	G, SS

	Type of error
D: She has been noted to have recurrent very low nadirs in the 30 to 40 range with some altered mental status, and then blood pressures as high as the 300s. **T:** ... very low nadirs in the 30 to 40 range with some altered mental status, and then blood <u>sugars</u> as high as the 300s.	DN, IW

(NOTE: In a patient with diabetes, the chief complaint is dictated "Low blood sugar.")

D: ...with a heavy history of smoking. **T:** ...with a history of heavy smoking.	SS
D: The attendant <u>that</u> is with the patient... **T:** The attendant <u>who</u> is with the patient...	G
D: No history of <u>self-injurous</u> behavior. **T:** No history of <u>self-injurious</u> behavior.	IW
D: The patient was very <u>tangental</u> in his thinking. **T:** The patient was very <u>tangential</u> in his thinking.	IW
D: They were placed parallel, starting about a centimeter and a half above the plafond... **T:** They were placed parallel, starting about 1.5 cm above the plafond...	STY
D: ... most likely long-standing <u>fungus</u> changes. **T:** ... most likely long-standing <u>fungal</u> changes.	G
D: Status post rollover <u>ATM</u> resulting in an open right tib/fib fracture. **T:** Status post rollover <u>ATV</u> resulting in an open right <u>tibia/fibula</u> fracture.	IW, STY
D: Creatinine kinase 39. **T:** <u>Creatine</u> kinase 39.	IW
D: The patient moves all four upper extremities freely. **T:** The patient moves _____ freely. (There is no way to check this dictation other than by asking the dictator of the report. The report should be flagged using the medical transcriptionist's normal procedure for flagging reports.)	IW

APPENDIX B

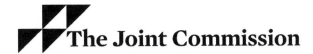

The Joint Commission

May 2005

Official "Do Not Use" List[1]

Do Not Use	Potential Problem	Use Instead
U (unit)	Mistaken for "0" (zero), the number "4" (four) or "cc"	Write "unit"
IU (International Unit)	Mistaken for IV (intravenous) or the number 10 (ten)	Write "International Unit"
Q.D., QD, q.d., qd (daily)	Mistaken for each other	Write "daily"
Q.O.D., QOD, q.o.d, qod (every other day)	Period after the Q mistaken for "I" and the "O" mistaken for "I"	Write "every other day"
Trailing zero (X.0 mg)* Lack of leading zero (.X mg)	Decimal point is missed	Write X mg Write 0.X mg
MS	Can mean morphine sulfate or magnesium sulfate	Write "morphine sulfate" Write "magnesium sulfate"
MSO_4 and $MgSO_4$	Confused for one another	

[1] Applies to all orders and all medication-related documentation that is handwritten (including free-text computer entry) or on pre-printed forms.

*Exception: A "trailing zero" may be used only where required to demonstrate the level of precision of the value being reported, such as for laboratory results, imaging studies that report size of lesions, or catheter/tube sizes. It may not be used in medication orders or other medication-related documentation.

Additional Abbreviations, Acronyms and Symbols
(For possible future inclusion in the Official "Do Not Use" List)

Do Not Use	Potential Problem	Use Instead
> (greater than) < (less than)	Misinterpreted as the number "7" (seven) or the letter "L" Confused for one another	Write "greater than" Write "less than"
Abbreviations for drug names	Misinterpreted due to similar abbreviations for multiple drugs	Write drug names in full
Apothecary units	Unfamiliar to many practitioners Confused with metric units	Use metric units
@	Mistaken for the number "2" (two)	Write "at"
cc	Mistaken for U (units) when poorly written	Write "ml" or "milliliters"
µg	Mistaken for mg (milligrams) resulting in one thousand-fold overdose	Write "mcg" or "micrograms"

APPENDIX C
AUDIO RUN TIMES

ID #	REPORT TITLE	PHYSICIAN	TIME
M-1	Bone Marrow Transplant Clinic	Fisher	05:42
M-2	Physical Medicine and Rehabilitation Consultation	Mooney	06:19
M-3	Orthopedic Clinic	Rodriguez	02:28
M-4	Emergency Department Treatment Record	Ernest	05:17
M-5	Vascular Surgery Clinic Followup Note	Tabor	03.37
M-6	Orthopedic Services Preoperative History and Physical	Rodriguez	04:57
M-7	Colorectal Surgery Consultation	McClure	04:37
M-9	Radiation Oncology Consultation	Erwin	04:21
M-10	Bone Marrow Transplant Clinic Followup Note	Fisher	04:24
M-11	Orthopedic Clinic Consultation	Rodriquez	05:55
M-12	Vascular Surgery Clinic Followup Note	Tabor	03:17
M-13	Emergency Department Treatment Record	Ernest	04:25
M-14	Pediatrics Consultation	Fry	07:21
M-15	Radiation Oncology Clinic Followup Note	Erwin	03:26
M-16	Vascular Surgery Followup Note	Tabor	03:13
M-17	Vascular and Neurovascular Surgery Followup Note	Tabor	04:25
M-18	Hematology/Oncology Bone Marrow Transplant Note	Fisher	05:12
M-19	Internal Medicine Clinic Note	Mooney	06:50
M-20	Emergency Department Treatment Record	Ernest	04:25
M-21	Bone Marrow Clinic History and Physical Examination	Fisher	07:54
M-23	Internal Medicine Followup Note	Mooney	04:41
M-24	Hematology/Oncology Clinic Outpatient Progress Note	Fisher	03:31
M-25	Physical Medicine and Rehabilitation Consultation	Mooney	06:06
M-26	Emergency Room Treatment Record	Ernest	06:13
M-27	Orthopedic Clinic Consultation	Rodriquez	03:50
M-28	Bone Marrow Transplant Clinic Followup Note	Fisher	02:23
M-29	Internal Medicine Clinic Followup Note	Mooney	05:04
M-30	Physical Medicine and Rehabilitation Followup Note	Mooney	05:37
M-31	Colorectal Surgery Consultation	McClure	02:21
M-32	Vascular Surgery Consultation	Tabor	03:27

ID #	REPORT TITLE	PHYSICIAN	TIME
M-34	Orthopedic Surgery Followup Note	Rodriquez	04:56
M-36	Orthopedic Followup Note	Fields	01:37
M-37	Emergency Room Treatment Record	Ernest	04:16
M-38	Hematology/Oncology Followup Note	Fisher	02:16
M-39	Vascular Surgery Followup Note	Tabor	02:58
M-40	Orthopedic Surgery History and Physical Examination	Rodriquez	07:39
M-41	Colorectal Surgery Consultation	McClure	02:50
M-42	Emergency Room Treatment Record	Ernest	08:13
M-43	Radiation Oncology Followup Note	Erwin	02:22
M-44	Emergency Department Treatment Record	Ernest	06:46
M-45	Bone Marrow Followup Note	Fisher	05:44
M-46	Emergency Room Treatment	Ernest	04:12
M-47	Orthopedic Surgery Followup Note	Fields	01:34
M-48	Vascular Surgery Consultation	Tabor	04:12
M-50	Emergency Department Treatment Record	Ernest	05:24
M-51	Orthopedic Clinic Consultation	Rodriquez	04:51
M-52	Emergency Department Treatment Record	Rodriquez	05:26
M-54	Oromaxillofacial Surgery Consultation	Pivari	06:48
M-55	Discharge Summary	Fisher	04:41
M-56	Preop History and Physical Examination	Rodriquez	03:42
M-57	Emergency Department Treatment Record	Ernest	06:44
M-59	Internal Medicine Clinic Followup Note	Panagides	06:05
M-60	Plastic Surgery Clinic Followup Note	Fry	02:36
M-61	Nephrology Clinic Followup Note	Panagides	08:16
M-62	Vascular Clinic Followup Note	Tabor	02:51
M-63	Neurology/Orthopedics Surgery Discharge Summary	Fields	02:57
M-64	Radiation Oncology Clinic History and Physical Examination	Erwin	05:57
M-65	Radiation Oncology Clinic Note	Erwin	04:32
M-66	Emergency Department Treatment Record	Ernest	04:43
M-67	Vascular Surgery Clinic Consult	Tabor	03:23
M-68	General Surgery Clinic Consult	McClure	03:19
M-69	Emergency Department Treatment Record	Ernest	03:44
M-70	Orthopedic Discharge Summary	Fields	03:18
M-71	Orthopaedic Clinic Followup Note	Fields	02:04
M-72	Radiation Oncology Clinic Followup Note	Erwin	04:03
M-73	Vascular Surgery Clinic Consultation	Tabor	03:57
M-74	General Surgery Consultation	McClure	03:26

ID #	REPORT TITLE	PHYSICIAN	TIME
M-75	Orthopedic Clinic Followup Note	Fields	02:24
M-76	Initial Colorectal Surgery Clinic Initial Consultation	McClure	03:45
M-77	Internal Medicine Clinic Followup Note	Panagides	07:32
M-78	Orthopaedic Clinic Followup Note	Fields	02:17
M-79	Hematology/Oncology Clinic Followup Note	Fisher	02:56
M-80	Internal Medicine Clinic Followup	Panagides	07:04
M-81	Orthopedic Surgery Hand Team Preoperative History and Physical Examination	Rodriguez	02:52
M-82	Hematology/Oncology Clinic Followup Note	Fisher	04:14
M-83	Orthopedic Clinic Preop History & Physical	Fields	02:10
M-84	Emergency Department Treatment Record	Ernest	05:06
M-85	Hematology/Oncology Clinic Followup Note	Fisher	05:30
M-86	Orthopaedic Surgery Spine Consultation	Fields	05:34
M-87	Emergency Department Treatment Record	Ernest	04:52
M-88	Internal Medicine Initial Visit	Panagides	09:08
M-89	Orthopedics Shoulder Clinic Consult	Rodriguez	05:54
M-90	Emergency Department Clinic Record	Ernest	03:48
M-91	Internal Medicine Clinic Followup Note	Mooney	03:35
M-92	Orthopedic Spine Clinic Followup Note	Fields	03:16
M-93	Emergency Department Treatment Record	Ernest	05:32
M-94	Internal Medicine Geriatrics Clinic Followup Note	Mooney	05:33
M-95	Orthopedic Clinic Followup Note	Rodriguez	02:22
M-96	Emergency Department Treatment Record	Ernest	03:14
M-97	Internal Medicine Clinic Followup Note	Mooney	06:35
M-99	Orthopedic Spine Clinic Followup Note	Fields	02:39
M-100	Emergency Department Treatment Record	Ernest	05:05

R-1	CT Brain Scan	Murray	01:07
R-2	Bilateral Low-Dose Mammograms	Murray	01:02
R-3	Right Breast Mammogram	Murray	01:09
R-4	Pain Management	Murray	01:25
R-5	MRI, Left Knee	Murray	02:47
R-6	Carotid Ultrasound	Murray	01:36
R-7	Bilateral Mammograms	Murray	01:20
R-8	Right Upper Quadrant Sonogram	Murray	01:10
R-9	Acute Abdominal Series	Murray	00:49
R-10	Ultrasound-Guided Left Hip Aspiration	Murray	01:31

ID #	REPORT TITLE	PHYSICIAN	TIME
R-11	Whole Body Bone Scan	Murray	03:15
R-12	CT of Left Hip	Murray	03:19

S-1	Oromaxillofacial Surgery	Pivari	04:38
S-2	Orthopedic Surgery	Fields	04:19
S-3	Genitourinary Surgery	Mendesz	05:48
S-4	Plastic Surgery	Fry	04:17
S-5	Obstetrics/Gynecology Surgery	Risha	03:47
S-6	General/Plastic Surgery	Fry	05:21
S-7	General Surgery	McClure	03:44
S-8	Orthopedics/Plastic Surgery	Rodriguez	05:18
S-9	Oromaxillofacial Surgery	Pivari	04:15
S-10	Ophthalmologic Surgery	Naimi	03:35
S-11	Obstetrics/Gynecology Surgery	Risha	07:24
S-12	Orthopedic Surgery	Rodriguez	08:51
S-13	Genitourinary Surgery	Mendesz	06:03
S-14	Oromaxillofacial Surgery	Pivari	04:35
S-15	Genitourinary Surgery	Mendesz	02:58
S-16	General Surgery	McClure	06:07
S-17	Orthopedic Surgery	Fields	03:46
S-18	Genitourinary Surgery	Mendesz	04:40
S-19	Ear, Nose, and Throat Surgery	Pivari	07:48
S-20	Ophthalmologic Surgery	Naimi	04:00
S-21	General Surgery Report	McClure	04:19
S-23	Plastic Surgery Report	Fry	03:50
S-24	Ear, Nose, and Throat Surgery	Pivari	04:10
S-25	Obstetrics/Gynecology Surgery	Risha	04:28
S-26	Gastroenterology Surgical Procedure	Panagides	03:37
S-27	General Surgery Report	McClure	03:36
S-28	General Surgery Report	McClure	03:46
S-29	Orthopaedic Surgical Report	Fields	04:15
S-30	Orthopaedic Surgical Report	Fields	02:22
S-31	Plastic Surgery Report	Fry	08:11
S-32	General Surgery Report	McClure	07:13
S-33	Genitourinary Surgery Report	Mendesz	07:49
S-34	Orthopedic Surgery Report	Rodriguez	06:11
S-36	General Surgery Report	McClure	07:04

ID #	REPORT TITLE	PHYSICIAN	TIME
S-37	Orthopaedic Surgery Report	Fields	05:37
S-38	Obstetrics/Gynecology Surgery	Risha	03:12
S-39	Genitourinary Surgery	Mendesz	05:52
S-40	Ear, Nose, and Throat Surgery	Pivari	05:37
S-42	General Surgery Report	McClure	13:17
S-43	Orthopedic Surgery Report	Fields	05:50
S-44	Ear, Nose, and Throat Surgical Report	Pivari	04:00
S-45	General Surgery Report	McClure	04:10
S-46	Orthopedic Surgical Report	Rodriguez	08:28
S-47	Ear, Nose, and Throat Surgical Report	Pivari	02:40
S-49	General Surgery Report	McClure	08:51
S-50	Orthopedic Surgical Report	Rodriguez	06:17
S-52	Ophthalmologic Surgery	Naimi	03:54
S-54	General Surgery	McClure	04:09
S-56	General Surgery	McClure	04:24
S-58	General Surgery	McClure	04:20
S-59	Orthopedic Spine Surgery	Fields	08:16
S-60	Ear, Nose, and Throat Surgery	Pivari	03:20
S-61	Obstetrics/Gynecology Surgery	Risha	05:47
S-62	Ophthalmologic Surgery	Naimi	06:25
S-63	Genitourinary Surgery	Mendesz	17:35
S-64	Vascular Surgery	Tabor	13:13
S-65	Oromaxillofacial Surgery	Pivari	06:21
S-66	General Surgery	McClure	03:25
S-67	Gastroenterology Surgery	Panagides	07:46
S-68	General Surgery	McClure	04:07
S-70	Vascular Surgery	Tabor	02:47
S-71	Ear, Nose, and Throat Surgery	Pivari	04:35
S-72	Orthopedic Surgery	Fields	07:56
S-73	Plastic Surgery	Fry	04:11
S-74	Obstetrics/Gynecology Surgery	Risha	04:08
S-75	General Surgery	McClure	03:46
S-76	Genitourinary Surgery	Mendesz	03:23
S-77	General Surgery	McClure	05:08
S-78	Ear, Nose, and Throat Surgery	Pivari	02:30
S-79	Orthopedic Surgery	Fields	04:07
S-80	General Surgery	McClure	02:44

ID #	REPORT TITLE	PHYSICIAN	TIME
S-81	Genitourinary Surgery	Mendesz	03:20
S-82	Obstetrics/Gynecology Surgery	Risha	03:00
S-83	Nephrology Surgery	Mendesz	04:35
S-84	Plastic Surgery	Fry	03:36
S-85	Ear, Nose, and Throat Surgery	Pivari	05:20
S-86	Genitourinary Surgery	Mendesz	05:31
S-87	Orthopedic Surgery	Rodriguez	06:32
S-88	Obstetrics/Gynecology Surgery	Risha	05:29
S-89	Plastic Surgery	Fry	03:08
S-90	Genitourinary Surgery	Mendesz	06:30
S-91	Ear, Nose, and Throat Surgery	Pivari	03:55
S-92	Orthopedic Surgery	Rodriguez	04:49
S-93	Obstetrics/Gynecology Surgery	Risha	04:22
S-94	Nephrology Surgery	Mendesz	04:35
S-95	Orthopedic Surgery	Fields	08:18
S-96	Ear, Nose, and Throat Surgery	Pivari	04:13
S-97	Obstetrics/Gynecology Surgery	Risha	03:56
S-98	Genitourinary Surgery	Mendesz	05:32
S-99	Orthopedic Surgery	Fields	07:44
S-100	Genitourinary Surgery	Mendesz	04:02

REPORTS BY SPECIALTY

Neurosurgery

M-50 (Emergency Department Treatment Record)

M-66 (Emergency Department Treatment Record)

Obstetrics/Gynecology

S-5 (Surgery Report)

S-11 (Surgery Report)

S-25 (Surgery Report)

S-38 (Surgery Report)

S-61 (Surgery Report)

S-74 (Surgery Report)

S-82 (Surgery Report)

S-88 (Surgery Report)

S-93 (Surgery Report)

S-97 (Surgery Report)

Ophthalmology

M-37 (Emergency Room Treatment Record)

M-46 (Emergency Room Treatment Record)

S-10 (Surgery Report)

S-20 (Surgery Report)

S-52 (Surgery Report)

S-62 (Surgery Report)

Oromaxillofacial Surgery

M-54 (Consultation)

S-1 (Surgery Report)

S-9 (Surgery Report)

S-14 (Surgery Report)

S-65 (Surgery Report)

Orthopedics

M-3 (Followup Note)

M-6 (Preoperative History and Physical)

M-11 (Consultation)

M-27 (Consultation)

M-34 (Followup Note)

M-36 (Followup Note)

M-40 (History and Physical Examination)

M-47 (Followup Note)

M-51 (Consultation)

M-52 (Emergency Department Treatment Record)

M-56 (Preoperative History and Physical Examination)

M-63 (Discharge Note)

M-70 (Discharge Summary)

M-71 (Followup Note)

M-75 (Followup Note)

M-78 (Followup Note)

M-81 (History and Physical Examination)

M-83 (Preop History and Physical)

M-86 (Consultation)

M-89 (Consult)

M-92 (Followup Note)

M-95 (Followup Note)

M-99 (Followup Note)

R-4 (Pain Management)

R-5 (MRI, Left Knee)

R-10 (Ultrasound-Guided Left Hip Aspiration)

R-12 (CT of Left Hip)

S-2 (Surgery Report)

S-8 (Surgery Report)

S-12 (Surgery Report)

S-17 (Surgery Report)

S-29 (Surgery Report)

S-30 (Surgical Report)

S-34 (Surgery Report)

S-37 (Surgery Report)

S-43 (Surgery Report)

S-46 (Surgical Report)

S-50 (Surgical Report)

S-59 (Surgery Report)

S-72 (Surgery Report)

S-79 (Surgery Report)

S-87 (Surgery Report)

S-92 (Surgery Report)

S-95 (Surgery Report)

S-99 (Surgery Report)

Pediatrics

M-14 (Consultation)

M-87 (Emergency Department Treatment Record)

M-100 (Emergency Department Treatment Record)

Physical Medicine/Rehab

M-2 (Consultation)

M-25 (Consultation)

M-30 (Followup Note)

Plastic Surgery

M-60 (Followup Note)

S-4 (Surgery Report)

S-23 (Surgery Report)

S-31 (Surgery Report)

S-73 (Surgery Report)

S-84 (Surgery Report)

S-89 (Surgery Report)

Psychiatry

M-57 (Emergency Department Treatment Record)

Radiation Oncology

M-9 (Consultation)

M-15 (Followup Note)

M-43 (Followup Note)

M-64 (History and Physical Examination)

M-65 (Note)

M-72 (Followup Note)

Trauma Surgery

M-44 (Emergency Department Treatment Record)

M-69 (Emergency Department Treatment Record)

M-93 (Emergency Department Treatment Record)

M-96 (Emergency Department Treatment Record)

Vascular Surgery

M-5 (Followup Note)

M-12 (Followup Note)

M-16 (Followup Note)

M-32 (Consultation)

M-39 (Followup Note)

M-48 (Consultation)

M-62 (Followup Note)

M-67 (Consult)

M-73 (Consultation)

S-64 (Surgery Report)

S-70 (Surgery Report)

Vascular and Neurovascular

M-17 (Followup Note)

INDEX

SYSTEM REQUIREMENTS AND SETUP INSTRUCTIONS FOR CD

Audio Files to Accompany The Dictated Word

Minimum System Requirements

- These MP3 files are for use with digital transcription audio player software designed to assist the transcription of audio recordings. Please consult the software minimum system requirements and user instructions of the software of your choice to make sure they are compatible with MP3 files.
- These files will also play on a PC or Macintosh® computer using MP3 software such as Windows® Media Player or Apple® iTunes.

Setup Instructions for Use on a PC

1. Insert disc into CD-ROM drive. The CD directory for The Dictated Word should open. Click on the folder of your choice and double-click on the MP3 file of your choice.

Technical Support

Telephone: 1-800-648-7450
8:30 A.M.-6:30 P.M. Eastern Time
E-mail: delmar.help@cengage.com

Microsoft® and Windows® are registered trademarks of the Microsoft Corporation.

Apple® and iTunes® is a registered trademark of the Apple Corporation.

SINGLE USER LICENSE

IMPORTANT! READ CAREFULLY: This End User License Agreement ("Agreement") sets forth the conditions by which Cengage Learning will make electronic access to the Cengage Learning-owned licensed content and associated media, software, documentation, printed materials, and electronic documentation contained in this package and/or made available to you via this product (the "Licensed Content"), available to you (the "End User"). BY CLICKING THE "I ACCEPT" BUTTON AND/OR OPENING THIS PACKAGE, YOU ACKNOWLEDGE THAT YOU HAVE READ ALL OF THE TERMS AND CONDITIONS, AND THAT YOU AGREE TO BE BOUND BY ITS TERMS, CONDITIONS, AND ALL APPLICABLE LAWS AND REGULATIONS GOVERNING THE USE OF THE LICENSED CONTENT.

1.0 SCOPE OF LICENSE

1.1 <u>Licensed Content</u>. The Licensed Content may contain portions of modifiable content ("Modifiable Content") and content which may not be modified or otherwise altered by the End User ("Non-Modifiable Content"). For purposes of this Agreement, Modifiable Content and Non-Modifiable Content may be collectively referred to herein as the "Licensed Content." All Licensed Content shall be considered Non-Modifiable Content, unless such Licensed Content is presented to the End User in a modifiable format and it is clearly indicated that modification of the Licensed Content is permitted.

1.2 Subject to the End User's compliance with the terms and conditions of this Agreement, Cengage Learning hereby grants the End User, a nontransferable, nonexclusive, limited right to access and view a single copy of the Licensed Content on a single personal computer system for noncommercial, internal, personal use only. The End User shall not (i) reproduce, copy, modify (except in the case of Modifiable Content), distribute, display, transfer, sublicense, prepare derivative work(s) based on, sell, exchange, barter or transfer, rent, lease, loan, resell, or in any other manner exploit the Licensed Content; (ii) remove, obscure, or alter any notice of Cengage Learning's intellectual property rights present on or in the Licensed Content, including, but not limited to, copyright, trademark, and/or patent notices; or (iii) disassemble, decompile, translate, reverse engineer, or otherwise reduce the Licensed Content.

2.0 TERMINATION

2.1 Cengage Learning may at any time (without prejudice to its other rights or remedies) immediately terminate this Agreement and/or suspend access to some or all of the Licensed Content, in the event that the End User does not comply with any of the terms and conditions of this Agreement. In the event of such termination by Cengage Learning, the End User shall immediately return any and all copies of the Licensed Content to Cengage Learning.

3.0 PROPRIETARY RIGHTS

3.1 The End User acknowledges that Cengage Learning owns all rights, title and interest, including, but not limited to all copyright rights therein, in and to the Licensed Content, and that the End User shall not take any action inconsistent with such ownership. The Licensed Content is protected by U.S., Canadian and other applicable copyright laws and by international treaties, including the Berne Convention and the Universal Copyright Convention. Nothing contained in this Agreement shall be construed as granting the End User any ownership rights in or to the Licensed Content.

3.2 Cengage Learning reserves the right at any time to withdraw from the Licensed Content any item or part of an item for which it no longer retains the right to publish, or which it has reasonable grounds to believe infringes copyright or is defamatory, unlawful, or otherwise objectionable.

4.0 PROTECTION AND SECURITY

4.1 The End User shall use its best efforts and take all reasonable steps to safeguard its copy of the Licensed Content to ensure that no unauthorized reproduction, publication, disclosure, modification, or distribution of the Licensed Content, in whole or in part, is made. To the extent that the End User becomes aware of any such unauthorized use of the Licensed Content, the End User shall immediately notify Cengage Learning. Notification of such violations may be made by sending an e-mail to infringement@cengage.com.

5.0 MISUSE OF THE LICENSED PRODUCT

5.1 In the event that the End User uses the Licensed Content in violation of this Agreement, Cengage Learning shall have the option of electing liquidated damages, which shall include all profits generated by the End User's use of the Licensed Content plus interest computed at the maximum rate permitted by law and all legal fees and other expenses incurred by Cengage Learning in enforcing its rights, plus penalties.

6.0 FEDERAL GOVERNMENT CLIENTS

6.1 Except as expressly authorized by Cengage Learning, Federal Government clients obtain only the rights specified in this Agreement and no other rights. The Government acknowledges that (i) all software and related documentation incorporated in the Licensed Content is existing commercial computer software within the meaning of FAR 27.405(b)(2); and (2) all other data delivered in whatever form, is limited rights data within the meaning of FAR 27.401. The restrictions in this section are acceptable as consistent with the Government's need for software and other data under this Agreement.

7.0 DISCLAIMER OF WARRANTIES AND LIABILITIES

7.1   Although Cengage Learning believes the Licensed Content to be reliable, Cengage Learning does not guarantee or warrant (i) any information or materials contained in or produced by the Licensed Content, (ii) the accuracy, completeness or reliability of the Licensed Content, or (iii) that the Licensed Content is free from errors or other material defects. THE LICENSED PRODUCT IS PROVIDED "AS IS," WITHOUT ANY WARRANTY OF ANY KIND AND CENGAGE LEARNING DISCLAIMS ANY AND ALL WARRANTIES, EXPRESSED OR IMPLIED, INCLUDING, WITHOUT LIMITATION, WARRANTIES OF MERCHANTABILITY OR FITNESS FOR A PARTICULAR PURPOSE. IN NO EVENT SHALL CENGAGE LEARNING BE LIABLE FOR: INDIRECT, SPECIAL, PUNITIVE OR CONSEQUENTIAL DAMAGES INCLUDING FOR LOST PROFITS, LOST DATA, OR OTHERWISE. IN NO EVENT SHALL CENGAGE LEARNING'S AGGREGATE LIABILITY HEREUNDER, WHETHER ARISING IN CONTRACT, TORT, STRICT LIABILITY OR OTHERWISE, EXCEED THE AMOUNT OF FEES PAID BY THE END USER HEREUNDER FOR THE LICENSE OF THE LICENSED CONTENT.

8.0 GENERAL

8.1   Entire Agreement. This Agreement shall constitute the entire Agreement between the Parties and supercedes all prior Agreements and understandings oral or written relating to the subject matter hereof.

8.2   Enhancements/Modifications of Licensed Content. From time to time, and in Cengage Learning's sole discretion, Cengage Learning may advise the End User of updates, upgrades, enhancements and/or improvements to the Licensed Content, and may permit the End User to access and use, subject to the terms and conditions of this Agreement, such modifications, upon payment of prices as may be established by Cengage Learning.

8.3   No Export. The End User shall use the Licensed Content solely in the United States and shall not transfer or export, directly or indirectly, the Licensed Content outside the United States.

8.4   Severability. If any provision of this Agreement is invalid, illegal, or unenforceable under any applicable statute or rule of law, the provision shall be deemed omitted to the extent that it is invalid, illegal, or unenforceable. In such a case, the remainder of the Agreement shall be construed in a manner as to give greatest effect to the original intention of the parties hereto.

8.5   Waiver. The waiver of any right or failure of either party to exercise in any respect any right provided in this Agreement in any instance shall not be deemed to be a waiver of such right in the future or a waiver of any other right under this Agreement.

8.6   Choice of Law/Venue. This Agreement shall be interpreted, construed, and governed by and in accordance with the laws of the State of New York, applicable to contracts executed and to be wholly preformed therein, without regard to its principles governing conflicts of law. Each party agrees that any proceeding arising out of or relating to this Agreement or the breach or threatened breach of this Agreement may be commenced and prosecuted in a court in the State and County of New York. Each party consents and submits to the nonexclusive personal jurisdiction of any court in the State and County of New York in respect of any such proceeding.

8.7   Acknowledgment. By opening this package and/or by accessing the Licensed Content on this Web site, THE END USER ACKNOWLEDGES THAT IT HAS READ THIS AGREEMENT, UNDERSTANDS IT, AND AGREES TO BE BOUND BY ITS TERMS AND CONDITIONS. IF YOU DO NOT ACCEPT THESE TERMS AND CONDITIONS, YOU MUST NOT ACCESS THE LICENSED CONTENT AND RETURN THE LICENSED PRODUCT TO CENGAGE LEARNING (WITHIN 30 CALENDAR DAYS OF THE END USER'S PURCHASE) WITH PROOF OF PAYMENT ACCEPTABLE TO CENGAGE LEARNING, FOR A CREDIT OR A REFUND. Should the End User have any questions/comments regarding this Agreement, please contact Cengage Learning at Delmar.help@cengage.com.